AF749351

Gastrointestinal Stromal Tumors

Charles R. Scoggins • Chandrajit P. Raut
John T. Mullen
Editors

Gastrointestinal Stromal Tumors

Bench to Bedside

Springer

Editors
Charles R. Scoggins
School of Medicine
University of Louisville
Louisville, Kentucky
USA

John T. Mullen
Harvard Medical School
Boston, Massachusetts
USA

Chandrajit P. Raut
Brigham & Women's Hospital
Harvard Medical School
Boston, Massachusetts
USA

ISBN 978-3-319-42630-3 ISBN 978-3-319-42632-7 (eBook)
DOI 10.1007/978-3-319-42632-7

Library of Congress Control Number: 2016960587

© Springer International Publishing Switzerland 2017
This work is subject to copyright. All rights are reserved by the Publisher, whether the whole or part of the material is concerned, specifically the rights of translation, reprinting, reuse of illustrations, recitation, broadcasting, reproduction on microfilms or in any other physical way, and transmission or information storage and retrieval, electronic adaptation, computer software, or by similar or dissimilar methodology now known or hereafter developed.
The use of general descriptive names, registered names, trademarks, service marks, etc. in this publication does not imply, even in the absence of a specific statement, that such names are exempt from the relevant protective laws and regulations and therefore free for general use.
The publisher, the authors and the editors are safe to assume that the advice and information in this book are believed to be true and accurate at the date of publication. Neither the publisher nor the authors or the editors give a warranty, express or implied, with respect to the material contained herein or for any errors or omissions that may have been made.

Printed on acid-free paper

This Springer imprint is published by Springer Nature
The registered company is Springer International Publishing AG Switzerland
The registered company is Gewerbestrasse 11, 6330 Cham, Switzerland

Preface

Like all aspects of modern medicine, the field of oncology is expanding at an alarming rate. One needs only to search PubMed on any given topic to quickly realize just how daunting a task it is to stay current. In oncology, the explosion of information regarding gastrointestinal stromal tumors is no exception. Gastrointestinal stromal tumor (GIST) is a relatively new diagnosis, borne out of a deeper understanding of gastrointestinal sarcoma biology and characterized by a distinctive immunohistochemical phenotype.

We intend this book to serve as a reference for training and practicing medical oncologists, surgical oncologists, general surgeons, and gastroenterologists. It is to serve as the backbone of a deeper understanding of GIST so that we can better care for the patients afflicted with this malignancy. These patients are our inspiration, our raison d'etre. Advanced surgical techniques are often required, and novel chemotherapeutic options are being developed daily. This book is dedicated to the patients that we care for and to the researchers who continuously push knowledge forward.

We greatly appreciate the time and effort of all authors who contributed to this book. Their dedication is a reflection to their professionalism and passion for the study of GIST. We would also like to thank our teachers and mentors for their direction and our families for their support that allowed this book to come to fruition.

Louisville, KY, USA — Charles R. Scoggins, MD, MBA
Boston, MA, USA — Chandrajit P. Raut, MD
Boston, MA, USA — John T. Mullen, MD

Contents

Contributors

Vedra A. Augenstein, MD, FACS Carolinas Medical Center, Division of Gastrointestinal and Minimally Invasive Surgery, Carolinas Laparoscopic and Advanced Surgery Program, Charlotte, NC, USA

William R. Brugge, MD Gastrointestinal Unit, Massachusetts General Hospital, Boston, MA, USA

Odise Cenaj Department of Pathology, Brigham and Women's Hospital, Harvard Medical School, Boston, MA, USA

Haesun Choi, MD Department of Diagnostic Radiology, Division of Diagnostic Imaging, The University of Texas, MD Anderson Cancer Center, Houston, TX, USA

S. Chopra Department of Pathology, Keck School of Medicine, University of Southern California, Los Angeles, CA, USA

Taylor M. Coe, BS School of Medicine, University of California, San Diego, La Jolla, CA, USA

Tiffany C. Cox, MD Carolinas Medical Center, Division of Gastrointestinal and Minimally Invasive Surgery, Carolinas Laparoscopic and Advanced Surgery Program, Charlotte, NC, USA

Leona A. Doyle Department of Pathology, Brigham and Women's Hospital, Boston, MA, USA

Harvard Medical School, Boston, MA, USA

B.L. Eisenberg Department of Surgery, Keck School of Medicine, University of Southern California, Los Angeles, CA, USA

Hoag Family Cancer Institute, Hoag Memorial Presbyterian Hospital, Newport Beach, CA, USA

Barry W. Feig, MD Department of Surgical Oncology, The University of Texas M.D. Anderson Cancer Center, Houston, TX, USA

Zhi Ven Fong, MD Division of Surgical Oncology, Department of Surgery, Massachusetts General Hospital, Harvard Medical School, Boston, MA, USA

B. Todd Heniford, MD, FACS Carolinas Medical Center, Division of Gastrointestinal and Minimally Invasive Surgery, Carolinas Laparoscopic and Advanced Surgery Program, Charlotte, NC, USA

Guozhi Hu, MD Department of Medicine, Division of Hematology Oncology, University of Miami, Sylvester Cancer Center, Miami, FL, USA

Katherine A. Janeway, MD, MMSc Harvard Medical School, Boston, MA, USA

Pediatric Oncology, Dana-Farber/Boston Children's Cancer and Blood Disorders Center, Boston, MA, USA

Vickie Y. Jo Department of Pathology, Brigham and Women's Hospital, Boston, MA, USA

Harvard Medical School, Boston, MA, USA

E. Jung Department of Surgery, Keck School of Medicine, University of Southern California, Los Angeles, CA, USA

Emily Z. Keung, MD Department of Surgery, Brigham and Women's Hospital, Center for Sarcoma and Bone Oncology, Dana-Farber Cancer Institute, Harvard Medical School, Boston, MA, USA

David A. Kooby, MD Division of Surgical Oncology, Winship Cancer Institute, Atlanta, GA, USA

David A. Mahvi, MD Department of Surgery, Brigham and Women's Hospital, Center for Sarcoma and Bone Oncology, Dana-Farber Cancer Institute, Harvard Medical School, Boston, MA, USA

Shishir K. Maithel, MD, FACS Division of Surgical Oncology, Department of Surgery, Winship Cancer Institute, Emory University, Atlanta, GA, USA

Christian F. Meyer, MD, PhD Medical Oncology, Sidney Kimmel Cancer Center Johns Hopkins, Baltimore, MD, USA

Thomas J. Miner, MD The Department of Surgery, Alpert Medical School of Brown University, Rhode Island Hospital, Providence, Rhode Island, USA

Andrew D. Morris, MD Division of Surgical Oncology, Department of Surgery, Winship Cancer Institute, Emory University, Atlanta, GA, USA

John T. Mullen, MD Division of Surgical Oncology, Massachusetts General Hospital, Boston, MA, USA

Kavitha M. Nair, MD Department of Medicine, Emory University School of Medicine, Atlanta, GA, USA

Ana Paz-Mejía Department of Medicine, Division of Hematology Oncology, University of Miami, Sylvester Cancer Center, Miami, FL, USA

Prejesh Philips, MD Department of Surgery, Division of Surgical Oncology, University of Louisville, Louisville, KY, USA

Brittany A. Potz, MD The Department of Surgery, Alpert Medical School of Brown University, Rhode Island Hospital, Providence, Rhode Island, USA

Chandrajit P. Raut, MD, MSc Department of Surgery, Brigham and Women's Hospital, Center for Sarcoma and Bone Oncology, Dana-Farber Cancer Institute, Harvard Medical School, Boston, MA, USA

Christina L. Roland, MD Department of Surgical Oncology, The University of Texas M.D. Anderson Cancer Center, Houston, TX, USA

Jack W. Rostas, MD Department of Surgery, Division of Surgical Oncology, University of Louisville, Louisville, KY, USA

Sam Schell Carolinas Medical Center, Division of Gastrointestinal and Minimally Invasive Surgery, Carolinas Laparoscopic and Advanced Surgery Program, Charlotte, NC, USA

Sooyoung Shin, MD Department of Diagnostic Radiology, MD Anderson Cancer Center, Houston, TX, USA

Jason K. Sicklick, MD, FACS Division of Surgical Oncology, Moores UCSD Cancer Center, University of California, San Diego, UC San Diego Health System, La Jolla, CA, USA

Gabriel Tinoco, MD Department of Medicine, Division of Hematology Oncology, University of Miami, Sylvester Cancer Center, Miami, FL, USA

Jonathan Trent, MD, PhD Department of Medicine, Division of Hematology Oncology, University of Miami, Sylvester Cancer Center, Miami, FL, USA

W.W. Tseng Department of Surgery, Keck School of Medicine, University of Southern California, Los Angeles, CA, USA

Hoag Family Cancer Institute, Hoag Memorial Presbyterian Hospital, Newport Beach, CA, USA

Field F. Willingham, MD, MPH Emory University Hospital, Atlanta, GA, USA

Osman Yuksel, MD Pancreas Biliary Center, Gastrointestinal Unit, Massachusetts General Hospital, Boston, MA, USA

Department of Gastroenterology, University of Hacettepe, Ankara, Turkey

History of GIST

Christina L. Roland and Barry W. Feig

Abbreviations

GIST Gastrointestinal stromal tumor
TKI Tyrosine kinase inhibitor

Gastrointestinal stromal tumors (GISTs) are the most common mesenchymal tumor of the gastrointestinal tract, accounting for 18 % of all sarcomas [1]. At least 50 % of all GISTs arise in the stomach, but these tumors can arise anywhere along the gastrointestinal tract. GISTs have historically been associated with a poor prognosis with a median survival for patients with primary disease of 60 months and 19 months for those with metastatic disease [2]. Advances in the last 20 years in the diagnosis and treatment of GISTs have led to significant improvements in outcomes, making the treatment of GIST a model for the development of targeted therapy for solid tumors.

Historically, mesenchymal tumors of the GI tract were inconsistently classified as either gastrointestinal sarcoma, gastrointestinal leiomyoma, leiomyosarcoma, leiomyoblastomas, plexosarcoma, or malignant fibrous histiocytoma [3]. In the 1980s, careful pathologic assessment of gastric wall tumors demonstrated variable immunohistochemical staining patterns within these different diagnoses [3, 4]. Whereas typical leiomyomas express the traditional smooth muscle cell markers, desmin and muscle actin, and gastric schwannomas tended to express the S100 marker [3, 4], a 3rd group of tumors (GIST) rarely expressed desmin, while actin expression was highly variable. This unique immunohistochemical profile brought into question the true cell of origin of these tumors, suggesting the possibility of this being a distinctive clinical entity. It is important to remember that reviews on gastrointestinal sarcomas published prior to 1998 included patients with tumors that would currently be classified as GISTs but were not a pathologic-described entity at that time [5, 6].

C.L. Roland, MD • B.W. Feig, MD (✉)
Department of Surgical Oncology, The University of Texas M.D. Anderson Cancer Center, 1400 Pressler St. Unit 1484, Houston 77030, TX, USA
e-mail: clroland@mdanderson.org; bwfeig@mdanderson.org

© Springer International Publishing Switzerland 2017

C.R. Scoggins et al. (eds.), *Gastrointestinal Stromal Tumors*,
DOI 10.1007/978-3-319-42632-7_1

A breakthrough in our understanding of the pathogenesis of GIST came in 1998. Hirota et al. [7] elegantly demonstrated several critical features that would change the way we diagnose and treat patients with mesenchymal tumors of the GI tract. Initially, KIT (CD 117) expression by immunohistochemistry was evaluated on 58 mesenchymal tumors of the GI tract. 78 % of suspected GIST were positive for KIT and CD34 (the known marker for GIST at that time), whereas 0 % of leiomyomas and schwannomas expressed KIT. Next, KIT and CD34 expression in these tumors were compared to expression in the interstitial cells of Cajal, the intestinal pacemaker cells located in and near the circular muscle layer of intestine. They found that these cells also co-expressed KIT and CD34, indicating this as the likely cell of origin of the GIST. Reverse-transcriptase-polymerase chain reaction of c-kit clones demonstrated activating mutations in the juxtamembrane domain of the c-kit gene (on exon 9, 11, 13, or 17), resulting in constitutive activation of the c-kit receptor tyrosine kinase. Finally, injection of mutant c-kit cells into nude mice resulted in tumor formation, whereas cells with wild-type c-kit did not. Based on these experiments, it is now established that GIST arise from the interstitial cells of Cajal and activating mutations in the transmembrane domain of the tyrosine kinase leads to activation of the receptor, resulting in tumor formation [7].

Around the same time that Hirota and colleagues were investigating c-kit in GIST, groundbreaking work was being done in the treatment of chronic myelogenous leukemia. Identification of the Philadelphia chromosome (BCR-ABL) led to the development of a tyrosine kinase inhibitor (TKI) and imatinib (Gleevec) which was under clinical trial for treatment of BCR-ABL+ CML [8]. Fortunately, it was noted that KIT and ABL share many structural similarities and imatinib was specific not only for the TK ABL, but KIT and platelet-derived growth factor receptor (PDGFR) as well. Two years after the identification of c-kit as the activating mutation in GIST, the first patient with advanced GIST was treated on a clinical trial with imatinib [9]. This led to phase I, II, and two phase III trials evaluating the effect of imatinib in patients with advanced and metastatic GIST [10, 11]. Median overall survival in these trials ranged from 55 to 57 months, compared to 9 months in historical controls (Fig. 1). The prognosis for patients with GIST had been significantly altered and the FDA first granted approval for the use of imatinib in patients with advanced GIST in February 2002.

Following the initial FDA approval for metastatic and advanced GIST, investigations into the use of imatinib for adjuvant therapy were undertaken. A multi-institutional, double blind randomized controlled trial (ACOSOG Z9001) demonstrated 1 year of adjuvant imatinib after complete surgical resection was associated with improved 1-year recurrence-free survival compared to placebo for patients with GIST >3 cm [12]. Based on these findings, the FDA approved imatinib for use in the adjuvant setting in 2012. Current data suggest that 3 years of adjuvant imatinib is associated with improved recurrence-free and overall survival compared with 1 year of imatinib (Fig. 2) [13]. At the present time, there is a phase II, multi-

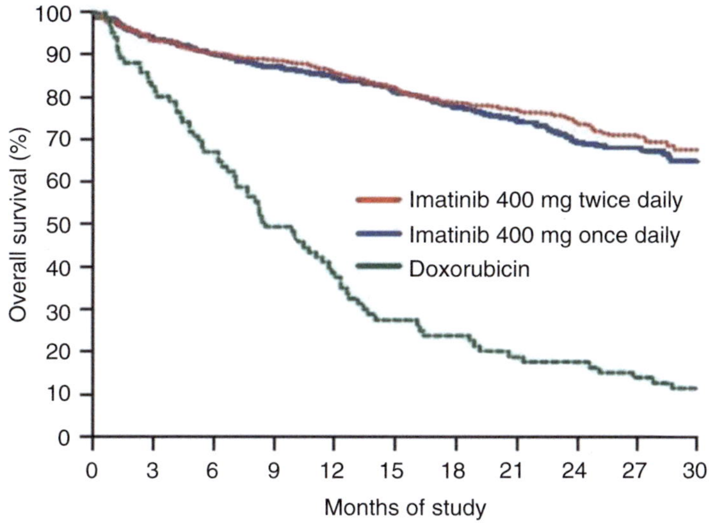

Number at risk						
Imatinib 400 mg once daily	473	423	387	315	192	49
Imatinib 400 mg twice daily	473	427	399	323	201	51
Doxorubicin	86	57	31	19	14	8

Fig. 1 Overall survival for total study population (EORTC 62005) with historical (GIST) controls from EORTC database (From Verweijet et al. [11], 1331; with permission)

center trial evaluating outcomes following 5 years of imatinib following after surgical resection [14], demonstrating that the duration of adjuvant TKI is yet to be fully elucidated.

Although the outcomes for patients with GIST have changed dramatically with the advent of imatinib, approximately 10 % of patients have primary resistance to imatinib and ~50 % will acquire secondary resistance, resulting in the need for second line therapies. Sunitinib is a TKI that inhibits KIT, PDGFRA, PDGFRB, and other TKs and was the second TKI approved for treatment of metastatic GIST after demonstrating prolonged progression-free survival in patients with imatinib-resistant GIST compared to placebo [15]. Regorafenib is the most recent FDA-approved TKI for patients with advanced/metastatic GIST, based on a phase III trial demonstrating improved median progression-free survival by 3.9 months compared to placebo [16].

The past 20 years has been a remarkable time in our understanding of the pathogenesis and treatment of GIST. Identification of (1) the cell of origin, (2) a targetable mutation, and (3) drug discovery has changed the outcome for thousands of patients with GIST. Future advances require an understanding of the molecular biology of when imatinib is ineffective, which will open opportunities for new treatments. It remains an exciting time in the study of these unique tumors, with endless possibilities.

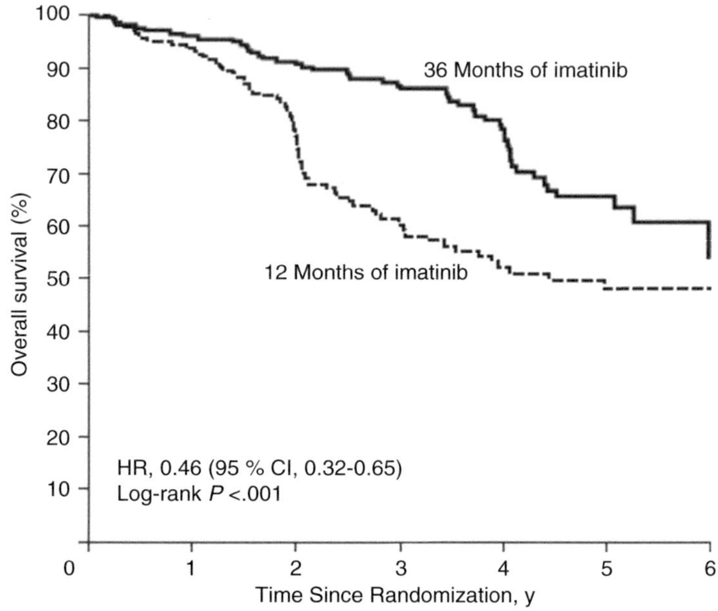

No. of patients							
36 Months of imatinib	198	184	173	133	82	39	8
12 Months of imatinib	199	177	137	88	49	27	10

Fig. 2 Recurrence-free survival in patients treated with 1 vs 3 years of adjuvant imatinib after surgical resection (From Joensuu et al. [13]; with permission)

References

1. Ducimetiere F, Lurkin A, Ranchere-Vince D, Decouvelaere AV, Peoc'h M, Istier L, et al. Incidence of sarcoma histotypes and molecular subtypes in a prospective epidemiological study with central pathology review and molecular testing. PLoS One. 2011;6(8):e20294.
2. DeMatteo RP, Lewis JJ, Leung D, Mudan SS, Woodruff JM, Brennan MF. Two hundred gastrointestinal stromal tumors: recurrence patterns and prognostic factors for survival. Ann Surg. 2000;231(1):51–8.
3. Mazur MT, Clark HB. Gastric stromal tumors. Reappraisal of histogenesis. Am J Surg Pathol. 1983;7(6):507–19.
4. Miettinen M. Gastrointestinal stromal tumors. An immunohistochemical study of cellular differentiation. Am J Clin Pathol. 1988;89(5):601–10.
5. Ng EH, Pollock RE, Munsell MF, Atkinson EN, Romsdahl MM. Prognostic factors influencing survival in gastrointestinal leiomyosarcomas. Implications for surgical management and staging. Ann Surg. 1992;215(1):68–77.
6. Conlon KC, Casper ES, Brennan MF. Primary gastrointestinal sarcomas: analysis of prognostic variables. Ann Surg Oncol. 1995;2(1):26–31.
7. Hirota S, Isozaki K, Moriyama Y, Hashimoto K, Nishida T, Ishiguro S, et al. Gain-of-function mutations of c-kit in human gastrointestinal stromal tumors. Science. 1998;279(5350):577–80.
8. O'Brien SG, Guilhot F, Larson RA, Gathmann I, Baccarani M, Cervantes F, et al. Imatinib compared with interferon and low-dose cytarabine for newly diagnosed chronic-phase chronic myeloid leukemia. N Engl J Med. 2003;348(11):994–1004.

9. Joensuu H, Roberts PJ, Sarlomo-Rikala M, Andersson LC, Tervahartiala P, Tuveson D, et al. Effect of the tyrosine kinase inhibitor STI571 in a patient with a metastatic gastrointestinal stromal tumor. N Engl J Med. 2001;344(14):1052–6.
10. Blanke CD, Rankin C, Demetri GD, Ryan CW, von Mehren M, Benjamin RS, et al. Phase III randomized, intergroup trial assessing imatinib mesylate at two dose levels in patients with unresectable or metastatic gastrointestinal stromal tumors expressing the kit receptor tyrosine kinase: S0033. J Clin Oncol Off J Am Soc Clin Oncol. 2008;26(4):626–32.
11. Verweij J, Casali PG, Zalcberg J, LeCesne A, Reichardt P, Blay JY, et al. Progression-free survival in gastrointestinal stromal tumours with high-dose imatinib: randomised trial. Lancet. 2004;364(9440):1127–34.
12. Dematteo RP, Ballman KV, Antonescu CR, Maki RG, Pisters PW, Demetri GD, et al. Adjuvant imatinib mesylate after resection of localised, primary gastrointestinal stromal tumour: a randomised, double-blind, placebo-controlled trial. Lancet. 2009;373(9669):1097–104.
13. Joensuu H, Eriksson M, Sundby Hall K, Hartmann JT, Pink D, Schutte J, et al. One vs three years of adjuvant imatinib for operable gastrointestinal stromal tumor: a randomized trial. JAMA. 2012;307(12):1265–72.
14. NCT00867113. Five year adjuvant imatinib mesylate (Gleevec®) in Gastrointestinal Stromal Tumor (GIST). 2015. Available from: https://clinicaltrials.gov/ct2/show/NCT00867113?term=GIST+5+year&rank=2.
15. Demetri GD, van Oosterom AT, Garrett CR, Blackstein ME, Shah MH, Verweij J, et al. Efficacy and safety of sunitinib in patients with advanced gastrointestinal stromal tumour after failure of imatinib: a randomised controlled trial. Lancet. 2006;368(9544):1329–38.
16. Demetri GD, Reichardt P, Kang YK, Blay JY, Rutkowski P, Gelderblom H, et al. Efficacy and safety of regorafenib for advanced gastrointestinal stromal tumours after failure of imatinib and sunitinib (GRID): an international, multicentre, randomised, placebo-controlled, phase 3 trial. Lancet. 2013;381(9863):295–302.

Epidemiology of GIST

Taylor M. Coe and Jason K. Sicklick

1 Historical Review of GIST Epidemiology

Gastrointestinal stromal tumors (GISTs) are mesenchymal tumors that are found throughout the gastrointestinal (GI) tract. Historically, they have been reported by several other names, including plexosarcoma and GI autonomic tumor [1–3]. Furthermore, they were often misclassified as several other tumor types including leiomyomas, leiomyosarcomas, neurofibromas, and schwannomas, because microscopic evaluation in the 1980s demonstrated that these tumors contained both myogenic and neural features [1–3]. In 1998, it was discovered that these tumors were molecularly characterized by a gain-of-function mutation in the *KIT* (*c-KIT*) gene [4]. Given these characteristics, it was postulated that these tumors arise from the interstitial cells of Cajal, which also express the KIT protein (also known as CD117) [4–7]. Prior to the implementation of these well-defined pathologic criteria, it was difficult to describe the epidemiology of these tumors due to their misclassification as many of the aforementioned tumor types. This lack of uniform nomenclature and histologic distinction resulted in frequent misdiagnoses by pathologists, as well as miscoding by cancer registrars [8, 9]. In turn, a complete understanding of the epidemiology of GIST was somewhat limited in many studies.

T.M. Coe, MD
Department of Surgery, Massachusetts General Hospital, Harvard Medical School, Boston, MA, USA
e-mail: tcoe@mgh.harvard.edu

J.K. Sicklick, MD, FACS (✉)
School of Medicine, University of California, San Diego, La Jolla, CA, USA

Division of Surgical Oncology and Department of Surgery, Moores UCSD Cancer Center, University of California, San Diego, UC San Diego Health System, 3855 Health Sciences Drive, Mail Code 0987, La Jolla, CA 92093-0987, USA
e-mail: jsicklick@ucsd.edu

© Springer International Publishing Switzerland 2017

C.R. Scoggins et al. (eds.), *Gastrointestinal Stromal Tumors*,
DOI 10.1007/978-3-319-42632-7_2

1.1 US Studies

The first national epidemiological study from the United States was completed in 2005 [10]. Utilizing the National Cancer Institute's Surveillance, Epidemiology, and End Results (SEER) database, which consists of 18 regional cancer registries across the United States and covers approximately 28 % of the US population, Tran et al. analyzed 1458 patients diagnosed with malignant GIST from 1992 to 2000. They found an age-adjusted annual incidence rate of 6.8 cases per million persons. Demographically, men were 1.5 times more likely to be affected than women and GISTs were most prevalent among African Americans. The mean age at diagnosis was 62.9 years old. The most common tumor location was the stomach (51 %), followed by the small intestine (36 %). At the time of diagnosis, 53 % of patients had localized, 19 % had regional disease, and 23 % had distant disease.

Subsequently, a separate analysis in 2006 utilized both the SEER database and the Florida Cancer Data System [11]. This study demonstrated a 25 % increase in GIST diagnoses from 1992 to 2002, which correlated with a decrease in reporting of smooth-muscle neoplasms (e.g., leiomyosarcoma). This was most likely due to pathologic reclassification, and less likely due to a true increase in the incidence of GIST. According to this study, the age-adjusted incidence of GIST was 6.88 cases per million persons [11]. The median age at diagnosis was 63 years old in both registries. Finally, the tumors were again noted to be more common in African Americans, corroborating the findings in the initial SEER study.

Five years later, in 2011, the SEER database was again queried between 1993 and 2002 [12]. In this study, the authors were expanding our understanding of the economic burden of GIST in the United States. In characterizing the patient cohort, the average annual incidence of surgically resected, localized GIST was 3.2 cases per million persons. This reported incidence was likely lower than prior studies because it was restricted to patients with localized diseases that were treated surgically. Moreover, they found that the economic burden of GIST was $23,300 in the first year after surgical resection while the 5-year cumulative cost of resected GIST for patients without a recurrence was $83,400, as compared to $185,100 for patients with a recurrence. This was important, because for the first time, they also reported that the 15-year limited-duration prevalence of GIST was 16.2 cases per million persons, suggesting that patients with GIST were living for many years following resection.

Taken together, the SEER database was analyzed several times in the early 2000s, providing relatively similar data on the incidence, demographics, and economic burden of GIST, but also being confounded by the presence of other sarcoma types in the analyses. Studies a decade later would clarify these issues and provide new insights into the epidemiology of GIST.

1.2 European Studies

In Europe, a number of retrospective population-based studies were conducted to identify the incidence of GIST based upon positive immunohistochemical staining for KIT. In Western Sweden, the tumors of 288 patients with KIT^+ primary GIST were retrospectively reviewed from 1983 to 2000 [13]. In this study, the annual incidence of GIST in Sweden was 14.5 cases per million persons and the prevalence was 129 cases per million persons. They found that the risk factors associated with mortality included tumor size, degree of cellular pleomorphism, mitotic index and the Ki-67 proliferative index. Another Northern European study investigated the populace of Iceland, which has a robust population-based database for the study of diseases. Tryggvason et al. analyzed 114 cases from 1990 to 2003 [14]. Of those cases, 57 were defined as GIST by positive KIT staining. The incidence of GIST was 11 cases per million persons with an average age of 65.8 years old. Tumors were more common in males (57.9 %) and most tumors were located in the stomach (61.4 %) or the small intestine (29.8 %). A separate retrospective in the Netherlands analyzed the Pathological Anatomy National Automated Archive (PALGA) registry, a nationwide network and registry of histopathology and cytopathology [15]. The authors reported an increase in the annual incidence of GIST from 2.1 cases per million persons to 12.7 cases per million persons from 1995 to 2003, which was explained by the advances in the histopathologic diagnosis of GIST. In the United Kingdom, Ahmed et al. retrospectively reviewed all possible GIST specimens from the Nottingham City Hospital and the Queens Medical Centre [16]. From 1987 to 2003, 225 patients with GIST were identified, however only 185 patients had complete histopathological and clinical data, as well as follow-up data. In this study, the annual incidence was 13.2 cases per million persons, while the average age at diagnosis was 64.4 years old. Consistent with all prior studies, the majority of tumors were found in the stomach (51.9 %). Looking southward, similar findings continued to be made. In an Italian study, Mucciarini et al. identified 124 patients with GIST within the Modena Cancer Registry from 1991 to 2004 [17]. The age-standardized incidence rate was found to be 6.6 cases per million persons. The median age at presentation was 69 years old with the stomach being the most common site. Finally, in France, a prospective study was performed in which pathologists reported all GIST cases during 2005 [18]. The estimated incidence was 8.5–10 cases per million persons with a mean age at diagnosis of 65 years old. Taken together, these six European studies analyzing immunohistochemically confirmed GIST demonstrated that: (1) annual incidence was 2.1–14.5 cases per million persons; (2) the disease was more common in males in these countries; (3) the average age of disease diagnosis was mid to late 60s; (4) and the stomach was the most common site of disease in more than half of cases.

1.3 Asian Studies

Like several European countries, the epidemiology of GIST has also been studied in individual Asian countries. In Taiwan, all GI tract surgical specimens at the Mackay Memorial Hospital were studied from 1998 to 2004 [19]. Mesenchymal lesions were evaluated with KIT (CD117) immunohistochemical analysis and KIT/PDGFRα mutational analyses. The annual incidence was estimated at 13.74 cases per million persons with the stomach being the most common site of disease (50.5 %). A second study from Taiwan analyzed the Taiwan Cancer Registry (TCR) from 1998 to 2008 [20]. Chiang et al. found that the incidence increased from 11.3 cases per million persons in 1998 to 19.7 cases per million persons in 2008. The median age range at diagnosis was 62–64 years old and there was a slight male predominance. In China, Chan et al. analyzed 47 patients from the Yan Chai Hospital who were diagnosed with GIST between 1995 and 2003 [21]. They described an annual incidence of 16.8–19.6 cases per million persons. The mean age at diagnosis was 66.6 years old and the stomach was again the most common site of disease (72.3 %). Taken together, these studies from Asia confirmed many of the aforementioned findings in the North American and European studies, while perhaps suggesting that the annual incidence of disease in Asian countries may be slightly higher than in non-Asian countries.

1.4 Summary of Studies in the 1990s–2000s

Overall, the 12 studies reported from the United States, as well as European and Asian countries collectively estimated an annual incidence of GIST between 2.1 and 19.7 cases per million persons. However, the reported rates in the United States appeared to fall on the lower end of this range. This is likely because SEER only includes "malignant" tumors (i.e., predates current-day GIST risk assessment stratifications), while the European and Asian studies outlined above included both "benign" and "malignant" cases that were also immunohistochemically confirmed to express KIT protein. But, it is now more accurate to consider every GIST as having malignant potential, and therefore stratify them as very low, low, intermediate, and high risk [22].

2 Recent Review of GIST Epidemiology in the United States

As previously discussed, coding in SEER historically did not distinguish GIST from other GI sarcoma types, including leiomyosarcoma. Thus, the implementation of a GIST-specific histology code in 2001 allowed for more accurate population-based epidemiological assessments. A contemporary analysis of the SEER database from 2001 to 2011 found that the US incidence of "malignant" GIST was 6.8 cases per million persons [23]. In this study, the age-adjusted incidence rose 42 % over the decade, from 5.5 cases per million persons in 2001 to 7.8 cases per million persons in 2011, with a peak incidence of 8.2 cases per million persons in 2010 [23]. While this incidence is comparable to prior SEER analyses, it is likely more accurate given the adoption of the GIST-specific histology code. However, due to the exclusion of "benign" GIST, it still likely underestimates the incidence in the United States. In this study, the median age at diagnosis was 64 years old and GIST was 36 % more common in males than females. Additionally, African Americans and Asians/Pacific Islanders were 2.07 and 1.5 times more likely to be diagnosed with GIST when compared to Caucasians. Consistent with all prior studies, tumors were most commonly located in the stomach (55 %) and small intestine (29 %), followed by the colon (2.9 %) and rectum (2.7 %). Risk factors associated with mortality included increased age at diagnosis, male sex, Black race, and regional or metastatic disease. It is noteworthy that this did not include tumor size. Given that SEER does not include "benign" GIST, which are often small and classified as very low or low risk by current risk stratification schema, Coe et al. performed a subset analysis of the SEER database to define the annual incidence of GIST that are smaller than 2 cm in diameter [24]. The authors found that the annual incidence was 0.42 cases per million persons. Unlike essentially all earlier reports of GIST, these small GISTs were equally distributed between the sexes. But, similar to GIST of all sizes, they were 2.1 times more common in African Americans than Caucasians and the most common sites remained the stomach (62.2 %) and the small intestine (23.3 %). Interestingly, the presence of additional cancers in these patients was associated with a 63 % increased risk of death on multivariate analysis controlling for age, sex, race, ethnicity, and tumor location. The underlying reasons for this remain to be determined. But, despite these increased insights into the epidemiology of GIST in the United States, the data remain limited because the SEER database only includes tumors that are labeled as "malignant" and therefore reported to respective cancer registries, leading to an underestimation of the true incidence of disease. In fact, Choi et al. recently demonstrated that only 38.8 % of GIST diagnosed at their institution were subsequently reported to a cancer registry [25]. Therefore, the true incidence of all GIST, both "benign" and "malignant," is likely higher than what is appreciated through these analyses of national cancer registries in the United States. In fact, while not population-based, and clearly subject to several biases, it has been reported that up to 30 % of people have small GIST based upon autopsy studies and retrospective pathological series, which include incidentally discovered asymptomatic tumors identified during endoscopic procedures or cross-sectional radiologic studies [26–34].

3 Additional Cancers in Patients with GISTs

GISTs have often been associated with additional cancers. Approximately 5 % of GISTs are due to hereditary syndromes while the remainder are considered sporadic

[35]. The most common hereditary syndromes include neurofibromatosis type I (NF-1), Carney's triad, Carney-Stratakis syndrome, and familial syndromes with germline mutations in *KIT* or *PDGFRAα* [35–39].

Among the remaining sporadic cases, it has been reported that the frequency of additional malignancies ranges from 4.5 to 33 % [40]. Recently, analysis of SEER demonstrated that 17.1 % of patients with GIST developed an additional cancer [41]. Cancers with significantly increased occurrence before and after GIST diagnosis included other sarcomas, neuroendocrine-carcinoid tumors, non-Hodgkin lymphoma, and colorectal adenocarcinoma. Prior to GIST diagnosis, esophageal, bladder and prostate adenocarcinoma, as well as melanoma were significantly more common. After GIST diagnosis, ovarian carcinoma, small intestine adenocarcinoma, papillary thyroid cancer, renal cell carcinoma, hepatobiliary adenocarcinoma, gastric adenocarcinoma, pancreatic adenocarcinoma, uterine adenocarcinoma, non-small cell lung cancer, and transitional cell carcinoma of the bladder were all significantly more common. Risk factors for additional cancers prior to GIST diagnosis included being of non-Hispanic ethnicity, as well as having a GIST $\leq$10 cm. Consistent with the aforementioned study of small GIST, patients with GIST $\leq$2 cm had the highest likelihood of developing an additional malignancy before/after GIST. The underlying reason(s) for this association remain to be determined, and our understanding of the nongenetic factors (e.g., infectious causes, environmental risk factors, exposure to toxic chemicals, treatment-related toxicities, and detection bias) that may contribute to the development and diagnosis of GIST remains limited, warranting further epidemiological studies (Table 1).

4 Conclusion

In conclusion, many studies around the world have attempted to identify the incidence of GIST, ranging from national database analyses in the United States to retrospective pathological analyses conducted throughout Europe and Asia. The incidence of disease varies from 2.1 to 19.7 cases per million persons. GIST appears to be slightly more common in males than females with an average age range in the mid-60s and peak incidence in the 70s. For unclear reasons, race appears to be a factor in disease development with African Americans and Asian/Pacific Islanders being more commonly affected than Caucasians. As reported in every study, it is clear that the stomach is the most common tumor location followed by the small intestine. Finally, risk factors for death secondary to disease include increased age at diagnosis, male sex, Black race, and regional/metastatic disease. Despite increased understanding of the epidemiology of GIST over the last two decades, further studies are warranted to better define the incidence, prevalence, and risk factors for developing GIST.

Table 1 Incidence and study characteristics from epidemiologic studies

Authors	Year	Country	Study period	Study type	KIT immunohistochemistry	Peak incidence (per 1,000,000)	Median age at diagnosis (years)
Goettsch et al. [15]	2005	Netherlands	1995–2003	Retrospective pathology review	Partial (87 %)	12.7	Not reported
Tryggvason et al. [14]	2005	Iceland	1990–2003	Retrospective pathology review	Yes	11[a]	65.8
Tran et al. [10]	2005	United States	1992–2000	SEER analysis	No	6.8[a]	63
Nilsson et al. [13]	2005	Western Sweden	1983–2000	Retrospective pathology review	Yes	14.5	69
Chan et al. [21]	2006	China	1995–2003	Retrospective pathology review	Yes	19.6[a]	66.6
Perez et al. [11]	2006	United States	1992–2002	SEER analysis	No	6.88[a]	63
Mucciarini et al. [17]	2007	Italy	1991–2004	Modena Cancer Registry analysis	Yes	6.6	69
Tzen et al. [19]	2007	Taiwan	1998–2004	Retrospective pathology review	Yes	13.74	Not reported
Ahmed et al. [16]	2008	United Kingdom	1987–2003	Retrospective pathology review	Yes	13.2	64.4
Monges et al. [18]	2010	France	2005	Prospective pathology review	Yes	10	65
Rubin et al. [12]	2011	United States	1993–2002	SEER analysis	No	3.2[a]	75
Chiang et al. [20]	2014	Taiwan	1998–2008	Taiwan Cancer Registry analysis	No	19.7[a]	62–64
Ma et al. [23]	2015	United States	2001–2011	SEER analysis	No	7.8[a]	64

[a]Originally reported per 100,000 persons. Data standardized as cases per million persons

References

1. Mazur MT, Clark HB. Gastric stromal tumors. Reappraisal of histogenesis. Am J Surg Pathol. 1983;7(6):507–19.
2. Herrera GA, Pinto de Moraes H, Grizzle WE, Han SG. Malignant small bowel neoplasm of enteric plexus derivation (plexosarcoma). Light and electron microscopic study confirming the origin of the neoplasm. Dig Dis Sci. 1984;29(3):275–84.
3. Herrera GA, Cerezo L, Jones JE, et al. Gastrointestinal autonomic nerve tumors. 'Plexosarcomas'. Arch Pathol Lab Med. 1989;113(8):846–53.
4. Hirota S, Isozaki K, Moriyama Y, et al. Gain-of-function mutations of c-kit in human gastrointestinal stromal tumors. Science. 1998;279(5350):577–80.
5. Sircar K, Hewlett BR, Huizinga JD, Chorneyko K, Berezin I, Riddell RH. Interstitial cells of Cajal as precursors of gastrointestinal stromal tumors. Am J Surg Pathol. 1999;23(4):377–89.
6. Kindblom LG, Remotti HE, Aldenborg F, Meis-Kindblom JM. Gastrointestinal pacemaker cell tumor (GIPACT): gastrointestinal stromal tumors show phenotypic characteristics of the interstitial cells of Cajal. Am J Pathol. 1998;152(5):1259–69.
7. Miettinen M, Sarlomo-Rikala M, Lasota J. Gastrointestinal stromal tumors: recent advances in understanding of their biology. Hum Pathol. 1999;30(10):1213–20.
8. Fletcher CD, Berman JJ, Corless C, et al. Diagnosis of gastrointestinal stromal tumors: a consensus approach. Hum Pathol. 2002;33(5):459–65.
9. Erlandson RA, Klimstra DS, Woodruff JM. Subclassification of gastrointestinal stromal tumors based on evaluation by electron microscopy and immunohistochemistry. Ultrastruct Pathol. 1996;20(4):373–93.
10. Tran T, Davila JA, El-Serag HB. The epidemiology of malignant gastrointestinal stromal tumors: an analysis of 1,458 cases from 1992 to 2000. Am J Gastroenterol. 2005;100(1):162–8.
11. Perez EA, Livingstone AS, Franceschi D, et al. Current incidence and outcomes of gastrointestinal mesenchymal tumors including gastrointestinal stromal tumors. J Am Coll Surg. 2006;202(4):623–9.
12. Rubin JL, Sanon M, Taylor DCA, Coombs J, Bollu V, Sirulnik L. Epidemiology, survival, and costs of localized gastrointestinal stromal tumors. Int J Gen Med. 2011;4:121–30.
13. Nilsson B, Bumming P, Meis-Kindblom JM, et al. Gastrointestinal stromal tumors: the incidence, prevalence, clinical course, and prognostication in the preimatinib mesylate era–a population-based study in western Sweden. Cancer. 2005;103(4):821–9.
14. Tryggvason G, Gislason HG, Magnusson MK, Jonasson JG. Gastrointestinal stromal tumors in Iceland, 1990–2003: the icelandic GIST study, a population-based incidence and pathologic risk stratification study. Int J Cancer J Int du Cancer. 2005;117(2):289–93.
15. Goettsch WG, Bos SD, Breekveldt-Postma N, Casparie M, Herings RM, Hogendoorn PC. Incidence of gastrointestinal stromal tumours is underestimated: results of a nation-wide study. Eur J Cancer (Oxford, England : 1990). 2005;41(18):2868–72.
16. Ahmed I, Welch NT, Parsons SL. Gastrointestinal stromal tumours (GIST) – 17 years experience from Mid Trent Region (United Kingdom). Eur J Surg Oncol J Eur Soc Surg Oncol Br Assoc Surg Oncol. 2008;34(4):445–9.
17. Mucciarini C, Rossi G, Bertolini F, et al. Incidence and clinicopathologic features of gastrointestinal stromal tumors. A population-based study. BMC cancer. 2007;7:230.
18. Monges G, Bisot-Locard S, Blay JY, et al. The estimated incidence of gastrointestinal stromal tumors in France. Results of PROGIST study conducted among pathologists. Bull Cancer. 2010;97(3):E16–22.
19. Tzen CY, Wang JH, Huang YJ, et al. Incidence of gastrointestinal stromal tumor: a retrospective study based on immunohistochemical and mutational analyses. Dig Dis Sci. 2007;52(3):792–7.
20. Chiang NJ, Chen LT, Tsai CR, Chang JS. The epidemiology of gastrointestinal stromal tumors in Taiwan, 1998–2008: a nation-wide cancer registry-based study. BMC Cancer. 2014;14:102.
21. Chan KH, Chan CW, Chow WH, et al. Gastrointestinal stromal tumors in a cohort of Chinese patients in Hong Kong. World J Gastroenterol WJG. 2006;12(14):2223–8.

22. Sicklick JK, Lopez NE. Optimizing surgical and imatinib therapy for the treatment of gastrointestinal stromal tumors. J Gastrointest Surg Off J Soc Surg Aliment Tract. 2013;17(11):1997–2006.
23. Ma GL, Murphy JD, Martinez ME, Sicklick JK. Epidemiology of gastrointestinal stromal tumors in the era of histology codes: results of a population-based study. Cancer Epidemiol Biomarkers Prev Publ Am Assoc Cancer Res, cosponsored by the American Society of Preventive Oncology. 2015;24(1):298–302.
24. Coe TM, Fero KE, Fanta PT, et al. Population-Based Epidemiology and Mortality of Small Malignant Gastrointestinal Stromal Tumors in the USA. Journal of Gastrointestinal Surgery. 2016;20(6):1132–40.
25. Choi AH, Hamner JB, Merchant SJ, et al. Underreporting of gastrointestinal stromal tumors: is the true incidence being captured? J Gastrointest Surg Off J Soc Surg Aliment Tract. 2015;19(9):1699–703.
26. Rammohan A, Sathyanesan J, Rajendran K, et al. A gist of gastrointestinal stromal tumors: a review. World J Gastrointest Oncol. 2013;5(6):102–12.
27. Demetri GD, von Mehren M, Antonescu CR, et al. NCCN Task Force report: update on the management of patients with gastrointestinal stromal tumors. J Natl Compr Canc Netw JNCCN. 2010;8 Suppl 2:S1–41; quiz S42–44.
28. Miettinen M, Lasota J. Gastrointestinal stromal tumors. Gastroenterol Clin North Am. 2013;42(2):399–415.
29. Scherubl H, Faiss S, Knoefel WT, Wardelmann E. Management of early asymptomatic gastrointestinal stromal tumors of the stomach. World J Gastrointest Endosc. 2014;6(7):266–71.
30. Agaimy A, Wunsch PH, Hofstaedter F, et al. Minute gastric sclerosing stromal tumors (GIST tumorlets) are common in adults and frequently show c-KIT mutations. Am J Surg Pathol. 2007;31(1):113–20.
31. Abraham SC, Krasinskas AM, Hofstetter WL, Swisher SG, Wu TT. "Seedling" mesenchymal tumors (gastrointestinal stromal tumors and leiomyomas) are common incidental tumors of the esophagogastric junction. Am J Surg Pathol. 2007;31(11):1629–35.
32. Kawanowa K, Sakuma Y, Sakurai S, et al. High incidence of microscopic gastrointestinal stromal tumors in the stomach. Hum Pathol. 2006;37(12):1527–35.
33. Rossi S, Gasparotto D, Toffolatti L, et al. Molecular and clinicopathologic characterization of gastrointestinal stromal tumors (GISTs) of small size. Am J Surg Pathol. 2010;34(10):1480–91.
34. Chan CHF, Cools-Lartigue J, Marcus VA, Feldman LS, Ferri LE. The impact of incidental gastrointestinal stromal tumours on patients undergoing resection of upper gastrointestinal neoplasms. Can J Surg. 2012;55(6):366–70.
35. Agaimy A, Hartmann A. Hereditary and non-hereditary syndromic gastointestinal stromal tumours. Pathologe. 2010;31(6):430–7.
36. Neuhann TM, Mansmann V, Merkelbach-Bruse S, et al. A novel germline KIT mutation (p.L576P) in a family presenting with juvenile onset of multiple gastrointestinal stromal tumors, skin hyperpigmentations, and esophageal stenosis. Am J Surg Pathol. 2013;37(6):898–905.
37. Kuroda N, Tanida N, Hirota S, et al. Familial gastrointestinal stromal tumor with germ line mutation of the juxtamembrane domain of the KIT gene observed in relatively young women. Ann Diagn Pathol. 2011;15(5):358–61.
38. Ponti G, Luppi G, Martorana D, et al. Gastrointestinal stromal tumor and other primary metachronous or synchronous neoplasms as a suspicion criterion for syndromic setting. Oncol Rep. 2010;23(2):437–44.
39. Stratakis CA, Carney JA. The triad of paragangliomas, gastric stromal tumours and pulmonary chondromas (Carney triad), and the dyad of paragangliomas and gastric stromal sarcomas (Carney-Stratakis syndrome): molecular genetics and clinical implications. J Intern Med. 2009;266(1):43–52.
40. Agaimy A, Wunsch PH, Sobin LH, Lasota J, Miettinen M. Occurrence of other malignancies in patients with gastrointestinal stromal tumors. Semin Diagn Pathol. 2006;23(2):120–9.
41. Murphy JD, Ma GL, Baumgartner JM, et al. Increased risk of additional cancers among patients with gastrointestinal stromal tumors: a population-based study. Cancer. 2015;121(17):2960–7.

Surgical Pathology of Gastrointestinal Stromal Tumors: Correlation with Clinical and Molecular Subtypes

Odise Cenaj, Vickie Y. Jo, and Leona A. Doyle

1 Introduction

Gastrointestinal stromal tumor (GIST) is the most common clinically significant mesenchymal tumor of the gastrointestinal (GI) tract [1] with a worldwide incidence of 11–18 cases per million annually [2–4]. In the early literature, these tumors were believed to contain "myofibrils," which, along with their resemblance to normal smooth muscle cells, led to their incorrect classification as various smooth muscle tumors: leiomyoma, leiomyosarcoma, and "leiomyoblastoma," the latter being now an obsolete term. However, with the advent of immunohistochemistry and electron microscopy, it became clear that these tumors did not show pure smooth muscle differentiation, and the term GIST was introduced to separate this histologically distinct group of neoplasms of the bowel wall from true smooth muscle neoplasms. Electron microscopy and immunohistochemistry showed that the tumor cells of GIST instead displayed features similar to interstitial cells of Cajal [5–8], a population of cells which reside in the autonomic myenteric plexus between muscularis propria fibers. These cells function as pacemaker cells to coordinate gut peristalsis, and show expression of KIT, as well as CD34, DOG1 (ANO1), the intermediate filament nestin, and ETV1, a member of the ETS family of transcription factors, all of which were found to be expressed in the tumor cells of GIST. Around the same time, in 1998, Hirota and colleagues identified driver oncogenic mutations in the tyrosine kinase receptor gene *KIT* in GIST [9]. Mutations in *PDGFRA* were identified in a smaller subset of GIST several years later. KIT and PDGFRA are both members of the type III receptor tyrosine kinase family and have a similar structure, consisting of an extracellular

O. Cenaj, MD • V.Y. Jo, MD • L.A. Doyle, MD (✉)
Department of Pathology, Brigham and Women's Hospital, Harvard Medical School, Boston, MA, USA
e-mail: ocenaj@partners.org; vjo@partners.org; ladoyle@partners.org

© Springer International Publishing Switzerland 2017

C.R. Scoggins et al. (eds.), *Gastrointestinal Stromal Tumors*,
DOI 10.1007/978-3-319-42632-7_3

ligand-binding domain, a transmembrane domain, a juxtamembrane domain, and a cytoplasmic kinase domain. Binding of ligand to the extracellular domain results in receptor dimerization and signal transduction via phosphorylation reactions with target proteins in the MAPK, PI3K, and p90RSK pathways. Oncogenic mutations in *KIT* and *PDGFRA* result in constitutive kinase activation in the absence of their natural ligands (stem-cell factor (SCF) for KIT, and PDGFA for PDGFRA). These discoveries led to the development of now routinely available diagnostic immunohistochemical tests (KIT and more recently DOG1), allowing for more accurate diagnosis of GIST, and it soon became apparent that GIST was far more common than pure smooth muscle tumors of the GI tract (perhaps with the exception of small benign leiomyomas of the muscularis mucosa of the colon), particularly in the stomach where smooth muscle tumors are exceptionally rare. Along with the improved classification and diagnosis of GIST, these discoveries revolutionized the field of targeted molecular therapies in solid tumors, as the tyrosine kinase inhibitor imatinib was shown to produce dramatic responses in a large number of patients and became a widely available effective treatment. It is now known that different tumor genotypes are associated with variable responses to imatinib and second, third, and fourth generation compounds, and that these genotypes often correlate with clinical and histologic features. This chapter will review key histologic features of GIST with an emphasis on clinical subtypes and molecular correlates, immunohistochemical and molecular techniques used in the evaluation of GIST, genetic changes associated with tumor development, primary and secondary resistance to therapies, and treatment response in GIST.

1.1 Clinical Features and Patterns of Disease Spread

GIST most often presents in middle aged adults, but can manifest at any age [1, 10]. There is no overall apparent sex predilection. Tumors can arise anywhere along the GI tract, with stomach being the most common site (60 %), followed by small intestine (30 %), and less often colon and esophagus. Some primary tumors are found to be located in mesenteric fat or omentum without an obvious attachment to bowel wall, and such cases likely represent tumors that were initially predominantly serosal or subserosal in location and over time became detached from the bowel wall. Extremely rare cases of GIST occurring outside the GI tract, specifically in lung and in the female genital tract, have been reported in the literature and are collectively labeled as "extra-gastrointestinal" GIST [11–13]. Patients may present with GI bleeding (or its complications) due to ulceration of overlying mucosa, obstructive symptoms such as abdominal pain or vomiting due to gastric outlet obstruction, and less often with a palpable mass, with specific symptoms dependent on tumor location within the GI tract. Not uncommonly, tumors are detected incidentally by endoscopy, radiographic imaging, or surgery performed for other unrelated indications.

The pattern of disease spread is typically characterized by liver metastasis and/or intra-abdominal dissemination along peritoneal surfaces. Lymph node metastases are exceedingly rare, but when they do occur, they are strongly associated with the clinicopathologically and molecularly distinct group of succinate dehydrogenase (SDH)-deficient GIST (see discussion below). Metastases to bone and lung can occur, albeit very rarely. Pediatric GIST, which comprises less than 2 % of all cases, has a strong female predilection [14–16], and represents the majority of SDH-deficient GIST. Clinical tumor syndromes associated with GIST include Carney triad (gastric GIST, paraganglioma, and pulmonary chondroma) and Carney-Stratakis syndrome (gastric GIST and paraganglioma) [17–19]. GIST also occurs in patients with type 1 neurofibromatosis, in which context they present as multifocal small intestinal tumors [20, 21].

1.2 Gross Pathology

GIST can range in size from less than 1 cm, so-called "micro-GIST" to up to 40 cm in greatest dimension [22], with a median size of 6 cm in the stomach, 4.5 cm in the duodenum, and 7 cm in the jejunum and ileum [16, 23, 24]. GIST usually presents as a mass arising in the submucosa, muscularis propria, or subserosa of the GI wall (Fig. 1), and serosal extension and mucosal ulceration are common. Some tumors are predominantly serosal or subserosal in location, or are located in mesenteric fat or omentum

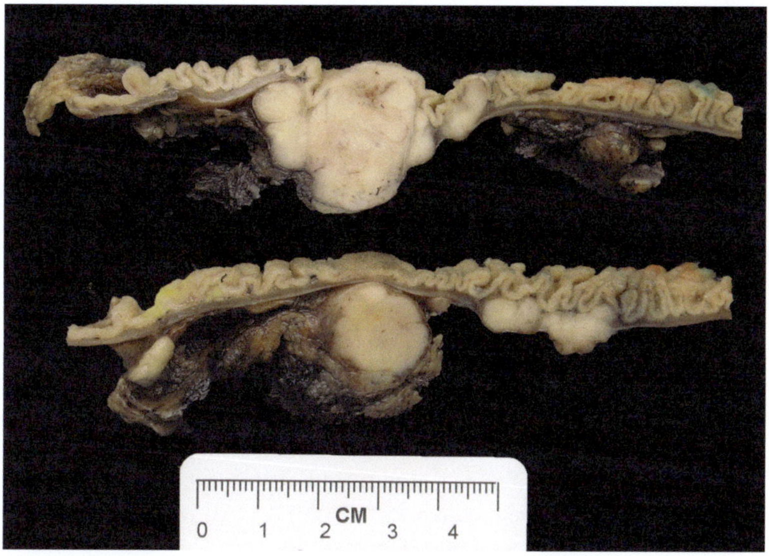

Fig. 1 Cross section through gastrointestinal stromal tumor involving the muscularis propria and subserosa of the duodenum and involvement of mesenteric fat, with an adjacent satellite tumor nodule

without an obvious attachment to bowel wall. The cut surface of GIST usually reveals a well-circumscribed fleshy (Fig. 1), fibrous, or gelatinous consistency, often with central cystic degeneration, hemorrhage, and less commonly frank necrosis.

1.3 Histopathology of GIST and Correlation with Clinical and Molecular Subtypes

1.3.1 Overview of Histologic Features

GIST has a relatively limited spectrum of histologic appearances. The majority are well-circumscribed, but some show infiltrative margins. Most (70 %) are composed of a relatively uniform population of spindle cells, and in 20 % of cases of a uniform population of epithelioid tumor cells; the remaining cases show mixed spindled and epithelioid cell morphology. The spindled tumor cells of GIST are arranged in short fascicles and appear bland (i.e., lack of significant cytologic atypia or pleomorphism) with indistinct cell borders, which imparts a syncytial appearance to the cytoplasm (Fig. 2a). The nuclei are elongated with tapered ends, vesicular chromatin, and inconspicuous nucleoli. The cells have moderate amounts of pale eosinophilic fibrillary cytoplasm (Fig. 2b). Paranuclear vacuoles are common in gastric GIST. Dense eosinophilic collagen fibrils, known as skenoid fibers, are often present in small bowel tumors. The vasculature can range from minimal to thick hyalinized hemangiopericytoma-like vessels. A lymphocytic infiltrate is often present, and nuclear palisading of tumor cells can be seen. Epithelioid GIST virtually always arises in the stomach, and is usually *PDGFRA*-mutant or less often SDH-deficient (see discussion below). These tumors have a nested or sheetlike growth pattern, and are composed of cells with round nuclei, vesicular chromatin, variably prominent nucleoli, and abundant cytoplasm which can be eosinophilic or less often clear, and may have distinct cell borders (Fig. 3a). A gastric tumor with a multinodular or plexiform growth pattern through the muscularis propria should raise suspicion for underlying SDH deficiency (discussed below). Some tumors, either epithelioid or spindled cell, may have a prominent myxoid stroma, making recognition of a tumor as GIST difficult.

1.3.2 KIT- and PDGFRA-Mutant GIST

Approximately 80 % of GIST harbor activating *KIT* mutations [1, 9, 10, 25] and 10 % mutations in *PDGFRA* [26], resulting in constitutive kinase activation independent of the presence of the receptor ligands (SCF for KIT and PDGFA for PDGFRA). KIT and PDGFRA are members of the type III receptor tyrosine kinase family and share a common structure that is comprised of an extracellular ligand-binding domain, a transmembrane domain, a juxtamembrane domain, and a cytoplasmic kinase domain. Ligand binding to the extracellular domain triggers receptor

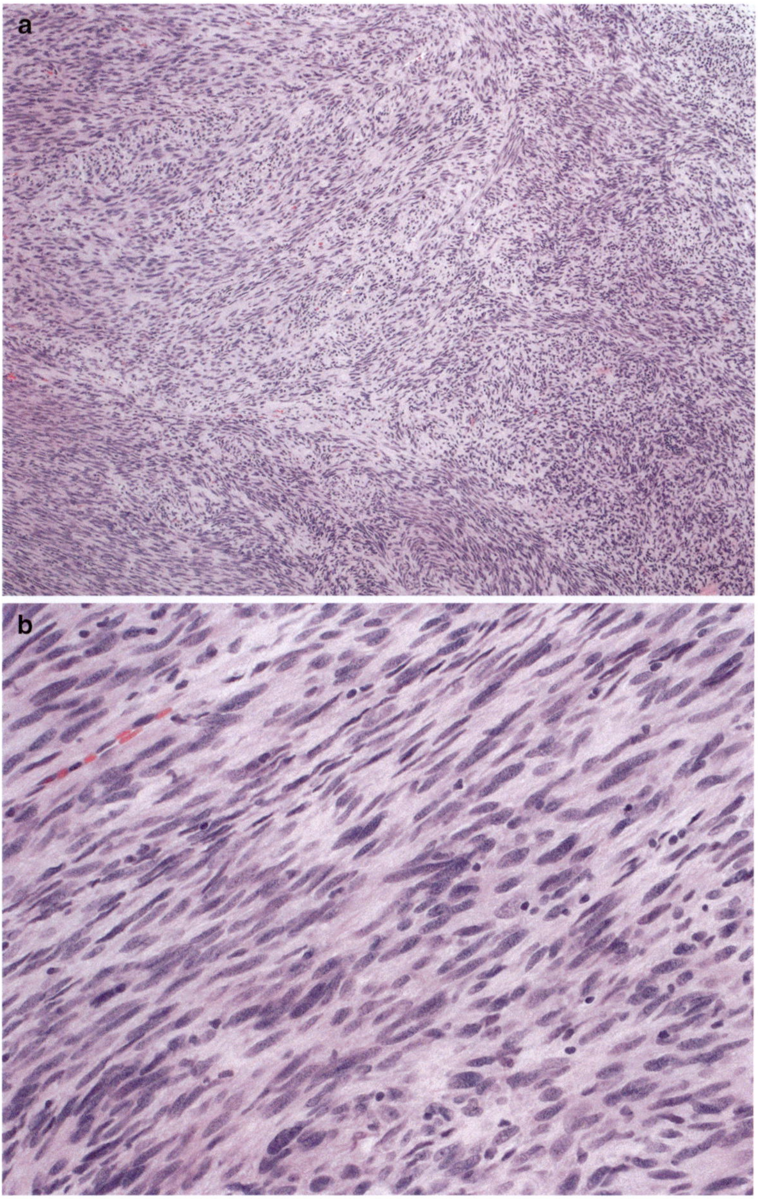

Fig. 2 Gastrointestinal stromal tumor, spindle cell type, is cellular and composed of fascicles of uniform spindle cells (**a**). On high power, the cells can be seen to have tapering nuclei with uniform fine chromatin and moderate amounts of cytoplasm with indistinct cell borders imparting a syncytial appearance (**b**). The majority of GISTs show diffuse cytoplasmic and membranous staining for KIT by immunohistochemistry (**c**)

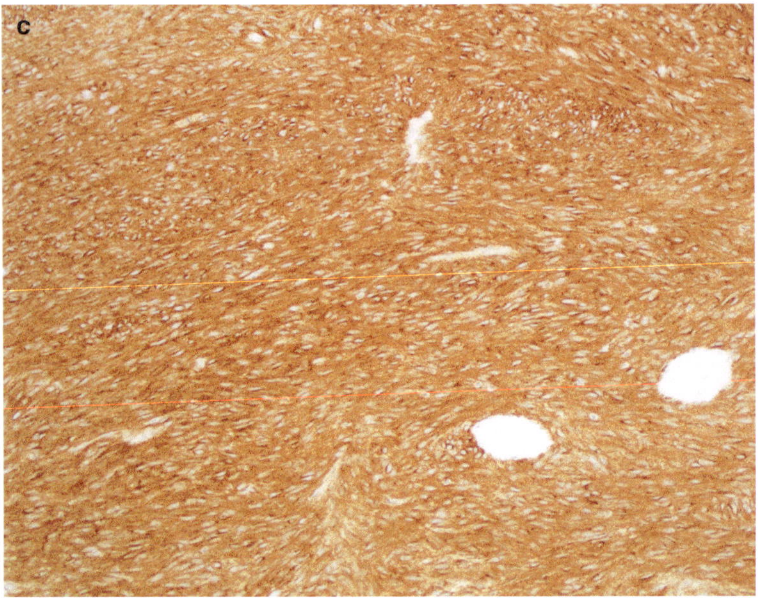

Fig. 2 (continued)

dimerization, phosphorylation, and signal transduction via MAPK, PI3K, and p90RSK pathways. It appears that *KIT* and *PDGFRA* mutations constitute the earliest molecular events detectable by current techniques in GIST tumorigenesis, and they are present in extremely small tumors [27].

The vast majority of *KIT*-mutant GIST harbors mutations in exon 11 (70 %), which encodes the juxtamembrane domain, whose normal function is to prevent the kinase activation loop from moving into the active conformation [9, 28]. Exon 11 mutations can result from substitutions, insertions, or in-frame deletions, and cause KIT to switch into an active conformation despite the absence of natural ligand SCF. Among the various mutagenic mechanisms, exon 11 deletions appear to portend a worse prognosis and are associated with shorter progression-free and overall survival compared to insertions or substitutions [29–32]. *KIT* exon 11-mutant GIST can arise anywhere in the GI tract, and are generally highly sensitive to imatinib, at least initially. The second largest group of *KIT*-mutant GIST harbors mutations in exon 9, which encodes the KIT extracellular domain, causing a conformational change that simulates ligand binding [33, 34]. Exon 9 mutations are seen in small and large intestinal GIST, but infrequently in gastric GIST. *KIT* exon 9-mutant GIST are less sensitive to tyrosine kinase inhibitors than exon 11-mutant tumors, largely because the kinase domain remains unaltered just as in wild-type *KIT,* and higher doses of imatinib are needed to achieve similar responses to those seen in exon 11-mutant tumors. Much rarer are mutations in *KIT* exon 17, which encodes the activation loop of the kinase domain, stabilizing KIT in its active conformation, and mutations in *KIT* exon 13, which encodes the adenosine triphosphate-binding

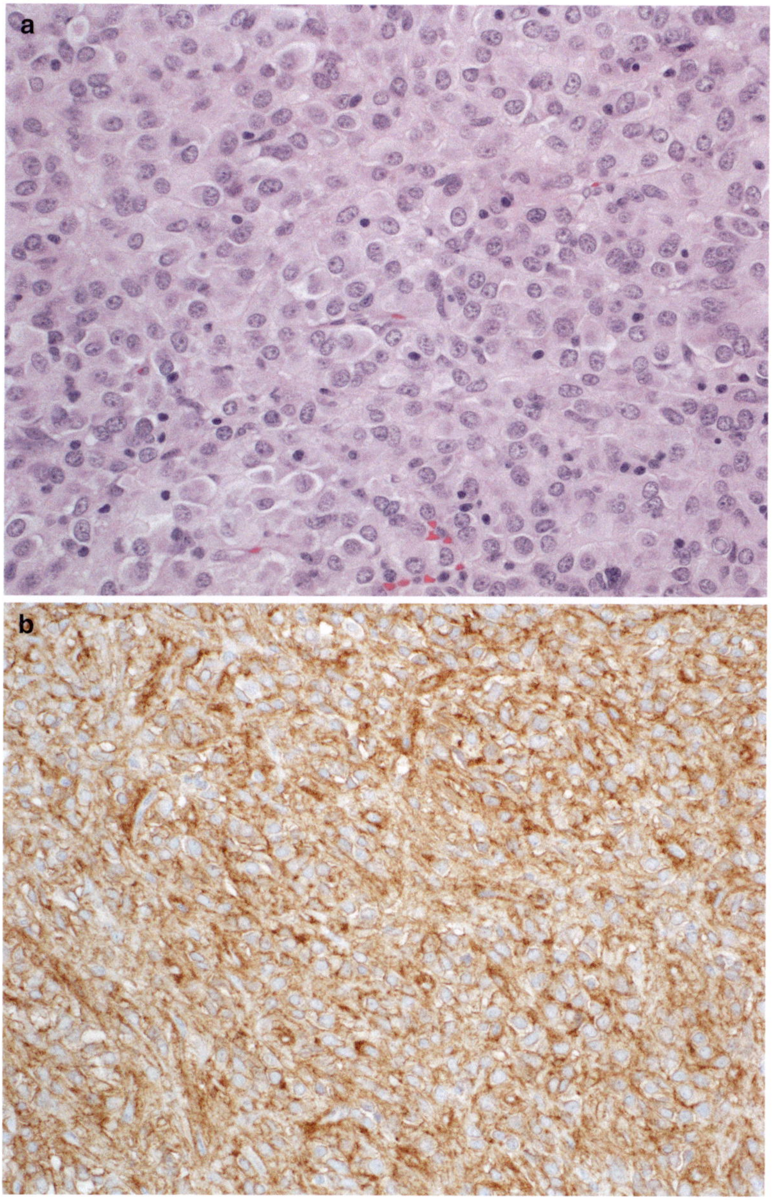

Fig. 3 Gastrointestinal stromal tumor, epithelioid type, is composed of sheets of cells with abundant pale eosinophilic cytoplasm and round to oval nuclei with variably prominent nucleoli (**a**). Some epithelioid GIST are negative for KIT, but the majority show cytoplasmic immunohistochemical expression of DOG1 (**b**)

region of the tyrosine kinase domain [35]. Both *KIT* exon 17-mutant and exon 13-mutant GIST are usually spindled in cytomorphology, and arise slightly more frequently in the small intestine than in the stomach [35]. *KIT* mutations occur extremely rarely in exon 8 [36, 37], and these tumors appear to have a predilection for the small intestine and show a mixed spindled and epithelioid morphology.

The most common *PDGFRA* mutations occur in exon 18, followed by exons 12 and 14. Exon 18 encodes the activation loop, while exons 12 and 14 encode the juxtamembrane domain and the adenosine triphosphate-binding domain, respectively [26, 38, 39]. *PDGFRA*-mutant GIST most often arises in the stomach and shows an epithelioid cytomorphology [40, 41]. Additionally, these tumors commonly have a myxoid stroma and may be negative for KIT expression by immunohistochemistry, making recognition difficult. The clinical behavior of *PDGFRA*-mutant GIST is generally more indolent compared to *KIT*-mutant GIST.

Familial GIST has been reported in multiple families [1, 25, 42]. These patients carry *KIT* or *PDGFRA* germline mutations and are affected with nearly 100 % penetrance. They present with tumors at multiple sites within the GI tract, often in a background of hyperplasia of the interstitial cells of Cajal.

1.3.3 Other Genomic Changes in GIST

In addition to oncogenic *KIT* and *PDGFRA* mutations, which are thought to represent early events in the molecular pathogenesis of GIST, comparative genomic hybridization analysis and cytogenetics studies have identified a signature of secondary chromosomal aberrations that are associated with disease progression, such as losses at 1p, 9p/9q, 11p, 15q, and gains at 5p, 8q, 17q, and 20q [43]. Chromosome 14 abnormalities occur in up to two-thirds of cases, predominantly monosomy or partial loss of 14q. Loss of the long arm of chromosome 22 is seen in approximately 50 % of tumors [35–38]. Losses at 14q and 22q do not appear to contribute to malignant behavior. However, gains on chromosome 8q (MYC locus), 3q (region of SMARCA3), and 17q have been associated with aggressive behavior [38, 39, 44, 45]. These findings are present in both *KIT* and *PDGFRA*-mutant GIST, as well as GIST that arises in patients with type 1 neurofibromatosis (NF1), but are not seen in SDH-deficient GIST. Gene expression profiling studies have identified genetic changes associated with an aggressive clinical course, including inactivation of the tumor suppressor gene *CDKN2A* [42, 46–48], *TP53* mutations [43, 49–51], abnormalities in genes involved in the PI3 kinase pathway [52], and rarely amplification of *MDM2* and *CCND1* [45, 53].

1.3.4 Micro-GIST

Tumors measuring less than 1 cm in greatest dimension are considered "micro-GIST." These small lesions are usually incidentally detected, if detected at all, and are in fact very common, as shown in systematic studies of stomachs at autopsy and surgical resection which estimate an overall frequency of 30 % among the general population [54, 55]. Micro-GIST typically shows a spindled cell morphology and has a hyalinized or calcified stroma. *KIT* mutations are detected in the vast majority of micro-GIST. The clinical course is benign and these tumors virtually never metastasize. Importantly, micro-GIST should not be confused with synchronous metastatic lesions measuring <1 cm and occurring in association with a larger dominant mass.

1.3.5 "Wild-Type" GIST

The term "wild-type" GIST is commonly used for tumors without identifiable *KIT* or *PDGFRA* mutations. This group accounts for approximately 10–15 % of adult GIST and 90 % of pediatric GIST. Recent advances in our understanding of the pathobiology of GIST have shown that this group of "wild-type" tumors actually represents a heterogeneous group of clinicopathologically and molecularly distinct GIST. This group includes not only sporadic tumors with distinct mutation signatures, but also lesions arising in patients with the nonhereditary Carney triad syndrome (gastric GIST, paraganglioma, and pulmonary chondroma) and the hereditary Carney-Stratakis syndrome (gastric GIST and paraganglioma), the latter two being part of the group of SDH-deficient GIST discussed in more detail below, NF1-associated GIST, *BRAF*-mutant GIST, and a small group whose molecular pathogenesis has yet to be elucidated. "Wild-type" GIST are largely resistant to imatinib, and therefore correct classification is paramount in order to select the appropriate therapy. Furthermore, since some of these tumors arise in association with inherited syndromes, correct classification is critical for clinical follow-up (i.e., detection of other tumor types), germline testing, and genetic counseling.

1.3.6 Succinate Dehydrogenase-Deficient GIST

This recently described clinicopathologically and molecularly distinct group of tumors includes the majority of pediatric GIST, GIST arising in patients with Carney triad, Carney-Stratakis syndrome, and a subset of apparently sporadic adult "wild-type" GIST (some previously referred to as "pediatric-type" GIST) [56, 57]. SDH-deficient GIST represents 7.5 % of all gastric GIST [58] and 42 % of all "wild-type" GIST. They have a female predilection, and arise exclusively in the stomach, usually in the antrum, where they may present as multiple discontiguous lesions. Histologically, this group of GIST shows a multinodular or plexiform growth pattern (Fig. 4a) and predominantly epithelioid morphology (Fig. 4b) [56, 57, 59]. In contrast to *KIT*- and *PDGFRA*-mutant GIST, vascular invasion may be seen and lymph node metastases are relatively more common. Although tumors lack *KIT* and *PDGFRA* mutations, immunoreactivity for KIT and DOG1 is usually strong. Additionally, tumor cells show loss of protein expression of SDHB (Fig. 4c), which is normally ubiquitously expressed in all cell types (see section "Immunohistochemistry in the Evaluation of GIST"); the mechanism underlying this "deficiency" of SDHB expression is discussed below. The above

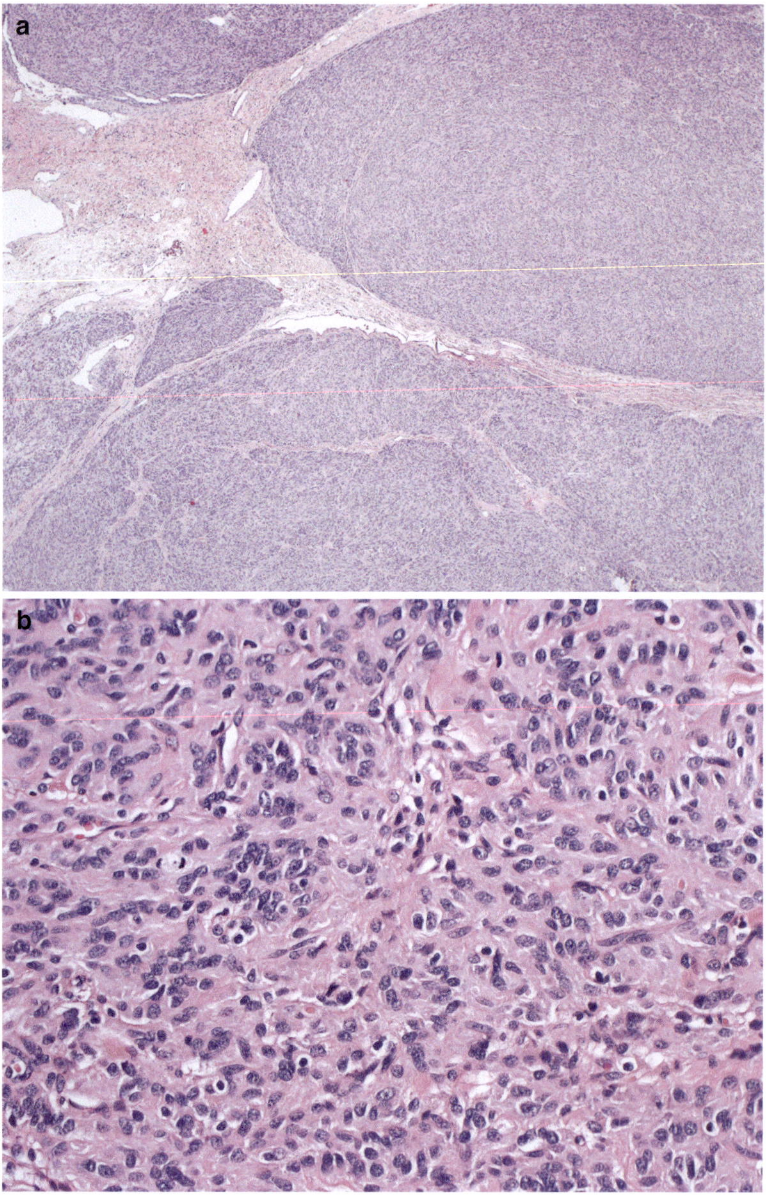

Fig. 4 Succinate dehydrogenase-deficient GIST arises in the stomach and has a characteristic plexiform or multinodular growth pattern, which can be appreciated on low power examination (**a**) or even on gross examination. The vast majority of tumors in this distinct group have an epithelioid morphology, usually purely but occasionally with a mixed spindle cell component (**b**). Like other GIST, the tumor cells express KIT and DOG1, but are distinguished by lack of expression of SDHB (**c**). SDHB is normally ubiquitously expressed, and therefore expression of SDHB within inflammatory cells, endothelium and stromal fibroblasts acts as an internal control, in contrast to the lack of staining in surrounding tumor cells, as illustrated in the image (**c**)

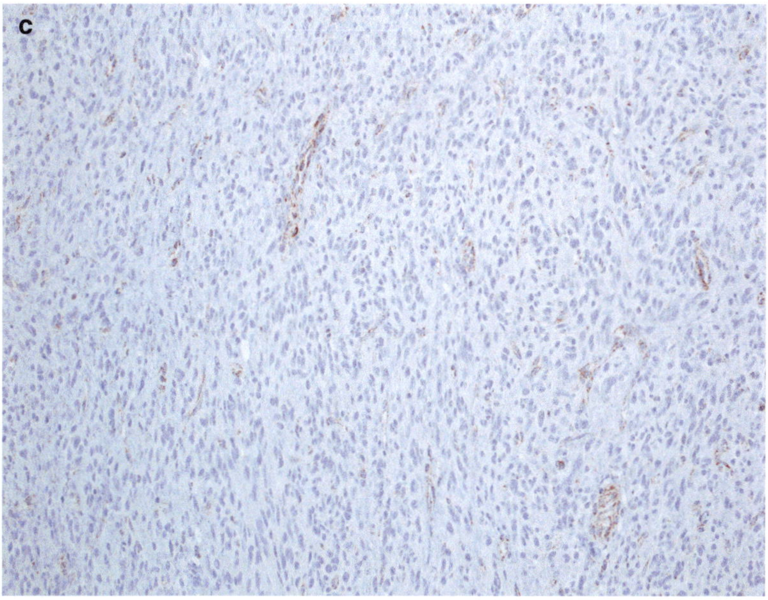

Fig. 4 (continued)

histologic and immunohistochemical features are all helpful clues to identify this distinct subgroup, which has important clinical and syndromic implications. SDH-deficient GIST tends to be resistant to imatinib, but may respond to second and third-generation tyrosine kinase inhibitors, and the clinical course of this group of tumors is relatively indolent, even in the setting of metastatic disease [56, 57].

The SDH enzyme complex is a member of the tricarboxylic acid cycle and electron transport chain that catalyzes the oxidation of succinate to fumarate, and is made of four normally and ubiquitously expressed subunit proteins SDHA, SDHB, SDHC, and SDHD [60]. Loss of SDHB expression in tumor cells reflects dysfunction of the entire SDH complex, which can be caused either by mutations in any of the genes coding for the four subunit proteins or by other functional deficiencies due to other mechanisms, such as hypermethylation or epigenetic events. In contrast, loss of SDHA expression is only seen in *SDHA*-mutated tumors. SDH complex dysfunction driven tumorigenesis is incompletely understood. Several studies have suggested that increased levels of the metabolite succinate alter the global gene methylation profile [61]. SDH-deficient GIST appears to have increased levels of methylated DNA when compared with *KIT*-mutant tumors. Succinate accumulation inhibits the TET family of DNA hydroxylases, which catalyze the production of the gene expression altering molecule 5-hydroxymethylcytosine (5-hmC). Reduced 5-hmC levels have been demonstrated in SDH-deficient GIST compared to *KIT*- and *PDGFRA*-mutant tumors [61, 62]. In addition, succinate accumulation stabilizes the hypoxia-inducible factor 1α, which enhances the transcription of target genes including vascular endothelial growth factor [63]. SDH-deficient GIST has also been strongly associated with overexpression of the type 1 insulin-like growth factor receptor (IGF1R) [64]. The mechanism underlying IGF1R overexpression is currently unknown.

The Carney-Stratakis syndrome is inherited in an autosomal dominant fashion with variable penetrance and young adulthood onset of gastric GIST and paraganglioma [18, 65]. Affected patients have loss-of-function germline mutations in *SDHB, SDHC,* or *SDHD* [65, 66]. The Carney triad syndrome is nonhereditary, usually affects young women, and manifests with gastric GIST, paraganglioma, and pulmonary chondroma [67]. GIST arising in the setting of Carney triad also shows SDH complex dysfunction reflected by loss of SDHB protein expression. However, these patients generally do not have *SDH* mutations [17, 19, 68, 69]. Recent evidence has demonstrated that the Carney triad is associated with hypermethylation of the *SDHC* promoter, resulting in loss of SDHC expression [70]. While only 20–25 % of patients with SDH-deficient GIST harbor mutations in *SDHB*, *SDHC*, or *SDHD*, mutations in *SDHA* have been found in one-third of these tumors, making *SDHA* the most commonly mutated subunit. SDH-deficient GIST with *SDHA* mutations have an older age distribution (third to fifth decades) and less female predominance compared to other SDH-deficient GIST [71–74]. Despite the presence of germline *SDHA* mutations, *SDHA*-mutant GIST is almost never familial and therefore has a low penetrance.

The diagnosis of SDH-deficient GIST has important clinical implications, both prognostically and predictively. These tumors pursue a relatively indolent clinical course, even in the presence of nodal and distant metastases. They respond poorly to imatinib, but many second- and third-generation tyrosine kinase inhibitors such as sunitinib, sorafenib, and dasatinib have greater efficacy [56, 75, 76]. Furthermore, the commonly used standard risk-stratification system (based on tumor site, tumor size, and mitotic index) for predicting malignant potential in GIST fails to predict clinical behavior for SDH-deficient tumors; thus it should not be applied [17, 56, 58]. Identifying SDH-deficient GIST also identifies a subset of patients who benefit from germline testing for *SDH* mutations and long-term clinical follow-up for the detection of the other aforementioned syndromic tumors [75, 77]. From a practical standpoint, we would advise that the possibility of SDH-deficient GIST should be considered when a gastric GIST with epithelioid morphology and multinodular plexiform architecture is encountered, and immunohistochemical loss of SDHB protein expression is an extremely useful screening tool in this regard.

1.3.7 BRAF-Mutant GIST

BRAF mutations in GIST may arise de novo or after treatment with tyrosine kinase inhibitors. Up to 13 % of "wild-type" GIST harbor the *BRAF* exon 15 V600E substitution mutation [78–80]. *BRAF*-mutant GIST have a slight female predilection, and most often arise in the small bowel. Their biological behavior and clinical course has not been well defined to date, but limited evidence suggests a high risk of malignancy based on risk-stratification criteria [78], with the caveat that *BRAF* mutations are also present in some micro-GIST with no mitotic activity [79]. *BRAF*-mutant GIST are typically composed of spindled cells and are morphologically indistinguishable from conventional *KIT*-mutant GIST

[80]. BRAF belongs to the RAF family of serine/threonine protein kinases in the RAS–RAF–ERK signaling pathway, which activates the MAPK pathway and controls cell cycle regulation and cellular response to growth signals. The V600E substitution activates the BRAF kinase domain. Thus, mutated *BRAF* may act as a primary oncogenic driver event. Moreover, since BRAF is located downstream of KIT, its activation leads to KIT-independent growth. Not surprisingly, *BRAF*-mutant "wild-type" GIST are resistant to imatinib, and *BRAF* mutations may contribute to the development of secondary resistance to imatinib in *KIT*- and *PDGFRA*-mutant GIST [78]. As a result, detection of this mutation also carries significant treatment implications. There is some evidence showing tumor regression in *BRAF*-mutant GIST treated with BRAF inhibitors [81].

1.3.8 GIST Associated with Neurofibromatosis

Patients with NF1 have a higher risk of developing GIST than the general population, and tumors usually occur at a younger age compared to cases of sporadic GIST [20, 23, 24]. NF1-associated GIST are "wild-type" and arise most frequently in the small intestine. They are usually small, almost always display a spindled cytomorphology with a low mitotic rate, and have a good prognosis [20]. In the GI tract of patients with NF1, GIST are more common than neurofibromas. Patients with NF1 typically present with multiple primary GIST, often arising in a background of hyperplasia of the interstitial cells of Cajal. The tumors display strong KIT immunoreactivity despite a lack of *KIT* mutations. The pathogenesis of GIST associated with NF1 remains unknown.

1.4 Immunohistochemistry in the Evaluation of GIST

KIT is strongly expressed in approximately 95 % of all GIST, in a diffuse cytoplasmic pattern (Fig. 2c) or, less frequently, with membranous or Golgi dot-like patterns [11]. The remaining 5 % of GIST that are KIT-negative tend to be gastric in location and epithelioid in morphology, and 70 % of this group has *PDGFRA* mutations [40]. Nearly all of the remaining 30 % of KIT-negative GIST are "wild-type." *KIT*-mutant GIST lacking KIT expression is rare [40, 82]. CD34 is positive in 70 % of GIST, h-caldesmon in 65 %, smooth muscle actin (SMA) in 30 %, and S-100 protein in 5 % (usually duodenal tumors). Desmin expression is seen in approximately 5 % of GIST, and is usually focal or multifocal in distribution (particularly gastric epithelioid GIST), and less than 1 % show focal positivity for cytokeratins. Diffuse KIT expression is uncommon in other tumor types, and is therefore helpful in confirming a diagnosis of GIST [83].

Discovered on GIST – 1, anoctamin 1 (DOG1) is a relatively new highly sensitive and specific marker for GIST [84]. DOG1 is a chloride channel protein whose overexpression was detected through gene expression profiling of GIST compared to other mesenchymal neoplasms. More than 95 % of GIST show diffuse cytoplasmic and membranous expression of DOG1 (Fig. 3b) [84–86]. DOG1 is useful to confirm a diagnosis of KIT-negative GIST as it is expressed in the majority of such tumors [82, 87, 88]. Challenging diagnostic cases of GIST that are negative for both DOG1 and KIT are rare (2.6 %) and therefore lack of expression of both markers may warrant further workup with mutational testing in order to confirm the diagnosis, as a significant subset of DOG1- and KIT-negative GIST will harbor *KIT* or *PDGFRA* mutations [86]. DOG1 is rarely expressed in other mesenchymal tumors; focal positivity has been reported in a small subset of leiomyosarcomas, uterine-type retroperitoneal leiomyomas, synovial sarcomas, and PEComas.

Immunohistochemistry for SDHB and SDHA is extremely valuable in the detection of SDH-deficient GIST [58, 59]. As discussed above, SDHB expression is lost in all SDH-deficient GIST. The diagnosis is established by the absence of SDHB staining in tumor cells and simultaneous intact staining in normal endothelial, epithelial and smooth muscle cells, which serve as an internal control (Fig. 4c). In contrast, SDHB expression is consistently intact in *KIT*- and *PDGFRA*- mutant GIST and NF1-associated GIST [89]. As discussed above, 30 % of SDH-deficient GIST has mutations in *SDHA*. These tumors exhibit loss of expression of both SDHA and SDHB [71, 72]. Loss of SDHB by immunohistochemistry should trigger reflex testing for SDHA expression. Germline mutational testing and careful family history should be obtained in patients with SDH-deficient GIST.

1.5 Prognosis and Risk Stratification

The spectrum of clinical/biological behavior of GIST ranges from "no risk" to "high risk" clinically aggressive tumors associated with widespread dissemination [90]. Most GIST have low mitotic activity. Risk stratification is performed by counting the number of mitoses in a 5 mm^2 area, which correlates to a variable number of high-power fields depending on the microscope used (in our institution this is approximately 20 high-power fields). The mitotic count is incorporated with primary tumor site and tumor size to determine risk of disease progression, based on data obtained from two large studies (Table 1) [90, 91]. As mentioned above, this

Table 1 Risk stratification of GIST by tumor size, mitotic index, and anatomic location

Mitoses (per 50 HPF)	Size (cm)	Risk of disease progression			
		Stomach	Duodenum	Jejunum/Ileum	Rectum
≤5	<2	None (0 %)	None (0 %)	None (0 %)	None (0 %)
≤5	2–5	Low (1.9 %)	Low (8.3 %)	Low (4.3 %)	Low (8.5 %)
≤5	5–10	Low (3.6 %)	Insufficient data	Moderate (24 %)	Insufficient data
≤5	>10	Moderate (10 %)	High (34 %)	High (52 %)	High (57 %)
>5	<2	None; small number of cases	Insufficient data	High; small number of cases	High (54 %)
>5	2–5	Moderate (16 %)	High (50 %)	High (73 %)	High (52 %)
>5	5–10	High (55 %)	Insufficient data	High (85 %)	Insufficient data
>5	>10	High (86 %)	High (86 %)	High (90 %)	High (71 %)

Adapted from Refs. [90, 91]

risk-stratification scheme does not apply to SDH-deficient GIST, for which clinical and histologic parameters do not seem to predict risk.

1.6 Evaluation of Treatment Response in GIST

The histologic response of GIST to tyrosine kinase inhibitors has been extensively studied. The features most commonly described are tumor necrosis, hyalinized stroma and reduction in overall tumor cellularity and mitotic activity (Fig. 5). However, none of these features seems to predict further response to therapy [92]. Marked nuclear pleomorphism may also occur in treated GIST [93, 94]. In contrast, de novo nuclear pleomorphism in GIST is very uncommon and its presence often raises the differential diagnosis of a high-grade spindle cell neoplasm. A rare effect of chronic imatinib therapy is dedifferentiation, a term used to describe tumor progression from a KIT-positive tumor to a highly pleomorphic or anaplastic KIT-negative tumor [41], which lacks the morphologic and immunophenotypic profile of conventional GIST and resembles undifferentiated pleomorphic sarcoma (Fig. 6a, b) [95]. Of note, the dedifferentiated component may show cytokeratin or desmin immunoreactivity, which can also be a diagnostic pitfall. Dedifferentiation in GIST can also occur de novo, albeit extremely rarely [96]. Dedifferentiated GIST is extremely aggressive and resistant to tyrosine kinase inhibitor therapy. Heterologous rhabdomyosarcomatous differentiation can also be seen in treated GIST, which is morphologically similar to embryonal or pleomorphic rhabdomyosarcoma [95].

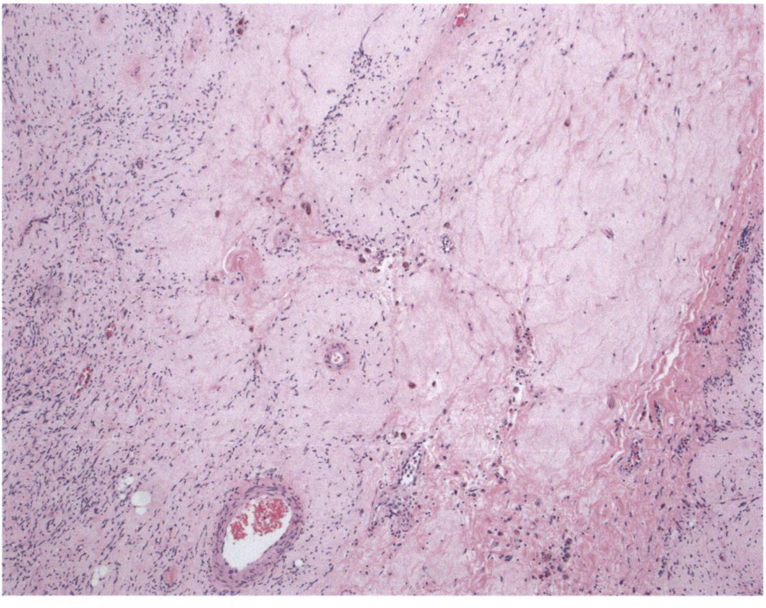

Fig. 5 The effect of tyrosine kinase inhibitors in GIST is manifested by hyalinization within the tumor, often accompanied by a reduction in tumor cellularity and mitotic activity

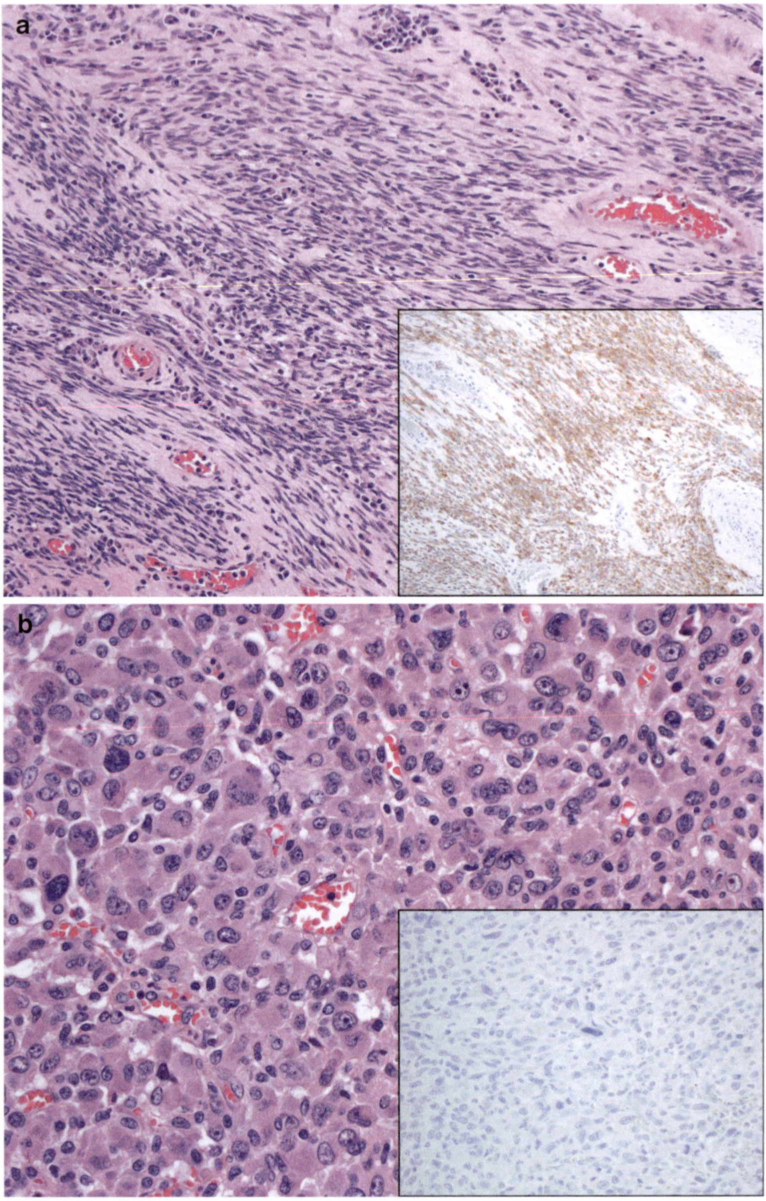

Fig. 6 Rarely, and usually after long-term treatment with tyrosine kinase inhibitors, GIST can undergo "dedifferentiation." This dedifferentiated GIST showed areas with typical spindle cell morphology, minimal atypia and some stromal hyalinization (**a**), but showed an abrupt transition to a high-grade sarcoma with marked cytologic atypia and pleomorphism (**b**), without any histologic features to suggest a diagnosis of GIST. Note the corresponding loss of expression of DOG1 in the dedifferentiated component (**b**, *inset*), in contrast to the conventional component that retains expression (**a**, *inset*). KIT usually shows a typical pattern of loss of expression in the dedifferentiated component

This phenomenon is thought to arise due to clonal evolution and has been associated with poor prognosis.

1.7 Primary and Secondary Resistance to Targeted Therapies

The two most commonly used small molecule inhibitors against KIT and PDGFRA are imatinib mesylate and sunitinib malate [91]. While imatinib is the first-line therapy for unresectable and/or metastatic GIST, sunitinib can be used for patients with progression on imatinib. Despite the success of imatinib with the vast majority of GIST, certain molecular variants show partial or no response to imatinib de novo, so-called primary resistance [97]. This group includes "wild-type" GIST (including SDH-deficient GIST), *KIT* exon 9-mutant GIST [98] (the vast majority of which is characterized by AY502-503 internal tandem duplication) and *PDGFRA* exon 18-mutant GIST (with D842V substitution being the most common alteration, which imparts complete resistance to imatinib). *KIT* exon 9-mutant GIST shows better response rates with higher dosing of imatinib, which is generally the first line of approach, whereas this effect is not seen in *PDGFRA*-mutant or "wild-type" GIST [97].

Approximately half of patients who initially respond to imatinib develop tumor progression after 6 months or more on therapy [91]. This phenomenon is termed secondary resistance and is thought to be due to secondary mutations in the KIT and PDGFRA kinase domain, leading to ineffective drug binding [25]. Most secondary KIT kinase mutations affect either the adenosine triphosphate-binding pocket of the kinase domain (V654A, T670I) or the kinase activation loop (C809G, D816H, D820A/E/G, N822K/Y, Y823D) [99]. Protein modeling studies show that these mutations induce protein conformational changes that reduce the affinity of KIT for the inhibitor [100]. In addition, it has been shown that different secondary mutations can be found in different tumor nodules within the same patient and even within different regions of the same nodule, highlighting the presence of resistant subclones and genetic diversity of disease progression, and potentially providing novel therapeutic approaches [97]. Alternative mechanisms of secondary resistance have been linked to *BRAF* mutations [78].

1.8 Role of KIT and PDGFRA Mutational Analysis

Molecular analysis of GIST is usually performed either through polymerase chain reaction or next-generation targeted exome sequencing assays and is useful in three settings. First, as discussed above, the mutational profile of GIST provides helpful prognostic information and determines the most appropriate type and dose of targeted therapy. In addition, mutational analysis can identify acquired mutations that confer secondary resistance to tyrosine kinase inhibitor therapy, thereby helping to modify the existing therapy regimen. Finally, identification of *KIT* and *PDGFRA* mutations can help in diagnostically challenging, but fortunately rare, cases of KIT- and DOG1-negative GIST and dedifferentiated GIST.

1.9 Differential Diagnosis and Histologic Mimics

The diagnosis of GIST is straightforward in most cases with characteristic morphologic features, and is aided by sensitive and specific immunohistochemical markers. However, for some cases, particularly small biopsy samples or those tumors with variant morphologic features such as marked cytologic pleomorphism or KIT negativity, the diagnosis may be more challenging. Tumors that fall into the differential diagnosis of spindle cell GIST include leiomyoma, schwannoma, desmoid fibromatosis, leiomyosarcoma, and inflammatory myofibroblastic tumor. Leiomyomas occur more frequently in the esophagus and rectum, whereas GIST is more common in the stomach and small intestine. Leiomyomas are composed of fascicles of spindle cells with cigar-shaped nuclei, bright eosinophilic cytoplasm, and distinct cell borders. Leiomyomas are negative for KIT and DOG1, but diffusely and strongly positive for SMA and desmin. Schwannomas of the GI tract typically arise in the stomach and have more stromal collagen and cytologic pleomorphism than GIST, and are surrounded by a cuff of lymphocytes. The tumor cells of schwannoma show diffuse positivity for S-100 protein and are negative for KIT. Primary GI leiomyosarcoma is exceedingly rare and typically has prominent cytologic atypia, bright eosinophilic cytoplasm, and a high mitotic rate. There is some histologic overlap between GIST and leiomyosarcoma: both exhibit a fascicular spindle cell cytomorphology and both may show variable expression of SMA and desmin. However, leiomyosarcoma shows greater atypia and is negative for KIT and DOG1. Desmoid fibromatosis is recognized by long fascicles of bland spindle cells in a background of dense stromal collagen. The tumor cells are positive for SMA and have aberrant nuclear beta-catenin staining in 80 % of cases, but are negative for KIT. Inflammatory myofibroblastic tumor is usually infiltrative and composed of fascicles of spindled myofibroblastic cells with tapered nuclei, small nucleoli, and variable amounts of pale indistinct cytoplasm. The stroma is myxoid or collagenous, with a prominent inflammatory infiltrate of plasma cells, lymphocytes, and eosinophils. Tumor cells are negative for KIT and DOG1, and express ALK in approximately 50 % of cases.

The differential diagnosis for epithelioid GIST includes carcinoid tumor and glomus tumor. Carcinoid tumors display a trabecular or nested architecture. The tumor cells have finely granular chromatin and variable amounts of cytoplasm, and immunohistochemically are positive for keratin, synaptophysin, and chromogranin, and negative for KIT. Glomus tumors are extremely rare and occur most often in the stomach. They are composed of sheets or nodules of monomorphic epithelioid cells with distinct cytoplasmic borders, similar to epithelioid GIST. Tumor cells typically show concentric growth around blood vessels. Glomus tumors are positive for SMA and caldesmon, but negative for KIT. Epithelioid GIST may resemble PEComa, but is usually readily distinguished by immunohistochemistry (the latter showing positivity for SMA, desmin, and melanocytic markers Melan A, HMB-45, and MiTF).

1.10 Fine Needle Aspiration Diagnosis of GIST and Molecular Cytopathology

Minimally invasive biopsy modalities, such as endoscopic ultrasound-guided fine needle aspiration (EUS-FNA) and intra-abdominal CT-guided FNA, have become increasingly employed in the evaluation of intra-abdominal and intrathoracic tumors, and often facilitate the initial diagnosis of GIST. Adequate sampling by endoscopic forceps can be technically challenging for tumors located submucosally or deeper within the wall of the GI tract. EUS-FNA and CT-guided FNA are inexpensive and less invasive compared to laparoscopic techniques, and have been proven to have minimal risk and yet the results can drastically alter patient management [101]. Many image-guided FNAs are performed with concurrent core needle biopsy; immunohistochemical and molecular studies can be performed both on the needle biopsy and on all cytologic preparations (aspirate smears, liquid-based preparation, and formalin-fixed paraffin-embedded cell blocks). While GIST were previously treated with resection alone in patients with localized disease, the discovery of KIT and advent of tyrosine kinase inhibitors allows the option of neoadjuvant therapy when a biopsy is diagnostic. EUS- and CT-guided FNA are therefore efficacious for patients with locally advanced unresectable tumors and patients with diffusely metastatic disease, as well as those who cannot tolerate invasive sampling procedures. In addition to establishing diagnosis, molecular testing of cytopathology specimens has become an indispensable tool in the prognostication of GIST. *KIT* and *PDGFRA* mutational analysis is feasible on routine FNA cell blocks, yielding comparable results to surgical biopsy and resection specimens [102, 103]. On-site assessment of specimen adequacy by a cytotechnologist or cytopathologist (which is routine at many institutions, including ours) can enhance diagnostic yield and ensure appropriate triage of the specimen for ancillary testing. However, it should be noted that risk stratification for malignant behavior is generally not possible in biopsy samples.

Smear preparations of spindle cell GIST tend to have moderate to high cellularity, with tumor cells arranged in cohesive clusters and sheets and singly dispersed (Fig. 7a). Within the larger fragments tumor cells are haphazardly arranged, and often associated with a prominent vascular network [104, 105]. The tumor cell population appears relatively uniform in size and shape, with spindle-shaped bland elongated nuclei having variably rounded or pointed ends (Fig. 7b). The chromatin is evenly dispersed and finely granular; nuclear membranes are smooth and nucleoli are inconspicuous. Cellular borders are usually indistinct, giving a characteristic syncytial appearance; the cytoplasm has a delicate fibrillary quality and wispy cytoplasmic projections can often be seen at the edges of the aggregates. Isolated nuclei with stripped cytoplasm are often seen in the background. For GIST with epithelioid predominant or mixed morphology, the cytologic features are overall similar but

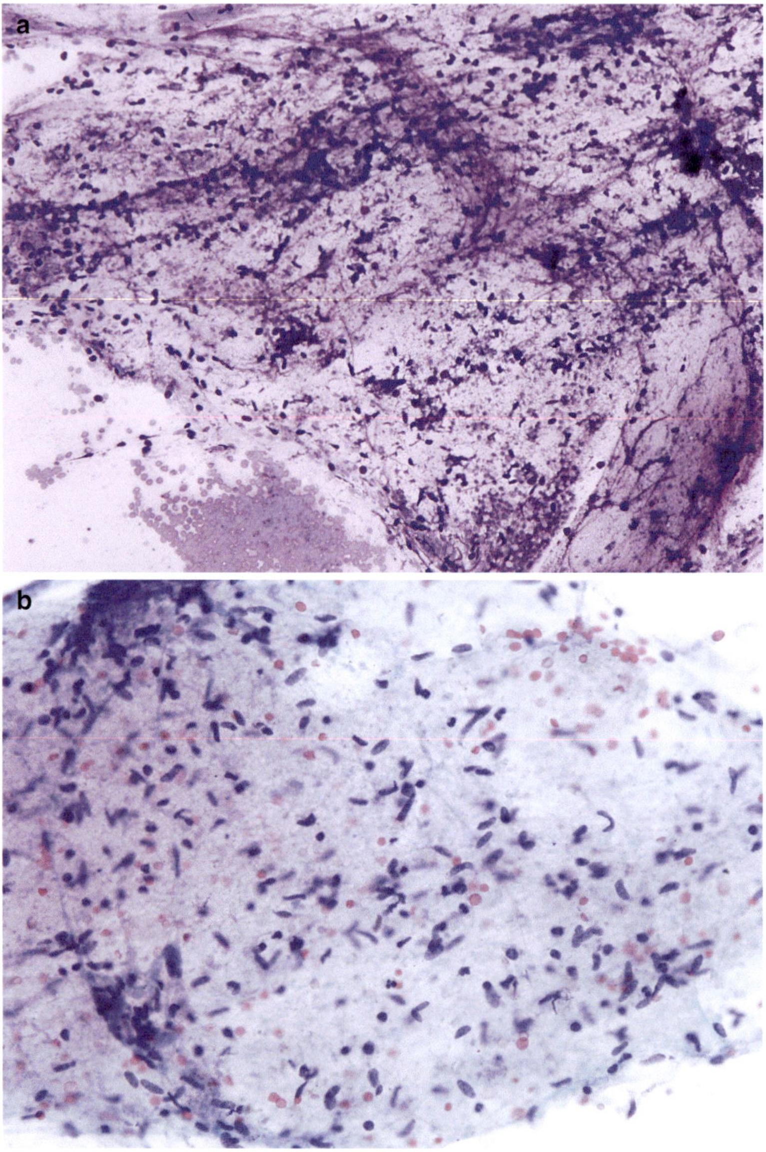

Fig. 7 Fine needle aspiration smears of GIST are cellular, with tumor cells in clusters or singly dispersed (**a**). The cells are spindled with tapering nuclei and mild cytologic atypia; cytoplasm is scant (or appears syncytial in groups) and naked nuclei are frequent (**b**)

variably round or polygonal nuclei are present. As expected, mitotic figures, necrosis and pleomorphism are rare in most GIST [106].

Similar to histologic preparations, immunohistochemistry can be used to help resolve differential diagnoses in certain cases, such as exclusion of smooth muscle tumors or schwannoma. However, in the evaluation of GIST in cytologic samples, it is important to note that the sensitivity of KIT may vary depending on the fixation method. Alcohol-fixed samples (which are usually collected by EUS-FNA) have a lower sensitivity for KIT than formalin-fixed samples [107]. However, DOG1 sensitivity remains high regardless of tissue fixative type [107]. Also noteworthy is that the presence of mast cells and the interstitial cells of Cajal, both of which express KIT, may be a diagnostic pitfall that can lead to false positive results. Therefore, the results of KIT staining should be interpreted in conjunction with cytomorphology and immunohistochemistry for DOG1, which is negative in these two cell populations.

2 Summary

Recent progress in our understanding of the pathobiology of GIST has led to an increasingly sophisticated subclassification of this molecularly heterogeneous group of tumors, with clinicopathologically distinct tumor subtypes recognized by a combination of clinical, histologic and molecular features. Knowledge of these subtypes allows pathologists to accurately diagnose and classify GIST, which in turn has significant implications for prognostication, therapeutics, and in some cases genetic counseling. The combination of histologic evaluation, immunohistochemistry, and mutational analysis therefore remains indispensable to the achievement of optimal clinical outcomes in patients with GIST.

References

1. Rubin BP. Gastrointestinal stromal tumours: an update. Histopathology. 2006;48:83–96.
2. Chan KH, Chan CW, Chow WH, Kwan WK, Kong CK, Mak KF, et al. Gastrointestinal stromal tumors in a cohort of Chinese patients in Hong Kong. World J Gastroenterol. 2006;12:2223–8.
3. Nilsson B, Bümming P, Meis-Kindblom JM, Odén A, Dortok A, Gustavsson B, et al. Gastrointestinal stromal tumors: the incidence, prevalence, clinical course, and prognostication in the preimatinib mesylate era – a population-based study in western Sweden. Cancer. 2005;103:821–9.
4. Goettsch WG, Bos SD, Breekveldt-Postma N, Casparie M, Herings RM, Hogendoorn PC. Incidence of gastrointestinal stromal tumours is underestimated: results of a nation-wide study. Eur J Cancer. 2005;41:2868–72.
5. Kindblom LG, Remotti HE, Aldenborg F, Meis-Kindblom JM. Gastrointestinal pacemaker cell tumor (GIPACT): gastrointestinal stromal tumors show phenotypic characteristics of the interstitial cells of Cajal. Am J Pathol. 1998;152:1259–69.
6. Maeda H, Yamagata A, Nishikawa S, Yoshinaga K, Kobayashi S, Nishi K, et al. Requirement of c-kit for development of intestinal pacemaker system. Development. 1992;116:369–75.
7. Huizinga JD, Thuneberg L, Klüppel M, Malysz J, Mikkelsen HB, Bernstein A. W/kit gene required for interstitial cells of Cajal and for intestinal pacemaker activity. Nature. 1995;373:347–9.
8. Robinson TL, Sircar K, Hewlett BR, Chorneyko K, Riddell RH, Huizinga JD. Gastrointestinal stromal tumors may originate from a subset of CD34-positive interstitial cells of Cajal. Am J Pathol. 2000;156:1157–63.

9. Hirota S, Isozaki K, Moriyama Y, Hashimoto K, Nishida T, Ishiguro S, et al. Gain-of-function mutations of c-kit in human gastrointestinal stromal tumors. Science. 1998;279:577–80.
10. Miettinen M, Lasota J. Gastrointestinal stromal tumors – definition, clinical, histological, immunohistochemical, and molecular genetic features and differential diagnosis. Virchows Arch. 2001;438:1–12.
11. Miettinen M, Sobin LH, Lasota J. Gastrointestinal stromal tumors presenting as omental masses – a clinicopathologic analysis of 95 cases. Am J Surg Pathol. 2009;33:1267–75.
12. Reith JD, Goldblum JR, Lyles RH, Weiss SW. Extragastrointestinal (soft tissue) stromal tumors: an analysis of 48 cases with emphasis on histologic predictors of outcome. Mod Pathol. 2000;13:577–85.
13. Yamamoto H, Oda Y, Kawaguchi K, Nakamura N, Takahira T, Tamiya S, et al. c-kit and PDGFRA mutations in extragastrointestinal stromal tumor (gastrointestinal stromal tumor of the soft tissue). Am J Surg Pathol. 2004;28:479–88.
14. Prakash S, Sarran L, Socci N, DeMatteo RP, Eisenstat J, Greco AM, et al. Gastrointestinal stromal tumors in children and young adults: a clinicopathologic, molecular, and genomic study of 15 cases and review of the literature. J Pediatr Hematol Oncol. 2005;27:179–87.
15. Pappo AS, Janeway KA. Pediatric gastrointestinal stromal tumors. Hematol Oncol Clin North Am. 2009;23:15–34.
16. Miettinen M, Lasota J, Sobin LH. Gastrointestinal stromal tumors of the stomach in children and young adults: a clinicopathologic, immunohistochemical, and molecular genetic study of 44 cases with long-term follow-up and review of the literature. Am J Surg Pathol. 2005;29:1373–81.
17. Zhang L, Smyrk TC, Young WF, Stratakis CA, Carney JA. Gastric stromal tumors in Carney triad are different clinically, pathologically, and behaviorally from sporadic gastric gastrointestinal stromal tumors: findings in 104 cases. Am J Surg Pathol. 2010;34:53–64.
18. Carney JA, Stratakis CA. Familial paraganglioma and gastric stromal sarcoma: a new syndrome distinct from the Carney triad. Am J Med Genet. 2002;108:132–9.
19. Stratakis CA, Carney JA. The triad of paragangliomas, gastric stromal tumours and pulmonary chondromas (Carney triad), and the dyad of paragangliomas and gastric stromal sarcomas (Carney-Stratakis syndrome): molecular genetics and clinical implications. J Intern Med. 2009;266:43–52.
20. Miettinen M, Fetsch JF, Sobin LH, Lasota J. Gastrointestinal stromal tumors in patients with neurofibromatosis 1: a clinicopathologic and molecular genetic study of 45 cases. Am J Surg Pathol. 2006;30:90–6.
21. Andersson J, Sihto H, Meis-Kindblom JM, Joensuu H, Nupponen N, Kindblom LG. NF1-associated gastrointestinal stromal tumors have unique clinical, phenotypic, and genotypic characteristics. Am J Surg Pathol. 2005;29:1170–6.
22. Miettinen M, Sobin LH, Lasota J. Gastrointestinal stromal tumors of the stomach: a clinicopathologic, immunohistochemical, and molecular genetic study of 1765 cases with long-term follow-up. Am J Surg Pathol. 2005;29:52–68.
23. Miettinen M, Kopczynski J, Makhlouf HR, Sarlomo-Rikala M, Gyorffy H, Burke A, et al. Gastrointestinal stromal tumors, intramural leiomyomas, and leiomyosarcomas in the duodenum. Am J Surg Pathol. 2003;27:625–41.
24. Miettinen M, Makhlouf H, Sobin LH, Lasota J. Gastrointestinal stromal tumors of the jejunum and ileum: a clinicopathologic, immunohistochemical, and molecular genetic study of 906 cases before imatinib with long-term follow-up. Am J Surg Pathol. 2006;30:477–89.
25. Rubin BP, Heinrich MC, Corless CL. Gastrointestinal stromal tumour. Lancet. 2007;369:1731–41.
26. Heinrich MC, Corless CL, Duensing A, McGreevey L, Chen CJ, Joseph N, et al. PDGFRA activating mutations in gastrointestinal stromal tumors. Science. 2003;299:708–10.
27. Corless CL, McGreevey L, Haley A, Town A, Heinrich MC. KIT mutations are common in incidental gastrointestinal stromal tumors one centimeter or less in size. Am J Pathol. 2002;160:1567–72.
28. Rubin BP, Singer S, Tsao C, Duensing A, Lux ML, Ruiz R, et al. KIT activation is a ubiquitous feature of gastrointestinal stromal tumors. Cancer Res. 2001;61:8118–21.

29. Cho S, Kitadai Y, Yoshida S, Tanaka S, Yoshihara M, Yoshida K, et al. Deletion of the KIT gene is associated with liver metastasis and poor prognosis in patients with gastrointestinal stromal tumor in the stomach. Int J Oncol. 2006;28:1361–7.
30. Andersson J, Bümming P, Meis-Kindblom JM, Sihto H, Nupponen N, Joensuu H, et al. Gastrointestinal stromal tumors with KIT exon 11 deletions are associated with poor prognosis. Gastroenterology. 2006;130:1573–81.
31. Taniguchi M, Nishida T, Hirota S, Isozaki K, Ito T, Nomura T, et al. Effect of c-kit mutation on prognosis of gastrointestinal stromal tumors. Cancer Res. 1999;59:4297–300.
32. Singer S, Rubin BP, Lux ML, Chen CJ, Demetri GD, Fletcher CD, et al. Prognostic value of KIT mutation type, mitotic activity, and histologic subtype in gastrointestinal stromal tumors. J Clin Oncol. 2002;20:3898–905.
33. Hirota S, Nishida T, Isozaki K, Taniguchi M, Nakamura J, Okazaki T, et al. Gain-of-function mutation at the extracellular domain of KIT in gastrointestinal stromal tumours. J Pathol. 2001;193:505–10.
34. Lux ML, Rubin BP, Biase TL, Chen CJ, Maclure T, Demetri GD, et al. KIT extracellular and kinase domain mutations in gastrointestinal stromal tumors. Am J Surg Pathol. 2000;156:791–5.
35. Lasota J, Corless CL, Heinrich MC, Debiec-Rychter M, Sciot R, Wardelmann E, et al. Clinicopathologic profile of gastrointestinal stromal tumors (GISTs) with primary KIT exon 13 or exon 17 mutations: a multicenter study on 54 cases. Mod Pathol. 2008;21:476–84.
36. Huss S, Künstlinger H, Wardelmann E, Kleine MA, Binot E, Merkelbach-Bruse S, et al. A subset of gastrointestinal stromal tumors previously regarded as wild-type tumors carries somatic activating mutations in KIT exon 8 (p.D419del). Mod Pathol. 2013;26:1004–12.
37. Hartmann K, Wardelmann E, Ma Y, Merkelbach-Bruse S, Preussner LM, Woolery C, et al. Novel germline mutation of KIT associated with familial gastrointestinal stromal tumors and mastocytosis. Gastroenterology. 2005;129:1042–6.
38. Hirota S, Ohashi A, Nishida T, Isozaki K, Kinoshita K, Shinomura Y, et al. Gain-of-function mutations of platelet-derived growth factor receptor α gene in gastrointestinal stromal tumors. Gastroenterology. 2003;125:660–7.
39. Kang HJ, Nam SW, Kim H, Rhee H, Kim N-G, Kim H, et al. Correlation of KIT and platelet-derived growth factor receptor alpha mutations with gene activation and expression profiles in gastrointestinal stromal tumors. Oncogene. 2005;24:1066–74.
40. Medeiros F, Corless CL, Duensing A, Hornick JL, Oliveira AM, Heinrich MC, et al. KIT-negative gastrointestinal stromal tumors: proof of concept and therapeutic implications. Am J Surg Pathol. 2004;28:889–94.
41. Debiec-Rychter M, Wasag B, Stul M, De Wever I, Van Oosterom A, Hagemeijer A, et al. Gastrointestinal stromal tumours (GISTs) negative for KIT (CD117 antigen) immunoreactivity. J Pathol. 2004;202:430–8.
42. Nishida T, Hirota S, Taniguchi M, Hashimoto K, Isozaki K, Nakamura H, et al. Familial gastrointestinal stromal tumours with germline mutation of the KIT gene. Nat Genet. 1998;19:323–4.
43. Wozniak A, Sciot R, Guillou L, Pauwels P, Wasag B, Stul M, et al. Array CGH analysis in primary gastrointestinal stromal tumors: cytogenetic profile correlates with anatomic site and tumor aggressiveness, irrespective of mutational status. Genes Chromosomes Cancer. 2007;46:261–76.
44. El-Rifai W, Sarlomo-Rikala M, Andersson LC, Miettinen M, Knuutila S. High-resolution deletion mapping of chromosome 14 in stromal tumors of the gastrointestinal tract suggests two distinct tumor suppressor loci. Genes Chromosomes Cancer. 2000;27:387–91.
45. Debiec-Rychter M, Lasota J, Sarlomo-Rikala M, Kordek R, Miettinen M. Chromosomal aberrations in malignant gastrointestinal stromal tumors: correlation with c-KIT gene mutation. Cancer Genet Cytogenet. 2001;128:24–30.
46. Chompret A, Kannengiesser C, Barrois M, Terrier P, Dahan P, Tursz T, et al. PDGFRA germline mutation in a family with multiple cases of gastrointestinal stromal tumor. Gastroenterology. 2004;126:318–21.

47. Perrone F, Tamborini E, Dagrada GP, Colombo F, Bonadiman L, Albertini V, et al. 9p21 locus analysis in high-risk gastrointestinal stromal tumors characterized for c-kit and platelet-derived growth factor receptor α gene alterations. Cancer. 2005;104:159–69.
48. Sabah M, Cummins R, Leader M, Kay E. Loss of heterozygosity of chromosome 9p and loss of p16INK4A expression are associated with malignant gastrointestinal stromal tumors. Mod Pathol. 2004;17:1364–71.
49. Astolfi A, Nannini M, Pantaleo MA, Di Battista M, Heinrich MC, Santini D, et al. A molecular portrait of gastrointestinal stromal tumors: an integrative analysis of gene expression profiling and high-resolution genomic copy number. Lab Invest. 2010;90:1285–94.
50. Feakins RM. The expression of p53 and bcl-2 in gastrointestinal stromal tumours is associated with anatomical site, and p53 expression is associated with grade and clinical outcome. Histopathology. 2005;46:270–9.
51. Romeo S, Diebiec-Rychter M, Van Glabbeke M, van Paassen H, Comite P, Van Eijk R, et al. Cell cycle/apoptosis molecules expression correlates with imatinib response in patients with advanced gastrointestinal stromal tumours. Clin Cancer Res. 2009;15:4191–8.
52. Hur K, Lee HJ, Woo JH, Kim JH, Yang HK. Gene expression profiling of human gastrointestinal stromal tumors according to its malignant potential. Dig Dis Sci. 2010;55:2561–7.
53. Tornillo L, Duchini G, Carafa V, Lugli A, Dirnhofer S, Di Vizio D, et al. Patterns of gene amplification in gastrointestinal stromal tumors (GIST). Lab Invest. 2005;85:921–31.
54. Kawanowa K, Sakuma Y, Sakurai S, Hishima T, Iwasaki Y, Saito K, et al. High incidence of microscopic gastrointestinal stromal tumors in the stomach. Hum Pathol. 2006; 37:1527–35.
55. Muenst S, Thies S, Went P, Tornillo L, Bihl MP, Dirnhofer S. Frequency, phenotype, and genotype of minute gastrointestinal stromal tumors in the stomach: an autopsy study. Hum Pathol. 2011;42:1849–54.
56. Rege TA, Wagner AJ, Corless CL, Heinrich MC, Hornick JL. "Pediatric-type" gastrointestinal stromal tumors in adults: distinctive histology predicts genotype and clinical behavior. Am J Surg Pathol. 2011;35:495–504.
57. Gill AJ, Chou A, Vilain RE, Clifton-Bligh RJ. "Pediatric-type" gastrointestinal stromal tumors are SDHB negative ("type 2") GISTs. Am J Surg Pathol. 2011;35:1245–7.
58. Miettinen M, Wang ZF, Sarlomo-Rikala M, Osuch C, Rutkowski P, Lasota J. Succinate dehydrogenase-deficient GISTs – a clinicopathologic, immunohistochemical, and molecular genetic study of 66 gastric GISTs with predilection to young age. Am J Surg Pathol. 2011;35:1712–21.
59. Doyle LA, Nelson D, Heinrich MC, Corless CL, Hornick JL. Loss of succinate dehydrogenase subunit B (SDHB) expression is limited to a distinctive subset of gastric wild-type gastrointestinal stromal tumours: a comprehensive genotype-phenotype correlation study. Histopathology. 2012;61:801–9.
60. Gottlieb E, Tomlinson IP. Mitochondrial tumour suppressors: a genetic and biochemical update. Nat Rev Cancer. 2005;5:857–66.
61. Killian JK, Kim SY, Miettinen M, Smith C, Merino M, Tsokos M, et al. Succinate dehydrogenase mutation underlies global epigenomic divergence in gastrointestinal stromal tumor. Cancer Discov. 2013;3:648–57.
62. Mason EF, Hornick JL. Succinate dehydrogenase deficiency is associated with decreased 5-hydroxymethylcytosine production in gastrointestinal stromal tumors: implications for mechanisms of tumorigenesis. Mod Pathol. 2013;26:1492–7.
63. Burnichon N, Brière JJ, Libé R, Vescovo L, Rivière J, Tissier F, et al. SDHA is a tumor suppressor gene causing paraganglioma. Hum Mol Genet. 2010;19:3011–20.
64. Lasota J, Wang Z, Kim SY, Helman L, Miettinen M. Expression of the receptor for type I insulin-like growth factor (IGF1R) in gastrointestinal stromal tumors: an immunohistochemical study of 1078 cases with diagnostic and therapeutic implications. Am J Surg Pathol. 2013;37:114–9.
65. Pasini B, McWhinney SR, Bei T, Matyakhina L, Stergiopoulos S, Muchow M, et al. Clinical and molecular genetics of patients with the Carney-Stratakis syndrome and germline mutations of the genes coding for the succinate dehydrogenase subunits SDHB, SDHC, and SDHD. Eur J Hum Genet. 2008;16:79–88.

66. McWhinney SR, Pasini B, Stratakis CA. Familial gastrointestinal stromal tumors and germline mutations. N Engl J Med. 2007;357:1054–6.
67. Carney JA, Sheps SG, Go VL, Gordon H. The triad of gastric leiomyosarcoma, functioning extra-adrenal paraganglioma and pulmonary chondroma. N Engl J Med. 1977;296:1517–8.
68. Gill AJ, Chou A, Vilain R, Clarkson A, Lui M, Jin R, et al. Immunohistochemistry for SDHB divides gastrointestinal stromal tumors (GISTs) into 2 distinct types. Am J Surg Pathol. 2010;34:636–44.
69. Matyakhina L, Bei TA, McWhinney SR, Pasini B, Cameron S, Gunawan B, et al. Genetics of Carney triad: recurrent losses at chromosome 1 but lack of germline mutations in genes associated with paragangliomas and gastrointestinal stromal tumors. J Clin Endocrinol Metab. 2007;92:2938–43.
70. Haller F, Moskalev EA, Faucz FR, Barthelmeß S, Wiemann S, Bieg M, et al. Aberrant DNA hypermethylation of SDHC: a novel mechanism of tumor development in Carney triad. Endocr Relat Cancer. 2014;21:567–77.
71. Wagner AJ, Remillard SP, Zhang YX, Doyle LA, George S, Hornick JL. Loss of expression of SDHA predicts SDHA mutations in gastrointestinal stromal tumors. Mod Pathol. 2013;26:289–94.
72. Miettinen M, Killian JK, Wang ZF, Lasota J, Lau C, Jones L, et al. Immunohistochemical loss of succinate dehydrogenase subunit A (SDHA) in gastrointestinal stromal tumors (GISTs) signals SDHA germline mutation. Am J Surg Pathol. 2013;37:234–40.
73. Oudijk L, Gaal J, Korpershoek E, van Nederveen FH, Kelly L, Schiavon G, et al. SDHA mutations in adult and pediatric wild-type gastrointestinal stromal tumors. Mod Pathol. 2013;26:456–63.
74. Dwight T, Benn DE, Clarkson A, Vilain R, Lipton L, Robinson BG, et al. Loss of SDHA expression identifies SDHA mutations in succinate dehydrogenase–deficient gastrointestinal stromal tumors. Am J Surg Pathol. 2013;37:226–33.
75. Agaram NP, Laquaglia MP, Ustun B, Guo T, Wong GC, Socci ND, et al. Molecular characterization of pediatric gastrointestinal stromal tumors. Clin Cancer Res. 2008;14:3204–15.
76. Marrari A, Wagner AJ, Hornick JL. Predictors of response to targeted therapies for gastrointestinal stromal tumors. Arch Pathol Lab Med. 2012;136:483–9.
77. Carney JA. Carney triad: a syndrome featuring paraganglionic, adrenocortical, and possibly other endocrine tumors. J Clin Endocrinol Metab. 2009;94:3656–62.
78. Agaram NP, Wong GC, Guo T, Maki RG, Singer S, DeMatteo RP, et al. Novel V600E BRAF mutations in imatinib-naive and imatinib-resistant gastrointestinal stromal tumors. Genes Chromosomes Cancer. 2008;47:853–9.
79. Agaimy A, Terracciano LM, Dirnhofer S, Tornillo L, Foerster A, Hartmann A, et al. V600E BRAF mutations are alternative early molecular events in a subset of KIT/PDGFRA wild-type gastrointestinal stromal tumours. J Clin Pathol. 2009;62:613–6.
80. Hostein I, Faur N, Primois C, Boury F, Denard J, Emile JF, et al. BRAF mutation status in gastrointestinal stromal tumors. Am J Clin Pathol. 2010;133:141–8.
81. Falchook GS, Trent JC, Heinrich MC, Beadling C, Patterson J, Bastida CC, et al. BRAF mutant gastrointestinal stromal tumor: first report of regression with BRAF inhibitor dabrafenib (GSK2118436) and whole exomic sequencing for analysis of acquired resistance. Oncotarget. 2013;4:310–5.
82. Kang GH, Srivastava A, Kim YE, Park HJ, Park CK, Sohn TS, et al. DOG1 and PKC-θ are useful in the diagnosis of KIT-negative gastrointestinal stromal tumors. Mod Pathol. 2011;24:866–75.
83. Hornick JL, Fletcher CD. Immunohistochemical staining for KIT (CD117) in soft tissue sarcomas is very limited in distribution. Am J Clin Pathol. 2002;117:188–93.
84. Espinosa I, Lee CH, Kim MK, Rouse BT, Subramanian S, Montgomery K, et al. A novel monoclonal antibody against DOG1 is a sensitive and specific marker for gastrointestinal stromal tumors. Am J Surg Pathol. 2008;32:210–8.
85. West RB, Corless CL, Chen X, Rubin BP, Subramanian S, Montgomery K, et al. The novel marker, DOG1, is expressed ubiquitously in gastrointestinal stromal tumors irrespective of KIT or PDGFRA mutation status. Am J Pathol. 2004;165:107–13.

86. Miettinen M, Wang ZF, Lasota J. DOG1 antibody in the differential diagnosis of gastrointestinal stromal tumors: a study of 1840 cases. Am J Surg Pathol. 2009;33:1401–8.
87. Liegl B, Hornick JL, Corless CL, Fletcher CD. Monoclonal antibody DOG1.1 shows higher sensitivity than KIT in the diagnosis of gastrointestinal stromal tumors, including unusual types. Am J Surg Pathol. 2009;33:437–46.
88. Yamamoto H, Kojima A, Nagata S, Tomita Y, Takahashi S, Oda Y. KIT-negative gastrointestinal stromal tumor of the abdominal soft tissue: a clinicopathologic and genetic study of 10 cases. Am J Surg Pathol. 2011;35:1287–95.
89. Doyle LA, Hornick JL. Gastrointestinal stromal tumours: from KIT to succinate dehydrogenase. Histopathology. 2014;64:53–67.
90. Miettinen M, Lasota J. Gastrointestinal stromal tumors: pathology and prognosis at different sites. Semin Diagn Pathol. 2006;23:70–83.
91. Demetri GD, von Mehren M, Antonescu CR, DeMatteo RP, Ganjoo KN, Maki RG, et al. NCCN Task Force report: update on the management of patients with gastrointestinal stromal tumors. J Natl Compr Canc Netw. 2010;8 suppl 2:S1–41.
92. Agaram NP, Besmer P, Wong GC, Guo T, Socci ND, Maki RG, et al. Pathologic and molecular heterogeneity in imatinib-stable or imatinib-responsive gastrointestinal stromal tumors. Clin Cancer Res. 2007;13:170–81.
93. Pauwels P, Debiec-Rychter M, Stul M, De Wever I, Van Oosterom AT, Sciot R. Changing phenotype of gastrointestinal stromal tumours under imatinib mesylate treatment: a potential diagnostic pitfall. Histopathology. 2005;47:41–7.
94. Liegl B, Kepten I, Le C, Zhu M, Demetri GD, Heinrich MC, et al. Heterogeneity of kinase inhibitor resistance mechanisms in GIST. J Pathol. 2008;216:64–74.
95. Liegl B, Hornick JL, Antonescu CR, Corless CL, Fletcher CD. Rhabdomyosarcomatous differentiation in gastrointestinal stromal tumors after tyrosine kinase inhibitor therapy: a novel form of tumor progression. Am J Surg Pathol. 2009;33:218–26.
96. Antonescu CR, Romeo S, Zhang L, Nafa K, Hornick JL, Nielsen GP, et al. Dedifferentiation in gastrointestinal stromal tumor to an anaplastic KIT-negative phenotype: a diagnostic pitfall: morphologic and molecular characterization of 8 cases occurring either de novo or after imatinib therapy. Am J Surg Pathol. 2013;37:385–92.
97. Heinrich MC, Corless CL, Demetri GD, Blanke CD, von Mehren M, Joensuu H, et al. Kinase mutations and imatinib response in patients with metastatic gastrointestinal stromal tumor. J Clin Oncol. 2003;21:4342–9.
98. Heinrich MC, Owzar K, Corless CL, Hollis D, Borden EC, Fletcher CD, et al. Correlation of kinase genotype and clinical outcome in the North American intergroup phase III trial of imatinib mesylate for treatment of advanced gastrointestinal stromal tumor: CALGB 150105 study by Cancer and Leukemia Group B and Southwest Oncology Group. J Clin Oncol. 2008;26:5360–7.
99. Heinrich MC, Corless CL, Blanke CD, Demetri GD, Joensuu H, Roberts PJ, et al. Molecular correlates of imatinib resistance in gastrointestinal stromal tumors. J Clin Oncol. 2006;24:4764–74.
100. Tamborini E, Pricl S, Negri T, Lagonigro MS, Miselli F, Greco A, et al. Functional analyses and molecular modeling of two c-Kit mutations responsible for imatinib secondary resistance in GIST patients. Oncogene. 2006;25:6140–6.
101. Akahoshi K, Sumida Y, Matsui N, Oya M, Akinaga R, Kubokawa M, et al. Preoperative diagnosis of gastrointestinal stromal tumor by endoscopic ultrasound-guided fine needle aspiration. World J Gastroenterol. 2007;13:2077–82.
102. Pang NK, Chin SY, Nga ME, Chang AR, Ismail TM, Omar SS, et al. Comparative validation of c-kit exon 11 mutation analysis on cytology samples and corresponding surgical resections of gastrointestinal stromal tumours. Cytopathology. 2009;20:297–303.
103. Gomes AL, Bardales RH, Milanezi F, Reis RM, Schmitt F. Molecular analysis of c-Kit and PDGFRA in GISTs diagnosed by EUS. Am J Clin Pathol. 2007;127:89–96.

104. Wieczorek TJ, Faquin WC, Rubin BP, Cibas ES. Cytologic diagnosis of gastrointestinal stromal tumor with emphasis on the differential diagnosis with leiomyosarcoma. Cancer. 2001;93:276–87.
105. Stelow EB, Stanley MW, Mallery S, Lai R, Linzie BM, Bardales RH. Endoscopic ultrasound-guided fine-needle aspiration findings of gastrointestinal leiomyomas and gastrointestinal stromal tumors. Am J Clin Pathol. 2003;119:703–8.
106. Layfield LJ, Wallander ML. Diagnosis of gastrointestinal stromal tumors from minute specimens: cytomorphology, immunohistochemistry, and molecular diagnostic findings. Diagn Cytopathol. 2012;40:484–90.
107. Hwang DG, Qian X, Hornick JL. DOG1 antibody is a highly sensitive and specific marker for gastrointestinal stromal tumors in cytology cell blocks. Am J Clin Pathol. 2011;135:448–53.

Inherited GIST

Katherine A. Janeway

1 Overview of Inherited GIST

1.1 Familial GIST due to Germline Mutations in KIT or PDGFRA

Germline mutations in KIT have been reported in about 25 families. These KIT germline mutations most often occur in exon 11 but can also occur in exons 8, 13, and 17. Inheritance is autosomal dominant. Gastrointestinal stromal tumors (GIST) diagnosis typically occurs in the fourth and fifth decade of life but diagnosis at ages as young as 15 years has also occurred. Other manifestations of *KIT* germline mutations include melanoma, lentigines, urticaria pigmentosa, perioral and perineal hyperpigmentation, and achalasia [1, 2]. A few families with germline mutations in PDGFRA and GIST have been described. Additional clinical features in familial GIST associated with germline PDGFRA mutation are variable and include lipomas, fibrous tumors in the gastrointestinal tract, and large hands [3, 4]. Treatment of familial GIST due to germline mutation in KIT or PDGFRA is similar to the approach for GIST tumors with somatic KIT or PDGFRA mutations. Interestingly, improvement in skin pigmentation has been observed in a patient with a KIT germline mutation with GIST treated with imatinib [5] (Table 1).

K.A. Janeway, MD, MMSc
Harvard Medical School, Dana-Farber/Boston Children's Cancer and Blood Disorders Center, 450 Brookline Ave, Boston, MA 02215, USA
e-mail: kjaneway@partners.org

© Springer International Publishing Switzerland 2017

C.R. Scoggins et al. (eds.), *Gastrointestinal Stromal Tumors*,
DOI 10.1007/978-3-319-42632-7_4

Table 1 Demographics and clinical features of inherited and syndromic GIST

GIST subtype	Molecular cause	Usual age GIST presentation	GIST location	Pathology of GIST tumors	Other cancers and clinical features
Familial GIST	Germline *KIT* or *PDGFRA* mutation	30–40 years	Stomach or small bowel	Spindle morphology KIT IHC present SDH IHC present	*KIT* mutation: melanoma, lentigen, uticaria pigmentosa, achalasia *PDGFRA* mutation: lipoma, fibrous tumor in the gastrointestinal tract and large hands
Neurofibromatosis 1	Germline mutation *NF1*	40–50 years	Small bowel	Spindle morphology KIT IHC present SDH IHC present	Neurofibroma, malignant peripheral nerve sheath tumor, optic glioma, café-au-lait macules, axillary freckling
Carney Triad	Somatic *SDHC* promoter hypermethylation or, less often *SDHX* mutation	20 years	Stomach	Epithelioid morphology KIT IHC present SDH IHC absent	Paraganglioma and pulmonary chondroma
Carney-Stratkis Dyad	*SDHX* mutation or, less often somatic *SDHC* promoter hypermethylation	20–30 years	Stomach	Epithelioid morphology KIT IHC present SDH IHC absent	Paraganglioma, renal cell carcinoma

1.2 Neurofibromatosis Type 1 (NF1)

GIST occurred in 7 % of patients with NF1 in a study utilizing Swedish health registry data [6, 7]. The median age of GIST diagnosis in NF1 patients is 49 years and it appears GIST occurs slightly more often in females than in males. GIST occurring in the setting of NF1 are located in the small bowel, have a spindle cell morphology, can be multiple, and often have a background of interstitial cells of Cajal hyperplasia. Prognosis is usually good when tumors are small and have a low mitotic rate which is the more common scenario [8]. There is little information to inform medical management of GIST occurring in patients with NF1. Imatinib does not seem to be effective. There is a case report with response to sunitinib [7, 9].

1.3 Succinate Dehydrogenase (SDH) Deficient GIST

Approximately 10 % of GIST occurring in adults [10] and 85 % of GIST occurring in children [11] lack an activating mutation in the tyrosine kinases – KIT, PDGFR, BRAF –typically mutated in GIST. This type of GIST has been called "wildtype GIST" or "pediatric GIST." Now that the biology of these GIST tumors is better understood, the preferred terminology for this group is "SDH-deficient GIST." As discussed in greater detail in the chapter "Surgical Pathology of Gastrointestinal Stromal Tumors: Correlation with Clinical and Molecular Subtypes," SDH-deficient GIST is defined by absence of immunohistochemical (IHC) staining for succinate dehydrogenase B (SDHB). The SDH-ubiquinone complex is a component of the Krebs cycle and the respiratory chain. It is a heteroligomer composed of subunits A, B, C, and D. Inactivation of any one of the three SDH subunits results in destabilization of the SDH complex, loss of enzymatic function, and absence of IHC staining for SDHB [12].

There appears to be two mechanisms through which SDH inactivation occurs, germline or somatic inactivating mutations [13] and methylation of the SDHC in this context refers to gene: succinate dehydrogenase complex (SDHC) promoter leading to silencing of SDHC expression [14]. We have called GIST with germline or somatic mutations in SDHA, SDHB, SDHC, or SDHD (also indicated by SDHX) SDH-mutant GIST and GIST with methylation of the SDHC promoter SDH-epimutant GIST [15]. As described in further detail below, it is important to recognize SDH-deficient GIST and to determine which subtype of SDH-deficient GIST a patient has because SDH-deficient GIST has unique epidemiologic (Fig. 1) and clinical features with implications for prognosis and clinical management.

1.4 SDH-Mutant GIST

Approximately 70 % of SDH-deficient GIST have an SDHX mutation and thus are best categorized as SDH-mutant GIST. The SDH subunit mutated in these

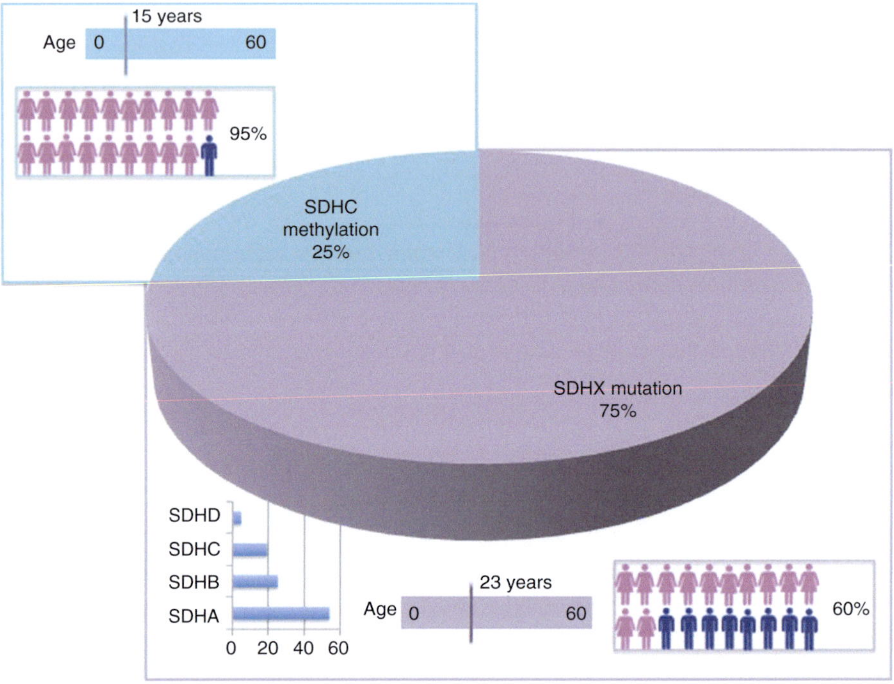

Fig. 1 SDH-deficient GIST subtypes. SDH-deficient GIST can be classified as SDH-epimutant (25 %) caused by methylation of the *SDHC* promoter region and SDH-mutant caused by mutation in one of the four SDH subunits. Average age of presentation and gender distribution are shown for both subtypes. For SDH-mutant GIST, the proportion of cases caused by *SDHA, SDHB, SDHC*, and *SDHD* mutations are shown (Adapted from Boikos et al. [15])

SDH-mutant GIST is *SDHA* in 54 % of cases, *SDHB* in 25 % of cases, *SDHC* in 19 % of cases, and *SDHD* in 2 % of cases. Approximately 80 % of patients with SDH-mutant GIST will have the identified SDHX mutation in the germline while the remaining 20 % appear to have the SDHX mutation present in the tumor only. The median age of GIST presentation in SDH-mutant GIST is 23 (range 7–58), much younger than the age of presentation for *KIT* and *PDGFRA* mutant GIST. About 60 % of patients presenting with SDH-mutant GIST are female. All SDH-mutant GIST occur in the stomach with 40 % of these gastric tumors being multifocal (more than one discrete gastric tumor) at the time of presentation. Approximately 30 % of patients with SDH-mutant GIST will have metastatic disease at presentation with lymph nodes being the most common site of metastatic disease followed by liver and peritoneum [15].

As discussed in much greater detail in the section SDH-deficient GIST, approach to cancer screening section later in this chapter, germline SDHX mutations cause hereditary paraganglioma, reviewed in [16]. Consequently, these patients are at risk for other cancers especially paraganglioma and pheochromocytoma.

1.5 SDH-Epimutant GIST

Approximately 30 % of SDH-deficient GIST have *SDHC* promoter hypermethylation and thus are best categorized as SDH-epimutant GIST. The median age of GIST presentation in SDH-epimutant GIST is 15 (range 8–50). Almost all of the patients presenting with SDH-epimutant GIST are female. Thus SDH-epimutant GIST is the predominant subtype occurring in young females. All SDH-epimutant GIST occur in the stomach with 72 % of these gastric tumors being multifocal at the time of presentation. Approximately 40 % of patients with SDH-epimutant GIST will have metastatic disease at presentation with liver and lymph nodes being the most common site of metastatic disease followed by peritoneum [15].

2 Overview of Syndromic GIST

2.1 Carney Triad and Carney-Stratakis Dyad

The Carney triad has been described as a sporadic syndrome defined by the association of GIST with paraganglioma and pulmonary chondroma. GIST in patients with Carney Triad tend to be multifocal and arise in the stomach, particularly in the antrum and lesser curvature. Eighty-five percent of patients with Carney triad are female and the mean age at presentation is 20.2 years. Local recurrence (46 %) and metastasis (55 %) to liver, lymph nodes, and peritoneum are common [17]. GIST tumors in patients with Carney Triad are SDH-deficient and have been found to have *SDHC* hypermethylation, identical to that seen in SDH-epimutant GIST [18]. *SDHC* hypermethylation appears to be the major mechanism of SDH inactivation in Carney Triad explaining the sporadic as opposed to inherited nature of this syndrome. However, one recent study reported that 10 % of patients with Carney Triad have germline mutations in *SDHA*, *SDHB*, or *SDHC* [19] and a comprehensive study of 95 patients with *KIT* and *PDGFRA* mutation negative GIST led by the NIH included 11 patients with Carney Triad, 5 of whom had *SDHA* or *SDHC* germline mutations. The remaining 6 had *SDHC* hypermethylation in the tumor [15]. Unlike the overall group of patients with Carney Triad, 50 % of patients with SDHX germline mutations and Carney Triad are male [19].

The Carney-Stratakis Dyad has been described as an autosomal-dominant inherited cancer predisposition syndrome caused by germline mutation in *SDHB*, *SDHC*, and *SDHD*. Patients with the Dyad are predisposed to paragangliomas, GIST, and other tumors. GIST in these patients is SDH-deficient and tends to be multifocal and located in the stomach. The median age of presentation in Carney-Stratakis Dyad is 19 years [20]. The comprehensive study of 95 patients with *KIT* and *PDGFRA* mutation negative GIST led by the NIH included 7 patients with Carney-Stratakis Dyad, 6 of whom had SDHX germline mutations and one of whom had *SDHC* hypermethylation in the tumor [15].

Although historically Carney Triad and Carney-Stratakis Dyad were recognized as distinct entities, a better understanding of the genomic and epigenomic mechanisms present in the GIST tumors in these syndromes and in *KIT* and *PDGFRA* mutation negative GIST reveals that these syndromes are part of a spectrum with SDH-deficient GIST characterized by SDH inactivation by either germline SDHX mutation or *SDHC* hypermethylation [15].

3 SDH-Deficient GIST Presentation and Staging

Like other GIST, SDH-deficient GIST arise from the interstitial cells of Cajal and, therefore, are in the muscularis propria layer of the gastrointestinal tract deep to the submucosa. In the case of SDH-deficient GIST, patients present with one or multiple intramural masses in the stomach. Because children with GIST essentially all have SDH-deficient GIST, information gleaned from case series of pediatric GIST has relevance to SDH-deficient GIST. In a summation of pediatric GIST series and case reports, by far the most common manifestations at the time of initial presentation are gastrointestinal bleeding and anemia or symptoms related to it such as fatigue. Patients can also have abdominal pain and a palpable abdominal mass or abdominal distension [21]. Staging which should be performed with ^{18}FDG-PET-CT reveals metastatic disease involving the gastric lymph nodes, liver, or peritoneum in 30–40 % of patients. If liver metastases are present, magnetic resonance imaging (MRI) can be helpful to establish a baseline appearance for correlation with later imaging assessment of response to treatment. Chest X-ray should be obtained at diagnosis to evaluate for the presence of pulmonary chondromas which occur in the setting of Carney Triad (Fig. 2).

4 SDH-Deficient GIST Diagnosis

The diagnosis of SDH-deficient GIST should be suspected in patients presenting with GIST at a young age (<40 years), whenever a patient presents with multifocal gastric tumors and when lymph nodes are involved with metastases at the time of diagnosis. The recommended approach for biopsy of SDH-deficient GIST is endoscopic, ultrasound-guided biopsy of the gastric masses except when presentation with massive hemorrhage or perforation necessitates emergency surgery. Endoscopic biopsy of GIST is discussed in detail in the chapter "Endoscopic Evaluation of Gastrointestinal Stromal Tumors."

The pathologic features of SDH-deficient GIST are discussed in detail in the chapter "Surgical Pathology of Gastrointestinal Stromal Tumors: Correlation with Clinical and Molecular Subtypes." Epitheilioid morphology and a multinodular or plexiform pattern are pathologic features suggesting a diagnosis of SDH-deficient GIST. In addition, SDH-deficient GIST should be considered when molecular testing

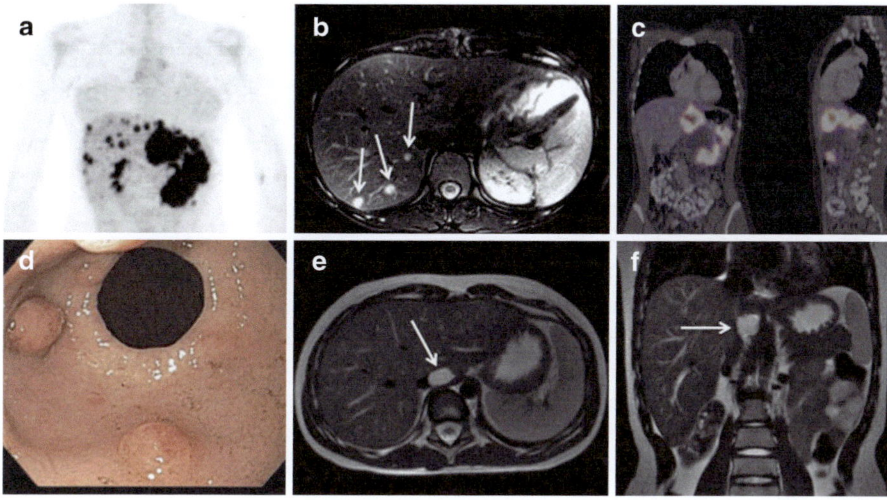

Fig. 2 Typical imaging characteristics of SDH-Deficient GIST. Patient with SDH-deficient GIST who presented with gastric GIST and liver metastases demonstrated on ^{18}FDG-PET (**a**), including a large gastric tumor (panel **c**, ^{18}FDG-PET), liver metastases which are best visualized with MRI (*arrows*, panel **b**), and multiple gastric tumors visualized with upper endoscopy (panel **d**). A different patient with SDH-deficient GIST with recurrence in a gastric lymph node (*arrows*, panels **e** and **f**, MRI)

of tumor reveals nosomatic mutations in *KIT*, *PDGFRA*, and *BRAF*. SDH-deficient GIST have strong membranous IHC staining for KIT and DOG1. The key pathologic feature confirming a diagnosis of SDH-deficient GIST is absence of IHC staining for SDHB [22]. SDHB IHC should be performed on GIST presenting in young patient, when multifocal GIST is present, when pathologic features are suggestive of SDH-deficient GIST, and when features of SDH-deficient GIST are not present but tumor sequencing does not reveal kinase mutations. It is also possible to perform IHC for SDHA. IHC staining for SDHA is absent in SDH-deficient GIST caused by germline or somatic mutations in *SDHA* [23, 24]. Sequencing tumor for mutations in *KIT*, *PDGFRA*, *BRAF*, *SDHA*, *SDHB*, *SDHC*, and *SDHD* can be very helpful in determining optimal treatment approaches, prognosis, and whether referral to a cancer predisposition program for genetic testing is indicated. Testing for mutations in *KIT* and *PDGFRA* and, when negative, for mutations in SDH genes is recommended in the National Comprehensive Cancer Network (NCCN) Guidelines [25].

5 SDH-Deficient GIST Clinical Course

As SDH-deficient GIST has only recently been identified as a distinct entity, there is limited data on the clinical course or prognosis of this entity. Because children with GIST essentially all have SDH-deficient GIST, information gleaned from case series of pediatric GIST has relevance to SDH-deficient GIST. A review of literature on pediatric GIST suggests that most SDH-deficient GIST have an indolent course. Despite the fact that many patients develop multiple disease recurrences or present with metastatic disease, patients can survive with active disease for many years [21]. In one of the largest series of pediatric GIST reported to date, with a mean duration of follow up of almost 5 years,10 of 12 patients (83 %) developed metastatic disease yet only one died as a consequence of GIST. Half of the patients were alive with disease and the mean duration of survival with disease was almost 6 years [26].

A comprehensive study of 84 patients with SDH-deficient GIST led by the NIH collected follow-up data on a cohort of patients who attended a clinic dedicated to assessment of patients with pediatric or wild-type GIST. In 63 patients with SDH-mutant GIST, after a median follow-up from diagnosis of 6 (range 1–44) years, 3 had died (8–24 years after initial diagnosis). In the 21 patients with SDH-epimutant GIST, after a median follow-up of 9 (range 1–32) years, 1 patient died 6 years after diagnosis [15]. Patients with *SDHA* mutant GIST appear to have an excellent prognosis [27].

6 SDH-Deficient GIST Medical Management

Given that SDH-deficient GIST has just been identified as a distinct entity, a few prospective clinical trials have been conducted in this patient population. Studies of kinase inhibitors in children with GIST and in adults with *KIT* and *PDGFRA* mutation negative or wild-type GIST can be illustrative of treatment response in SDH-deficient GIST.

Imatinib is the recommended therapy for *KIT* and *PDGFRA* mutation positive GIST when the disease is advanced or following completed resection when there is a high risk of recurrence [25]. But, response to imatinib in GIST varies by tumor genotype. The comprehensive cohort study of 84 patients with SDH-deficient GIST led by the NIH collected treatment data. In this cohort, only 1 of 49 patients with SDH-deficient GIST treated with imatinib had a partial response. In patients with wild-type advanced GIST, many of whom likely had SDH-deficient GIST, the objective response rate and median time to tumor progression (TTP) with imatinib therapy is significantly lower than is seen in patients with *KIT/PDGFRA* mutant GIST [28]. There are reports of imatinib administration in ten pediatric patients. One partial response and three stable diseases were observed [21]. Available evidence suggests adjuvant imatinib is not effective in GIST lacking *KIT* or *PDGFRA* mutations, most of which are SDH-deficient [29].

In patients with advanced imatinib-resistant GIST, sunitinib significantly prolongs TTP and survival [30]. Sunitinib is ten times more potent than imatinib with regard to inhibition of wild-type KIT [26]. Adult patients with wild-type GIST are among those achieving the greatest clinical benefit from sunitinib [31]. In the limited treatment data available from the NIH SDH-deficient GIST cohort study, 7 of 38 patients with SDH-deficient GIST treated with sunitinib had responses (1 complete, 3 partial, 3 mixed) [15]. In a compassionate access study, sunitinib was administered in seven pediatric patients with GIST who failed imatinib. One patient had a partial response and five had disease stabilization that lasted from 7–21+ months [32]. Combined, these data suggest modest activity of sunitinib in SDH-deficient GIST but with most patients having stable disease as their best response.

Pazopanib is a broad-spectrum tyrosine kinase inhibitor which has been evaluated in GIST that has progressed after imatinib and sunitinib. Two patients with SDH-deficient GIST participated in a phase II study of pazopanib. One of these patients had a 16 % reduction in tumor size and had been on pazopanib for 17 months at the time of study analysis and continued on treatment. The other patient stopped treatment because of side effects [33]. A similar case of prolonged disease stabilization in a patient with wild-type GIST is reported in a randomized phase II trial of pazopanib [34]. Sorafenib has been studied in phase II trials in advanced GIST refractory to imatinib and sunitinib. In one such study, five patients with wild-type GIST were enrolled. One of these five patients had a partial response, two had stable disease for greater than 6 months, and one had stable disease for less than 6 months [35]. Regorafenib is recommended as third-line therapy in advanced GIST. In an academic phase II trial of regorafenib, objective responses were reported in two patients with SDH-deficient GIST [36].

Due to the fact that SDH-deficient GIST has an indolent course and because medical therapies effective in SDH-deficient GIST appear to more frequently result in disease stabilization than objective response, it is helpful to document disease progression with a short interval scan prior to initiating medical treatment. After initial staging with ^{18}FDG-PET-CT and, if liver metastases are present, with an MRI of the abdomen, we suggest monitoring for disease progression or response on therapy with MRI of the abdomen and pelvis. One rationale for MRI as the primary modality to monitor for treatment response is the importance of minimizing radiation exposure as patients with SDH-deficient GIST are young and likely, given the disease course, to require multiple disease assessment with imaging over many years. In addition, abdominal and pelvis MRI are sensitive for detecting disease in sites where SDH-deficient GIST is most likely to recur; the liver, lymph nodes and peritoneum. Additional or recurrent gastric tumors are more difficult to detect with MRI and so monitoring with gastric endoscopy can be performed in patients considered to be at high risk for gastric recurrence. Unlike in *KIT* or *PDGFRA* mutant GIST, decrease in ^{18}FDG-PET has not been validated to be a reliable marker of disease response to therapy. In addition, ^{18}FDG-PET may reveal very small tumors without an anatomic correlate and the appropriate response to this type of lesion is not clear, given the lack of medical therapy with proven benefit in SDH-deficient GIST.

7 Unique Aspects of Surgical Management in SDH-Deficient GIST

NCCN guidelines for GIST recommend consideration of preoperative imatinib for tumors where surgical morbidity can be reduced by downstaging the tumor preoperatively [25]. Due to the apparent lack of efficacy of imatinib in SDH-deficient GIST, preoperative imatinib would not be recommended in patients with this GIST subtype. While sunitinib, sorafenib, and pazopanib appear to have more activity in SDH-deficient GIST, the available evidence, while limited in nature, suggests that significant tumor shrinkage is unlikely. Therefore, medical therapy alone is usually insufficient to alleviate symptoms such as bleeding or obstruction caused by a large gastric tumor and therefore, surgery should be considered to prevent or address tumor-related symptoms [37].

8 SDH-Deficient GIST Approach to Germline Genetic Testing and Cancer Screening

Referral to a genetic counselor is recommended for all patients with SDH-deficient GIST. Testing for mutations in SDHX genes should be performed in patients with SDHB IHC negative tumors [25]. As mentioned above, 80 % of patients with an SDHX mutation identified in the tumor will have the same mutation in the germline.

Hereditary paraganglioma syndromes 1, 3, 4, and 5 refer, respectively, to germline mutations in *SDHD*, *SDHC*, *SDHB*, and *SDHA*. As suggested by the name, the most common cancers occurring in those with SDHX germline mutations are paraganglioma and pheochromocytoma. The frequency and location of paragangliomas varies by genotype as does the frequency of other cancers. However, there is considerable variability in presentation between patients with the same genotype and penetrance is incomplete resulting in challenges for genetic counseling [38]. The other cancer that patients with hereditary paraganglioma are at increased risk of developing is renal cell carcinoma [16]. The renal cell carcinomas have a distinct morphology and are, like other tumors occurring in hereditary paraganglioma, SDHB IHC negative [39]. GIST is such an uncommon manifestation of SDHX germline mutations. Neuroblastoma and pituitary adenoma have rarely been reported in patients with hereditary paraganglioma [40].

Screening for paraganglioma/pheochromocytoma in patients with SDHX germline mutations has been recommended by some. The recommendation to screen is based on the presumption that, as surgical resection is the primary therapeutic modality for paraganglioma/pheochromocytoma, early detection will result in improved disease control [41]. At a minimum, screening should include biochemical evaluation and a history and physical exam for symptoms associated with catecholamine excess (hypertension). There is no consensus on the frequency and imaging modalities to be utilized for screening. While total body MRI appears to identify asymptomatic paragangliomas in a reasonable proportion of patients, some studies suggest functional imaging with ^{18}FDG-PET or somatostatin receptor scintography may improve tumor identification [42–45].

References

1. Neuhann TM, Mansmann V, Merkelbach-Bruse S, Klink B, Hellinger A, Hoffkes HG, et al. A novel germline KIT mutation (p.L576P) in a family presenting with juvenile onset of multiple gastrointestinal stromal tumors, skin hyperpigmentations, and esophageal stenosis. Am J Surg Pathol. 2013;37(6):898–905. Epub 2013/04/20.
2. McWhinney SR, Pasini B, Stratakis CA. Familial gastrointestinal stromal tumors and germline mutations. N Engl J Med. 2007;357(10):1054–6.
3. Pasini B, Matyakhina L, Bei T, Muchow M, Boikos S, Ferrando B, et al. Multiple gastrointestinal stromal and other tumors caused by platelet-derived growth factor receptor alpha gene mutations: a case associated with a germline V561D defect. J Clin Endocrinol Metab. 2007;92(9):3728–32. Epub 2007/06/15.
4. Ricci R, Martini M, Cenci T, Carbone A, Lanza P, Biondi A, et al. PDGFRA-mutant syndrome. Mod Pathol. 2015;28(7):954–64. Epub 2015/05/16.
5. Campbell T, Felsten L, Moore J. Disappearance of lentigines in a patient receiving imatinib treatment for familial gastrointestinal stromal tumor syndrome. Arch Dermatol. 2009;145(11):1313–6. Epub 2009/11/18.
6. Zoller ME, Rembeck B, Oden A, Samuelsson M, Angervall L. Malignant and benign tumors in patients with neurofibromatosis type 1 in a defined Swedish population. Cancer. 1997;79(11):2125–31. Epub 1997/06/01.
7. Patil S, Chamberlain RS. Neoplasms associated with germline and somatic NF1 gene mutations. Oncologist. 2012;17(1):101–16. Epub 2012/01/14.
8. Miettinen M, Fetsch JF, Sobin LH, Lasota J. Gastrointestinal stromal tumors in patients with neurofibromatosis 1: a clinicopathologic and molecular genetic study of 45 cases. Am J Surg Pathol. 2006;30(1):90–6.
9. Kalender M, Sevinc A, Tutar E, Sirikci A, Camci C. Effect of sunitinib on metastatic gastrointestinal stromal tumor in patients with neurofibromatosis type 1: a case report. World J Gastroenterol. 2007;13(18):2629–32. Epub 2007/06/07.
10. Agaram NP, Wong GC, Guo T, Maki RG, Singer S, Dematteo RP, et al. Novel V600E BRAF mutations in imatinib-naive and imatinib-resistant gastrointestinal stromal tumors. Genes Chromosomes Cancer. 2008;47(10):853–9.
11. Janeway KA, Liegl B, Harlow A, Le C, Perez-Atayde A, Kozakewich H, et al. Pediatric KIT wild-type and platelet-derived growth factor receptor alpha-wild-type gastrointestinal stromal tumors share KIT activation but not mechanisms of genetic progression with adult gastrointestinal stromal tumors. Cancer Res. 2007;67(19):9084–8.
12. van Nederveen FH, Gaal J, Favier J, Korpershoek E, Oldenburg RA, de Bruyn EM, et al. An immunohistochemical procedure to detect patients with paraganglioma and phaeochromocytoma with germline SDHB, SDHC, or SDHD gene mutations: a retrospective and prospective analysis. Lancet Oncol. 2009;10(8):764–71.
13. Janeway KA, Kim SY, Lodish M, Nose V, Rustin P, Gaal J, et al. Defects in succinate dehydrogenase in gastrointestinal stromal tumors lacking KIT and PDGFRA mutations. Proc Natl Acad Sci U S A. 2011;108(1):314–8. Epub 2010/12/22.
14. Killian JK, Miettinen M, Walker RL, Wang Y, Zhu YJ, Waterfall JJ, et al. Recurrent epimutation of SDHC in gastrointestinal stromal tumors. Sci Transl Med. 2014;6(268):268ra177. Epub 2014/12/30.
15. Boikos SA, Pappo AS, Killian JK, LaQuaglia MP, Weldon CB, George S, et al. Molecular subtypes of KIT/PDGFRA wild-type gastrointestinal stromal tumors: a report from the National Institutes of Health Gastrointestinal Stromal Tumor Clinic. JAMA Oncol. 2016;2(7):922–8. Epub 2016/03/25.
16. Benn DE, Robinson BG, Clifton-Bligh RJ. 15 years of paraganglioma: clinical manifestations of paraganglioma syndromes types 1–5. Endocr Relat Cancer. 2015;22(4):T91–103. Epub 2015/08/15.

17. Carney JA. Gastric stromal sarcoma, pulmonary chondroma, and extra-adrenal paraganglioma (Carney Triad): natural history, adrenocortical component, and possible familial occurrence. Mayo Clin Proc. 1999;74(6):543–52.
18. Haller F, Moskalev EA, Faucz FR, Barthelmess S, Wiemann S, Bieg M, et al. Aberrant DNA hypermethylation of SDHC: a novel mechanism of tumor development in Carney triad. Endocr Relat Cancer. 2014;21(4):567–77. Epub 2014/05/27.
19. Boikos SA, Xekouki P, Fumagalli E, Faucz FR, Raygada M, Szarek E, et al. Carney triad can be (rarely) associated with germline succinate dehydrogenase defects. Eur J Hum Genet. 2016;24(4):569–73. Epub 2015/07/16.
20. Pasini B, McWhinney SR, Bei T, Matyakhina L, Stergiopoulos S, Muchow M, et al. Clinical and molecular genetics of patients with the Carney-Stratakis syndrome and germline mutations of the genes coding for the succinate dehydrogenase subunits SDHB, SDHC, and SDHD. Eur J Hum Genet. 2008;16(1):79–88.
21. Janeway KA, Pappo AS. Pediatric gastrointestinal stromal tumors. Hematol Oncol Clin North Am. 2009;23(1):15–34.
22. Miettinen M, Wang ZF, Sarlomo-Rikala M, Osuch C, Rutkowski P, Lasota J. Succinate dehydrogenase-deficient GISTs: a clinicopathologic, immunohistochemical, and molecular genetic study of 66 gastric GISTs with predilection to young age. Am J Surg Pathol. 2011;35(11):1712–21. Epub 2011/10/15.
23. Oudijk L, Gaal J, Korpershoek E, van Nederveen FH, Kelly L, Schiavon G, et al. SDHA mutations in adult and pediatric wild-type gastrointestinal stromal tumors. Mod Pathol. 2013;26(3):456–63. Epub 2012/11/24.
24. Wagner AJ, Remillard SP, Zhang YX, Doyle LA, George S, Hornick JL. Loss of expression of SDHA predicts SDHA mutations in gastrointestinal stromal tumors. Mod Pathol. 2013;26(2):289–94. Epub 2012/09/08.
25. von Mehren M, Randall RL, Benjamin RS, Boles S, Bui MM, Casper ES, et al. Gastrointestinal stromal tumors, version 2.2014. J Natl Compr Canc Netw. 2014;12(6):853–62. Epub 2014/06/14.
26. Agaram NP, Laquaglia MP, Ustun B, Guo T, Wong GC, Socci ND, et al. Molecular characterization of pediatric gastrointestinal stromal tumors. Clin Cancer Res. 2008;14(10):3204–15.
27. Pantaleo MA, Lolli C, Nannini M, Astolfi A, Indio V, Saponara M, et al. Good survival outcome of metastatic SDH-deficient gastrointestinal stromal tumors harboring SDHA mutations. Genet Med. 2015;17(5):391–5. Epub 2014/09/05.
28. Heinrich MC, Owzar K, Corless CL, Hollis D, Borden EC, Fletcher CD, et al. Correlation of kinase genotype and clinical outcome in the North American Intergroup Phase III Trial of imatinib mesylate for treatment of advanced gastrointestinal stromal tumor: CALGB 150105 Study by Cancer and Leukemia Group B and Southwest Oncology Group. J Clin Oncol. 2008;26(33):5360–7. Epub 2008/10/29.
29. Corless CL, Ballman KV, Antonescu CR, Kolesnikova V, Maki RG, Pisters PW, et al. Pathologic and molecular features correlate with long-term outcome after adjuvant therapy of resected primary GI stromal tumor: the ACOSOG Z9001 trial. J Clin Oncol. 2014;32(15):1563–70. Epub 2014/03/19.
30. Demetri GD, van Oosterom AT, Garrett CR, Blackstein ME, Shah MH, Verweij J, et al. Efficacy and safety of sunitinib in patients with advanced gastrointestinal stromal tumour after failure of imatinib: a randomised controlled trial. Lancet. 2006;368(9544):1329–38.
31. Heinrich MC, Maki RG, Corless CL, Antonescu CR, Harlow A, Griffith D, et al. Primary and secondary kinase genotypes correlate with the biological and clinical activity of sunitinib in imatinib-resistant gastrointestinal stromal tumor. J Clin Oncol. 2008;26(33):5352–9.
32. Janeway KA, Albritton KH, Van den Abbeele AD, D'Amato GZ, Pedrazzoli P, Sienna S, et al. Sunitinib treatment in pediatric patients with advanced GIST following failure of imatinib. Pediatr Blood Cancer. 2009;52(7):767–71.
33. Ganjoo KN, Villalobos VM, Kamaya A, Fisher GA, Butrynski JE, Morgan JA, et al. A multicenter phase II study of pazopanib in patients with advanced gastrointestinal stromal tumors (GIST) following failure of at least imatinib and sunitinib. Ann Oncol. 2014;25(1):236–40. Epub 2013/12/21.

34. Mir O, Cropet C, Toulmonde M, Cesne AL, Molimard M, Bompas E, et al. Pazopanib plus best supportive care versus best supportive care alone in advanced gastrointestinal stromal tumours resistant to imatinib and sunitinib (PAZOGIST): a randomised, multicentre, open-label phase 2 trial. Lancet Oncol. 2016;17(5):632–41. Epub 2016/04/14.
35. Kindler HL, Campbell NP, Wroblewski K, Maki RG, D'Adamo DR, Chow WA, et al. Sorafenib (SOR) in patients (pts) with imatinib (IM) and sunitinib (SU)-resistant (RES) gastrointestinal stromal tumors (GIST): final results of a University of Chicago Phase II Consortium trial. J Clin Oncol. 2011;29(Suppl):Abstr 10009.
36. George S, Feng Y, von Mehren M, Choy E, Corless CL, Hornick JL, et al. Prolonged survival and disease control in the academic phase II trial of regorafenib in GIST: response based on genotype. J Clin Oncol. 2013;31(Suppl):Abstr 10511.
37. Janeway KA, Weldon CB. Pediatric gastrointestinal stromal tumor. Semin Pediatr Surg. 2012;21(1):31–43. Epub 2012/01/18.
38. Raygada M, King KS, Adams KT, Stratakis CA, Pacak K. Counseling patients with succinate dehydrogenase subunit defects: genetics, preventive guidelines, and dealing with uncertainty. J Pediatr Endocrinol Metab. 2014;27(9–10):837–44. Epub 2014/05/24.
39. Gill AJ, Hes O, Papathomas T, Sedivcova M, Tan PH, Agaimy A, et al. Succinate dehydrogenase (SDH)-deficient renal carcinoma: a morphologically distinct entity: a clinicopathologic series of 36 tumors from 27 patients. Am J Surg Pathol. 2014;38(12):1588–602. Epub 2014/07/16.
40. Tischler AS, deKrijger RR. 15 years of paraganglioma: pathology of pheochromocytoma and paraganglioma. Endocr Relat Cancer. 2015;22(4):T123–33. Epub 2015/07/03.
41. Malkin D, Nichols KE, Zelley K, Schiffman JD. Predisposition to pediatric and hematologic cancers: a moving target. Am Soc Clin Oncol Educ Book. 2014;2014:e44–55. Epub 2014/05/27.
42. Lepoutre-Lussey C, Caramella C, Bidault F, Deandreis D, Berdelou A, Al Ghuzlan A, et al. Screening in asymptomatic SDHx mutation carriers: added value of (1)(8)F-FDG PET/CT at initial diagnosis and 1-year follow-up. Eur J Nucl Med Mol Imaging. 2015;42(6):868–76. Epub 2015/02/14.
43. Anupindi SA, Bedoya MA, Lindell RB, Rambhatla SJ, Zelley K, Nichols KE, et al. Diagnostic performance of whole-body MRI as a tool for cancer screening in children with genetic cancer-predisposing conditions. AJR Am J Roentgenol. 2015;205(2):400–8. Epub 2015/07/24.
44. Jasperson KW, Kohlmann W, Gammon A, Slack H, Buchmann L, Hunt J, et al. Role of rapid sequence whole-body MRI screening in SDH-associated hereditary paraganglioma families. Fam Cancer. 2014;13(2):257–65. Epub 2013/08/13.
45. Gimenez-Roqueplo AP, Caumont-Prim A, Houzard C, Hignette C, Hernigou A, Halimi P, et al. Imaging work-up for screening of paraganglioma and pheochromocytoma in SDHx mutation carriers: a multicenter prospective study from the PGL.EVA Investigators. J Clin Endocrinol Metab. 2013;98(1):E162–73. Epub 2012/11/20.

Part I
Localized Disease

Natural History and Prognosis of Localized Gastrointestinal Stromal Tumors in the Pre- and Post-imatinib Eras

Zhi Ven Fong and John T. Mullen

1 Introduction

Gastrointestinal stromal tumors (GISTs), historically misclassified as leiomyomas, leiomyosarcomas, or schwannomas, are the most common mesenchymal neoplasms found in the gastrointestinal (GI) tract. The cornerstone in the treatment of GISTs has always been surgical resection, yet historically this has been associated with suboptimal overall survival and recurrence rates [1, 2]. However, there was a major breakthrough in 1998 when it was discovered that GISTs arise from the interstitial cell of Cajal and are molecularly characterized principally by mutations in the c-KIT and PDGFRA genes [3]. Since then, multiple clinical trials have evaluated the efficacy of imatinib mesylate, an oral tyrosine kinase inhibitor (TKI), as a treatment modality for GIST with excellent results [2, 4–7]. Today, imatinib plays a critical role in both the neoadjuvant and adjuvant treatment of GISTs, and in addition to other TKIs such as sunitinib and regorafenib, these drugs have fundamentally altered the natural history of both localized and metastatic GIST. Given that TKI therapy is costly and is associated with long-term adverse effects, it is critical to understand the natural history of localized GISTs as well as the prognostic factors for recurrence in order to identify those patients who would benefit most from TKI therapy. In this chapter, we review the natural history and prognosis of localized GISTs before the introduction of imatinib, the landmark trials demonstrating its efficacy, and the improved prognosis of localized GISTs after the introduction of imatinib.

Z.V. Fong, MD • J.T. Mullen, MD (✉)
Division of Surgical Oncology, Department of Surgery, Massachusetts General Hospital, Harvard Medical School, 55 Fruit St, Yawkey 7B, Boston, MA 02114, USA
e-mail: jmullen@partners.org

© Springer International Publishing Switzerland 2017

C.R. Scoggins et al. (eds.), *Gastrointestinal Stromal Tumors*,
DOI 10.1007/978-3-319-42632-7_5

2 The Pre-imatinib Era

2.1 Predictors of Disease Progression

Utilizing specimens submitted to the Armed Forces Institute of Pathology from 1970 to 1996, Miettinen and colleagues performed some of the most comprehensive analyses of the natural history of GIST in the pre-imatinib era. The authors identified GISTs from the stomach ($n=1765$) [8], duodenum ($n=156$) [9], jejunum and ileum ($n=1091$) [10], and the rectum and anus ($n=133$) [11] based on KIT and CD34 positivity. Imatinib therapy is costly and is associated with long-term adverse effects, precluding its widespread application. Therefore, Miettinen et al. sought to identify those pathological features of primary GISTs that predicted recurrence in an attempt to identify those patients who would benefit most from imatinib treatment.

Approximately 60–70 % of all GISTs arise in the stomach, and gastric GISTs generally exhibit the most favorable outcomes. In their series, Miettinen et al. found that the strongest predictors of disease progression (i.e., metastases) were tumor size and mitotic activity. The risk of metastases in patients with tumors less than 5 cm in size and with fewer than 5 mitoses/50 high-power fields (HPFs) is only 2–3 %. Conversely, this risk is as high as 86 % in patients with tumors greater than 10 cm in size with more than 10 mitoses/50 HPFs. Interestingly, patients with mixed pathologic features demonstrated rather favorable outcomes – patients with GISTs less than 5 cm in size with more than 5 mitoses/50 HPFs had a metastasis rate of 15 %, whereas those with tumors greater than 5 cm in size with fewer than 5 mitoses/50 HPFs had a metastasis rate of 11 % (Table 1) [8]. When stratified by location within the stomach, GISTs in the gastric fundus and cardia were associated with worse outcomes (36 % and 53 % rates of progression, respectively) than those in the gastric antrum or along the gastric curvatures. This was reasoned to be due to the predominantly malignant spindle histologic subtype of the proximal gastric GISTs, which generally confers a worse prognosis. Other unfavorable histologic factors included the presence of coagulative necrosis, ulceration, and mucosal invasion.

In an analysis of GISTs arising from other parts of the GI tract, it appears that the more distal the tumor is along the GI tract, the worse its prognosis (Table 1). Similar to gastric GISTs, GISTs in the duodenum, jejunum, ileum, rectum, and anus measuring less than 5 cm in size and with fewer than 5 mitoses/50 HPFs are associated with lower rates of progression (Table 1). However, in contrast to GISTs arising from the stomach, mixed pathologic features do not confer as favorable a prognosis in GISTs arising more distally in the GI tract. Notably, GISTs arising in the rectum and anus with a maximum diameter of less than 5 cm but harboring more than 5 mitoses/50 HPFs had a progression rate of 66 %, similar to those greater than 5 cm in size with fewer than 5 mitoses/50 HPFs (progression rate of 71 %), both no different than rectal or anal GISTs measuring greater than 5 cm in size and harboring more than 5 mitoses/50 HPFs (70 %) [9–11].

Table 1 Progression rate (defined by metastases) of GISTs based on location within the gastrointestinal tract and stratified by tumor size and mitotic rate

		Progression rate with full long-term follow-up			
		Size <5 cm	Size <5 cm	Size >10 cm	Size >10 cm
GIST location	*N*	<5 mitoses per 50 HPFs	>5 mitoses per 50 HPFs	< 5 mitoses per 50 HPFs	> 5 mitoses per 50 HPFs
Stomach [8]	1765	2–3 %	15 %	11 %	86 %
Duodenum [9]	156	8 %	50 %	34 %	100 %
Jejunum/Ileum [10]	1091	2–3 %	24 %	50 %	86 %
Rectum/Anus [11]	133	<1 %	66 %	71 %	70 %

HPFs high-power fields

2.2 "Small/Micro" GIST

The notion that all GISTs, irrespective of tumor size and mitotic rate, have a quantifiable risk of progression and malignant potential is controversial. Based on both autopsy and population level studies, incidentally identified "small" or "micro" GISTs, defined as GISTs measuring less than 1 cm in size, are quite common, occurring in the stomachs of 23 % of patients older than 50 years of age [12], in 35 % of patients with gastric cancer [13], and in 10 % of patients with gastroesophageal cancer [14]. Pathological analysis has demonstrated that these small GISTs already exhibit KIT and PDGFRA mutations in ~70–90 % of cases, but these tumors are clinically indolent [15, 16]. There are two retrospective analyses of small submucosal GISTs resected endoscopically, and both studies demonstrate stable disease on follow-up. Bai et al. analyzed 25 patients with small/micro-GISTs (84 % very low risk, 12 % low risk, and 4 % intermediate risk) and demonstrated no recurrence or metastasis with a mean follow-up of almost 12 months [17]. Similarly, Catalano and colleagues demonstrated a 5-year disease-free survival rate of 100 % in 10 patients with small GISTs that were resected endoscopically [15].

2.3 NIH and NCCN Classification Systems

In 2001, the NIH convened a GIST Workshop and established a NIH consensus classification system which risk stratifies GISTs based on tumor size and mitotic count (Table 2) [18]. Given the aforementioned progression risk of even small tumors with low mitotic counts (especially distal lesions with mixed pathologic features), this classification system does not dichotomize GISTs into benign and malignant lesions. Rather, it classifies GISTs into very low-, low-, intermediate-, and high-risk categories [18]. While the performance of this classification system has generally been demonstrated to be quite satisfactory [19–21], it is notable that the NIH classification schema does not take into consideration several other important predictors of aggressive tumor biology. The multiple series by Miettinen et al.

Table 2 The NIH consensus classification system of GIST, risk-stratifying lesions based on tumor size and mitotic count (per 50 high-power fields)

Risk category	Tumor size in largest dimension	Mitotic count
Very low	<2 cm	<5
Low	2–5 cm	<5
Intermediate	<5 cm	6–10
	5–10 cm	<5
High	>5 cm	>5
	>10 cm	Any mitotic count
	Any size	>10

Adapted from Fletcher et al. [18]

mentioned above highlight the biologic differences of GISTs based on tumor location, with small bowel GISTs demonstrating a more aggressive biology than gastric GISTs of equal size. The Memorial Sloan Kettering Cancer Center (MSKCC) group demonstrated that a nomogram that includes tumor location (small bowel versus stomach) in addition to tumor size and mitotic count performed better than the NIH classification system in predicting recurrence-free survival (concordance probability 0.76 vs. 0.70, $P=0.04$) [22].Based on MSKCC's report, the National Comprehensive Cancer Network (NCCN) adopted a more comprehensive risk stratification schema incorporating tumor location, as depicted in Table 3 [23, 24]. Inclusion of tumor location allows for more accurate risk classification given that extra-gastric GISTs have a poorer prognosis when compared to gastric GISTs.

It should be noted that the size and mitotic count thresholds of 5 cm and of 5 mitoses per 50 HPFs, respectively, first employed by Miettinen and colleagues and later adopted by the NIH and NCCN in their classification systems, were arbitrary and based on expert consensus. In a retrospective analysis of 929 resected GISTs in the pre-imatinib era (1980–2000), Rossi et al. constructed a risk stratification system that included tumor size and mitotic rate as continuous variables as opposed to arbitrarily dichotomized categorical variables [25]. The resultant nomogram demonstrates that the added risk of a GIST with 6 mitoses/50 HPFs is not equivalent to that of a GIST with 12 mitoses/50 HPFs, as would be the assumption of the prior risk stratification schema that uses them as categorical variables (Fig. 1). Their model demonstrated improved discriminative ability (C-index 0.72) when compared to the NIH (C-index 0.64) and the NCCN (C-index 0.63) risk stratification systems, suggesting that future risk prediction models should be constructed with continuous variables for better discriminative performance.

These same authors also proposed complementing the clinicopathologic risk stratification with the tumor's mutation profile [26]. Pathologic analysis of untreated GISTs demonstrates that tumors with KIT exon 9 and exon 11 mutations are biologically more aggressive than wild-type GISTs or those with PDGFRA mutations [27, 28].In studying 451 primary GISTs treated only with surgery and no neoadjuvant or adjuvant therapy, Rossi and colleagues corroborated these findings, prog-

Table 3 Risk stratification of primary GIST by mitotic index, tumor size, and tumor location

Tumor parameters		Risk of progressive disease (%)			
Mitotic index	Size	Gastric	Duodenum	Jejunum/ileum	Rectum
≤ 5/50 HPF	≤2 cm	None (0)	None (0)	None (0)	None (0)
≤ 5/50 HPF	>2 ≤ 5 cm	Very low (1.9)	Low (4.3)	Low (8.3)	Low (8.3)
≤ 5/50 HPF	>5 ≤ 10 cm	Low (3.6)	Moderate (24)	Insuff. data	Insuff. data
≤ 5/50 HPF	>10 cm	Moderate (10)	High (52)	High (34)	High (57)
> 5/50 HPF	≤2 cm	None	High	Insuff. data	High (54)
> 5/50 HPF	>2 ≤ 5 cm	Moderate (16)	High (73)	High (50)	High (52)
> 5/50 HPF	>5 ≤ 10 cm	High (55)	High (85)	Insuff. data	Insuff. data
> 5/50 HPF	>10 cm	High (86)	High (90)	High (86)	High (71)

Adapted from Demetri et al. [23]
HPFs high-power fields

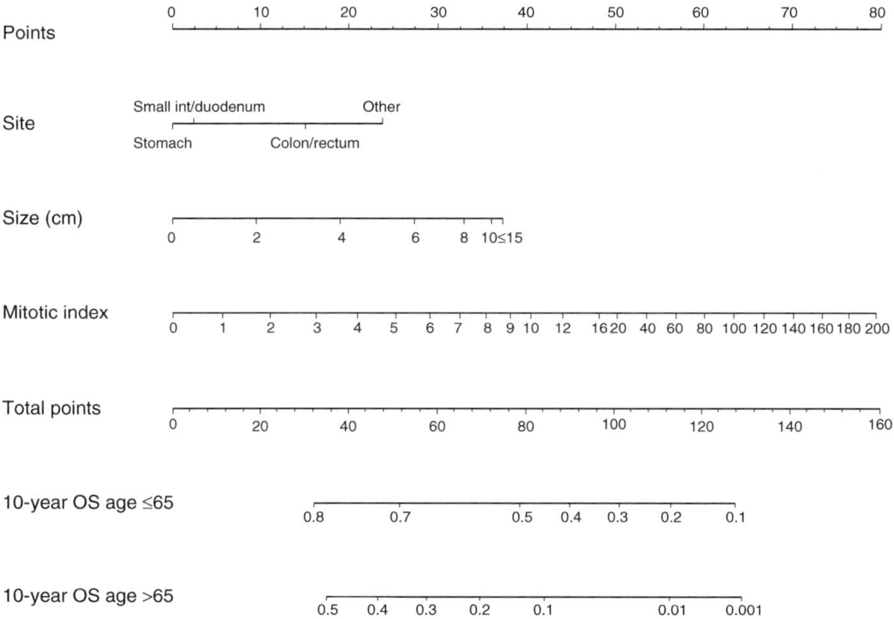

Fig. 1 Nomogram utilizing tumor size and mitotic index as continuous variables predicting 10-year overall survival in patients with GIST, stratified by age (Adapted from Rossi et al. [25])

nostically classifying GISTs into three distinct groups with decreasingly favorable biology: Group I, including GISTs with mutations in PDGFRA exon 13, KIT exon 17, and BRAF (reference group); Group II, including GISTs with mutations in KIT exon 17, PDGFRA exon 18 D842V, and PDGFRA exon 14, as well as triple-negative GISTs (HR 3.06, 95 % C.I. 1.09–8.58); and Group III, including GISTs with mutations in KIT exons 9 and 11 and PDGFRA exon 18 other than D842V (HR 4.52, 95 % C.I. 1.65–12.37) [26]. However, in current clinical practice, resected GISTs are not routinely submitted for mutational analysis, nor is it recommended by the NCCN GIST Task Force [24], as more data are needed to justify its added value in prognostication, taking into consideration the added cost and expertise required to do it.

It should also be noted that symptomatic presentation [29], tumor rupture [30, 31], cellularity, ulceration, and mucosal invasion [32] have all been shown to be important prognostic factors, but they are less commonly used for risk stratification.

3 Post-imatinib Era

3.1 Imatinib for Metastatic Disease

Imatinib mesylate is a molecular inhibitor of tyrosine kinases, which includes KIT, PDGFR, ABL, and BCR, and it was originally used to treat patients with chronic myelogenous leukemia via the inhibition of BCR-ABL oncoproteins. It was not until 2002 that imatinib was demonstrated to be effective in the treatment of metastatic GIST via the inhibition of KIT and PDGFR tyrosine kinases [33]. In a randomized controlled trial of 147 patients, Demetri and colleagues demonstrated partial responses in 53.7 % of patients and stable disease in 27.9 % of patients [2]. Subsequent randomized controlled trials have corroborated these results [7, 34], with a dose schedule of 400 mg twice a day demonstrating longer progression-free survival than a dose schedule of 400 mg once a day (HR 0.82, 95 % C.I. 0.69–0.98, $P=0.026$) [7].

3.2 Imatinib as an Adjuvant Therapy

Given its efficacy in the metastatic setting, imatinib was then investigated in the adjuvant setting in a randomized controlled trial by the American College of Surgeons Oncology Group Intergroup Adjuvant GIST Study Team (ACOSOG trial Z9001). ACOSOG trial Z9001 was a phase III, double-blind, placebo-controlled trial randomizing 703 patients with resected GISTs (at least 3 cm in size) to receive imatinib 400 mg once daily, or placebo once daily, for a year. The trial was terminated on interim analysis when the group receiving imatinib demonstrated a longer

1-year recurrence-free survival rate when compared with the placebo group (98 % vs. 83 %, overall HR 0.35, P <0.0001), and patients with KIT-mutated GISTs derived the most benefit from treatment [4]. Even when stratified by tumor size, the recurrence-free survival rate in the treatment group remained superior to the placebo group (Fig. 2). Based on these results from the Z9001 trial, the U.S. Food and Drug Administration (FDA) and the European Medicines Agency (EMEA) approved imatinib for the treatment of GIST in the adjuvant setting.

3.3 Duration of Imatinib Therapy

It should be noted that despite the recurrence-free survival benefit in the imatinib group, the overall survival rates were no different. Many patients in the group treated with imatinib for 12 months suffered disease recurrence within the first 2 years after discontinuation of imatinib. In fact, up to 54.8 % of disease recurrences occurred after the discontinuation of imatinib therapy (Fig. 2) [4]. This is consistent with the findings of the French Sarcoma group in their trial (BRF14) of imatinib treatment in patients with advanced GIST, comparing the interruption versus the continuation of imatinib therapy past 1 year. They found that the majority of disease progression occurred at a median of 6 months after the discontinuation of therapy [35]. These results suggested that the duration of imatinib treatment should be extended beyond 1 year, and this prompted the Scandinavian Sarcoma Group (SSG) trial XVIII.

The SSG trial XVIII was an open label, phase III study randomizing 400 patients with NIH high-risk classification GISTs within 12 weeks of surgery to 400 mg per day of imatinib for either 12 months or 36 months of treatment. At a median follow-up of 54 months, the group randomized to 36 months of imatinib therapy demonstrated a longer 5-year recurrence-free survival rate than those patients randomized to the 12-month arm (65.6 % vs. 47.9 %, HR 0.46, 95 % C.I. 0.32–0.65, P <0.001). Additionally, the 36-month group also enjoyed a longer 5-year overall survival rate compared to the 12-month group (92.0 % vs. 81.7 %, HR 0.45, 95 % C.I. 0.22–0.89, P =0.02) [36]. However, 25.8 % of the patients in the 36-month group had to discontinue imatinib for one or more reasons other than GIST recurrence, as compared to 12.6 % in the 12-month group. This trial concluded that the survival benefits of prolonged imatinib administration need to be balanced with the treatment-related toxicity. A phase II, nonrandomized, open-label trial evaluating the efficacy of 5 years of adjuvant imatinib treatment for patients status post resection of high-risk GISTs is currently underway (NCT00867113).

3.4 Imatinib Resistance

Unfortunately, approximately 5–15 % of all GISTs are primarily resistant to imatinib therapy [5, 6, 34]. Of patients who were initially responsive to imatinib

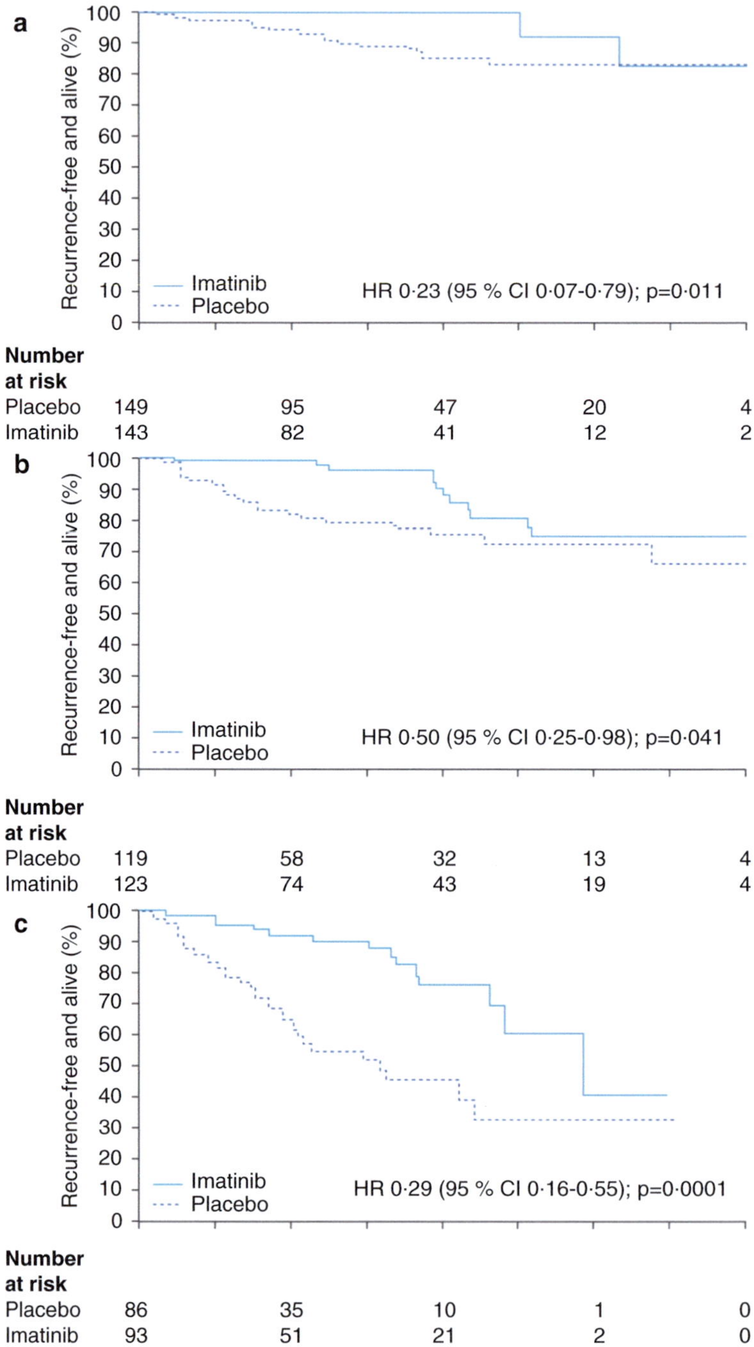

Fig. 2 Recurrence-free survival for patients with GIST with tumor size (**a**) 6 cm or greater, (**b**) less than 10 cm, and (**c**) 10 cm or greater (Adapted from Dematteo et al. [4])

therapy, another 14 % also eventually developed imatinib resistance and disease progression, although it is unclear if this resistance is a result of the development of a second mutation during treatment or if the mutation was present pretreatment but was not detected at the time of biopsy [37, 38].

Sunitinib, the current second-line treatment for imatinib-resistant GISTs, is a more broadly acting TKI, binding to RET, CD114, CD135, and VEGFR tyrosine kinases in addition to KIT and PDGFRA. In a double-blinded, randomized, placebo-controlled trial of 312 patients with advanced GIST failing initial imatinib treatment, Demetri and colleagues demonstrated a longer time to tumor progression (median 27.3 weeks vs. 6.4 weeks, HR 0.33, $P<0.0001$) and an improved overall survival rate (HR 0.49, 95 % C.I. 0.29–0.83, $P=0.007$) in the treatment group when compared to the placebo group [5]. However, imatinib therapy was discontinued at the time of randomization in the control group despite the fact that 34 % of these patients benefitted from a partial response to imatinib therapy and another 34 % had stable disease, which likely biased the outcome favoring the treatment group. The effect estimates might have been less significant if imatinib treatment was continued for the placebo group. The simultaneous inhibition of these receptors also led to many of its side effects, most notably dermatologic toxicities like hand-foot syndrome and stomatitis. Up to 83 % of sunitinib-treated patients reported treatment-related adverse events, but only 9 % discontinued treatment because of toxicity. Since then, several other TKIs, such as regorafenib [39], nilotinib [40], and masitinib [41], are being investigated for the treatment of imatinib-resistant GISTs, and further studies will be necessary to determine their long-term efficacy.

4 Conclusion

Imatinib has brought about dramatic improvements in the progression-free and overall survival of patients with both resectable and unresectable GIST. The current risk stratification system endorsed by the NCCN is based on tumor size, mitotic count, and tumor location, and it has demonstrated satisfactory prognostic performance. However, models incorporating tumor size and mitotic count as continuous variables as opposed to categorical variables have been shown to be more discriminatory and should be further explored. If known, the mutational profile of a GIST further serves as a valuable prognostic complement to the aforementioned clinicopathologic features. Improved risk stratification schemas will serve to help the clinician more accurately assess the risk of GIST tumor recurrence or progression and improve patient selection for TKI therapy, weighing the potential benefits against the costs and side effects of treatment. With our improved molecular understanding and risk stratification of patients with GISTs, the disease has evolved from a malignancy with high rates of tumor progression and death into a chronic disease manageable with long-term oral TKI therapy.

References

1. Dematteo RP, Heinrich MC, El-Rifai WM, et al. Clinical management of gastrointestinal stromal tumors: before and after STI-571. Hum Pathol. 2002;33:466–77.
2. Demetri GD, von Mehren M, Blanke CD, et al. Efficacy and safety of imatinib mesylate in advanced gastrointestinal stromal tumors. N Engl J Med. 2002;347:472–80.
3. Hirota S, Isozaki K, Moriyama Y, et al. Gain-of-function mutations of c-kit in human gastrointestinal stromal tumors. Science. 1998;279:577–80.
4. Dematteo RP, Ballman KV, Antonescu CR, et al. Adjuvant imatinib mesylate after resection of localised, primary gastrointestinal stromal tumour: a randomised, double-blind, placebo-controlled trial. Lancet. 2009;373:1097–104.
5. Demetri GD, van Oosterom AT, Garrett CR, et al. Efficacy and safety of sunitinib in patients with advanced gastrointestinal stromal tumour after failure of imatinib: a randomised controlled trial. Lancet. 2006;368:1329–38.
6. Blanke CD, Demetri GD, von Mehren M, et al. Long-term results from a randomized phase II trial of standard- versus higher-dose imatinib mesylate for patients with unresectable or metastatic gastrointestinal stromal tumors expressing KIT. J Clin Oncol. 2008;26:620–5.
7. Verweij J, Casali PG, Zalcberg J, et al. Progression-free survival in gastrointestinal stromal tumours with high-dose imatinib: randomised trial. Lancet. 2004;364:1127–34.
8. Miettinen M, Sobin LH, Lasota J. Gastrointestinal stromal tumors of the stomach: a clinicopathologic, immunohistochemical, and molecular genetic study of 1765 cases with long-term follow-up. Am J Surg Pathol. 2005;29:52–68.
9. Miettinen M, Kopczynski J, Makhlouf HR, et al. Gastrointestinal stromal tumors, intramural leiomyomas, and leiomyosarcomas in the duodenum: a clinicopathologic, immunohistochemical, and molecular genetic study of 167 cases. Am J Surg Pathol. 2003;27:625–41.
10. Miettinen M, Makhlouf H, Sobin LH, et al. Gastrointestinal stromal tumors of the jejunum and ileum: a clinicopathologic, immunohistochemical, and molecular genetic study of 906 cases before imatinib with long-term follow-up. Am J Surg Pathol. 2006;30:477–89.
11. Miettinen M, Furlong M, Sarlomo-Rikala M, et al. Gastrointestinal stromal tumors, intramural leiomyomas, and leiomyosarcomas in the rectum and anus: a clinicopathologic, immunohistochemical, and molecular genetic study of 144 cases. Am J Surg Pathol. 2001;25:1121–33.
12. Agaimy A, Wunsch PH, Hofstaedter F, et al. Minute gastric sclerosing stromal tumors (GIST tumorlets) are common in adults and frequently show c-KIT mutations. Am J Surg Pathol. 2007;31:113–20.
13. Kawanowa K, Sakuma Y, Sakurai S, et al. High incidence of microscopic gastrointestinal stromal tumors in the stomach. Hum Pathol. 2006;37:1527–35.
14. Abraham SC, Krasinskas AM, Hofstetter WL, et al. "Seedling" mesenchymal tumors (gastrointestinal stromal tumors and leiomyomas) are common incidental tumors of the esophagogastric junction. Am J Surg Pathol. 2007;31:1629–35.
15. Catalano F, Rodella L, Lombardo F, et al. Endoscopic submucosal dissection in the treatment of gastric submucosal tumors: results from a retrospective cohort study. Gastric Cancer. 2013;16:563–70.
16. Rossi S, Gasparotto D, Toffolatti L, et al. Molecular and clinicopathologic characterization of gastrointestinal stromal tumors (GISTs) of small size. Am J Surg Pathol. 2010;34:1480–91.
17. Bai J, Wang Y, Guo H, et al. Endoscopic resection of small gastrointestinal stromal tumors. Dig Dis Sci. 2010;55:1950–4.
18. Fletcher CD, Berman JJ, Corless C, et al. Diagnosis of gastrointestinal stromal tumors: a consensus approach. Hum Pathol. 2002;33:459–65.
19. Dematteo RP, Gold JS, Saran L, et al. Tumor mitotic rate, size, and location independently predict recurrence after resection of primary gastrointestinal stromal tumor (GIST). Cancer. 2008;112:608–15.

20. DeMatteo RP, Lewis JJ, Leung D, et al. Two hundred gastrointestinal stromal tumors: recurrence patterns and prognostic factors for survival. Ann Surg. 2000;231:51–8.
21. Langer C, Gunawan B, Schuler P, et al. Prognostic factors influencing surgical management and outcome of gastrointestinal stromal tumours. Br J Surg. 2003;90:332–9.
22. Gold JS, Gonen M, Gutierrez A, et al. Development and validation of a prognostic nomogram for recurrence-free survival after complete surgical resection of localised primary gastrointestinal stromal tumour: a retrospective analysis. Lancet Oncol. 2009;10:1045–52.
23. Demetri GD, Benjamin RS, Blanke CD, et al. NCCN Task Force report: management of patients with gastrointestinal stromal tumor (GIST)--update of the NCCN clinical practice guidelines. J Natl Compr Canc Netw. 2007;5 Suppl 2:S1–29; quiz S30.
24. Demetri GD, von Mehren M, Antonescu CR, et al. NCCN Task Force report: update on the management of patients with gastrointestinal stromal tumors. J Natl Compr Canc Netw. 2010;8 Suppl 2:S1–41; quiz S42-4.
25. Rossi S, Miceli R, Messerini L, et al. Natural history of imatinib-naive GISTs: a retrospective analysis of 929 cases with long-term follow-up and development of a survival nomogram based on mitotic index and size as continuous variables. Am J Surg Pathol. 2011;35:1646–56.
26. Rossi S, Gasparotto D, Miceli R, et al. KIT, PDGFRA, and BRAF mutational spectrum impacts on the natural history of imatinib-naive localized GIST: a population-based study. Am J Surg Pathol. 2015;39:922–30.
27. Andersson J, Bumming P, Meis-Kindblom JM, et al. Gastrointestinal stromal tumors with KIT exon 11 deletions are associated with poor prognosis. Gastroenterology. 2006;130:1573–81.
28. Antonescu CR, Sommer G, Sarran L, et al. Association of KIT exon 9 mutations with nongastric primary site and aggressive behavior: KIT mutation analysis and clinical correlates of 120 gastrointestinal stromal tumors. Clin Cancer Res. 2003;9:3329–37.
29. Hassan I, You YN, Shyyan R, et al. Surgically managed gastrointestinal stromal tumors: a comparative and prognostic analysis. Ann Surg Oncol. 2008;15:52–9.
30. Takahashi T, Nakajima K, Nishitani A, et al. An enhanced risk-group stratification system for more practical prognostication of clinically malignant gastrointestinal stromal tumors. Int J Clin Oncol. 2007;12:369–74.
31. Rutkowski P, Bylina E, Wozniak A, et al. Validation of the Joensuu risk criteria for primary resectable gastrointestinal stromal tumour – the impact of tumour rupture on patient outcomes. Eur J Surg Oncol. 2011;37:890–6.
32. Martin J, Poveda A, Llombart-Bosch A, et al. Deletions affecting codons 557-558 of the c-KIT gene indicate a poor prognosis in patients with completely resected gastrointestinal stromal tumors: a study by the Spanish Group for Sarcoma Research (GEIS). J Clin Oncol. 2005;23:6190–8.
33. Joensuu H, Roberts PJ, Sarlomo-Rikala M, et al. Effect of the tyrosine kinase inhibitor STI571 in a patient with a metastatic gastrointestinal stromal tumor. N Engl J Med. 2001;344:1052–6.
34. Blanke CD, Rankin C, Demetri GD, et al. Phase III randomized, intergroup trial assessing imatinib mesylate at two dose levels in patients with unresectable or metastatic gastrointestinal stromal tumors expressing the kit receptor tyrosine kinase: S0033. J Clin Oncol. 2008;26:626–32.
35. Blay JY, Le Cesne A, Ray-Coquard I, et al. Prospective multicentric randomized phase III study of imatinib in patients with advanced gastrointestinal stromal tumors comparing interruption versus continuation of treatment beyond 1 year: the French Sarcoma Group. J Clin Oncol. 2007;25:1107–13.
36. Joensuu H, Eriksson M, Sundby Hall K, et al. One vs three years of adjuvant imatinib for operable gastrointestinal stromal tumor: a randomized trial. JAMA. 2012;307:1265–72.
37. Wardelmann E, Merkelbach-Bruse S, Pauls K, et al. Polyclonal evolution of multiple secondary KIT mutations in gastrointestinal stromal tumors under treatment with imatinib mesylate. Clin Cancer Res. 2006;12:1743–9.

38. Heinrich MC, Maki RG, Corless CL, et al. Primary and secondary kinase genotypes correlate with the biological and clinical activity of sunitinib in imatinib-resistant gastrointestinal stromal tumor. J Clin Oncol. 2008;26:5352–9.
39. Demetri GD, Reichardt P, Kang YK, et al. Efficacy and safety of regorafenib for advanced gastrointestinal stromal tumours after failure of imatinib and sunitinib (GRID): an international, multicentre, randomised, placebo-controlled, phase 3 trial. Lancet. 2013;381:295–302.
40. Montemurro M, Schoffski P, Reichardt P, et al. Nilotinib in the treatment of advanced gastrointestinal stromal tumours resistant to both imatinib and sunitinib. Eur J Cancer. 2009;45:2293–7.
41. Le Cesne A, Blay JY, Bui BN, et al. Phase II study of oral masitinib mesilate in imatinib-naive patients with locally advanced or metastatic gastro-intestinal stromal tumour (GIST). Eur J Cancer. 2010;46:1344–51.

Imaging and Response Evaluation of Gastrointestinal Stromal Tumors

Sooyoung Shin and Haesun Choi

1 Introduction

Gastrointestinal stromal tumor (GIST) is the most common tumor of nonepithelial origin in the gastrointestinal (GI) tract and the most common neoplasm arising from mesenchymal tissue. Mazur and Clark first coined the term GIST in 1983 to distinguish an unusual type of nonepithelial GI tumor [1]. Recent findings indicate that more than 95 % of GIST express a transmembrane receptor tyrosine protein kinase (Kit, also known as CD117 or c-Kit proto-oncogene) encoded by the *KIT* gene; and an activating mutation of the KIT proto-oncogene has been thought as key in the pathogenesis of GIST, suggesting its origin from GI pacemaker cells called the interstitial cells of Cajal [2]. A minority of patients with clinicopathological features of GIST show a platelet-derived growth factor receptor (PDGFR)-alpha activating mutation and KIT negativity, which together result in consequences in the downstream signaling pathway similar to those noted with KIT mutation [3, 4]. These groundbreaking discoveries have contributed to the development of targeted therapy for GIST, thus changing the paradigm for the roles of imaging and treatment.

Imaging plays crucial roles in identifying the primary turmor, the disease staging and perhaps most importantly, in assessing treatment response following molecular targeted therapy for GIST. In this chapter, we review the various imaging features of GIST throught the course of the disease as well as the technical aspects of relevant imaging modalities in GIST management. New imaging techniques are also briefly discussed.

S. Shin, MD • H. Choi, MD (✉)
Department of Diagnostic Radiology, MD Anderson Cancer Center,
1515 Holcombe Blvd, Unit 1473, Houston, TX 77030, USA
e-mail: hchoi@mdanderson.org

© Springer International Publishing Switzerland 2017
C.R. Scoggins et al. (eds.), *Gastrointestinal Stromal Tumors*,
DOI 10.1007/978-3-319-42632-7_6

2 Endoscopy and Endoscopic Ultrasound

2.1 Endoscopy

GIST is often a mass found incidentally during routine endoscopy performed for other indications, such as vague GI symptoms or, less commonly, GI bleeding. On endoscopy, a mass protrudes into the lumen with an intact overlying mucosa unless the lesion ulcerates [5]. However, endoscopic findings alone cannot accurately differentiate GIST from other submucosal neoplasms such as leiomyoma. Endoscopic ultrasound (EUS) usually follows endoscopy to help better characterize and differentiate GIST from other possible diagnoses.

Mucosal biopsy guided by endoscopy carries the potential risk of intraoperative perforation of the bowel wall and generally is not useful for histologic diagnosis, since most mucosal tissue is intact. A mucosal biopsy is not recommended unless the mucosa is ulcerated [5].

2.2 Endoscopic Ultrasound

EUS is a hybrid imaging tool of endoscopy that uses an ultrasound probe (12–30 Hz) at the tip of the endoscope, allowing more accurate assessment of the origin of a mass and better characterization of submucosal tumors than does endoscopy alone. Generally, GIST arises from the fourth layer of the bowel wall, the muscularis propria layer. On EUS, GIST is usually observed as a homogeneous, hypoechoic mass with a smooth margin when it is small, but when the lesion is larger, it can develop an irregular margin or invade into the other layers [5].

In addition to its role in helping distinguish GIST from other submucosal tumors, EUS also plays a role in identifying the malignant potential of a GIST. Previous studies demonstrated that lesion size larger than 4–5 cm, irregular margins, existence of cystic portions or hyperechoic foci inside the tumor, lobulation, and extraluminal extension are features related to the malignant potential of GIST. Identification of various combinations of the above features by EUS imaging resulted in a sensitivity of between 80 and 100 % and a positive predictive value of up to 100 % using this modality [6–8].

With the fine-needle attachment on the transducer, EUS allows safe tissue sampling from the subepithelial layers, enabling a preoperative diagnosis. Cytology-based EUS-fine-needle aspiration (EUS-FNA) analysis has been reported to have a sensitivity of 78.4 % [9]. A combination of cytologic and immunohistochemical analysis has yielded a higher diagnostic accuracy in differentiating GIST from other submucosal tumors, with an accuracy ranging from 86 to 95.6 % [10–12]. However, owing to the nature of insufficient sampling and potential sampling errors by EUS-FNA, its use in this setting is limited [9, 13, 14]. Generally, preoperative biopsy is not recommended unless metastasis is suspected or neoadjuvant molecular therapy prior to surgery is planned. When preoperative biopsy is indicated, EUS-FNA when applicable is preferred over percutaneous biopsy owing to the risk of peritoneal seeding following the latter method.

Recently introduced contrast-enhanced harmonic EUS (CEH-EUS) has been shown to improve the diagnostics accuracy of submucosal tumors and has shown the ability to predict malignant potential by analyzing the pattern of tumor vascularity [15, 16].

The use of EUS imaging is limited to the esophagus, stomach, duodenum, and anorectum owing to the technical accessibility of there parts of the GI tract [17]. Also, because of EUS's limited ability for full assessment, especially of large tumors, and depending upon the operator's experience, additional imaging techniques such as computed tomography (CT) are recommended to further delineate the diagnosis and treatment plan.

3 Computed Tomography

With the introduction of molecular targeted therapy and the subsequent dramatic improvement in the survival of patients with GIST [18, 19], imaging not only has gained importance in the initial diagnosis but also plays a central role in assessing treatment response and surveillance. Contrast-enhanced CT is currently the imaging modality of choice owing to its universal availability, easy access to the standardized imaging protocol, and ability to assess the extent of disease beyond the primary site. For an accurate assessment of hypervascular tumors like GIST, a biphasic or triphasic technique including arterial and portal venous phases, is warranted [17].

3.1 Initial Imaging Presentation

Primary GIST can demonstrate various imaging features on CT, depending on the tumor size, location, and aggressiveness.

GISTs are typically highly vascular tumors with significant enhancement on contrast-enhanced CT images. GIST usually presents as a solitary mass with a smooth contour without a capsule. Small GIST are relatively hypoattenuating endoluminal, polypoid masses or intramural masses with homogeneous enhancement on contrast-enhanced CT. Tumors larger than 5 cm tend to grow exophytically, displacing the organs or vessels nearby. Large GIST are more heterogeneous due to hemorrhage, necrosis, or myxohyaline degeneration, resulting in a central hypodensity with peripheral enhancement from the viable soft tissue component. On occasion multiseptation in the center of the tumor due to tumor vessels can be observed. Calcification is uncommon before treatment. Large GIST can fistularize, to the lumen of the originating loop of bowel, and this is depicted on CT as air or oral contrast within the turmor [20, 21]. Local invasion or bowel obstruction is uncommon even in large GIST (Fig. 1).

Other submucosal, subepithelial tumors may be included in the differential diagnosis when GIST is suspected based on CT. Leiomyoma tends to be a hypoattenuating

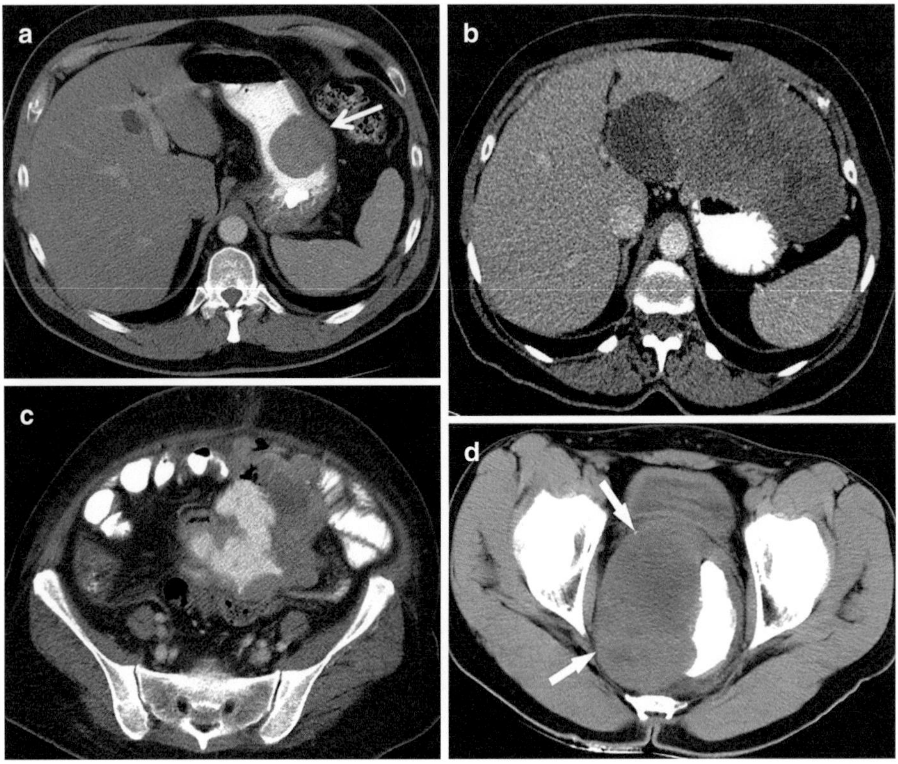

Fig. 1 CT characteristics of GISTs. (**a**) Polypoid gastric GIST (*arrow*), (**b**) Exophytic gastric GIST (**c**) Exophytic small bowel GIST fistulizing to the bowel lumen note the contrast within the tumor cavity. (**d**) Rectal GIST (*arrow*).

mass with a smooth margin, while leiomyosarcoma usually has variable density inside the lesion owing to internal necrosis, with or without calcification [22]. Carcinoid needs to be ruled out in the case of an intraluminal hypervascular mass. A diagnosis of lymphoma is favored especially in the presence of bulky adenopathy or marked mural thickening [20]. Due to its proximity to the pancreas, a large gastric GIST can mimica pancreatic neuroendocrine tumor [23].

Almost half of patients with GIST have metastasis at initial presentation [24]. GIST follows a hematogenous metastatic pattern, with the liver and peritoneum being the most common sites of metastasis. Less frequently, metastases can be found in the soft tissues, lungs, and pleura. Regional lymph node metastasis should raise the suspicion of other diagnoses [25].

Imaging features of metastatic lesions are similar to those of the primary lesion, including a hyperdense mass which enhances homogeneously to heterogeneously, depending on the presence of viable tumor tissue, necrosis, hemorrhage, or cystic elemenate within the tumor.

3.2 Monitoring Treatment Response

Traditionally, Response Evaluation Criteria in Solid Tumors (RECIST), which are based on changes in tumor size, have been universally used to measure tumor response following systemic treatment [26, 27] (Table 1). GIST responding to a targeted agent demonstrate homogeneous hypoattenuation, resolution of enhancing tumor nodules, and decreased tumor vascularity on contrast-enhanced CT compared with heterogeneous, hyperattenuating, enhancing lesions visualized on pre-treatment CT (Fig. 2).

CT imaging features correlate with pathologic change, characterized by necrosis with decreased cellularity inside the tumor, myxohyaline degeneration, and pseudo-

Table 1. Treatment response criteria

Criteria	Response	Description
RECIST 1.1	CR	No residual target lesions. All suspicious lymph nodes should be reduced to <10 mm in short axis
	PR	≥30 % reduction in sum of long axis diameter of target lesions compared with baseline sum of long axis diameter
	SD	Neither qualifying PD nor PR compared with the smallest sum of long axis diameter during the treatment period
	PD	≥20 % increase in sum of long axis diameter of target lesions with absolute increase of >5 mm in sum of long axis diameter, compared with the smallest sum of long axis diameter during treatment period
		Appearance of new lesion
Choi	CR	Disappearance of all lesions. No new lesion
	PR	≥10 % decrease in sum of long axis diameter of target lesions or ≥15 % decrease in tumor density on CT (HU) without evidence of new lesion or progression of nonmeasurable disease
	SD	Not satisfying CR, PR or PD. No evidence of worsening symptoms due to tumor progression
	PD	≥10 % increase in sum of long axis diameter of target lesions, and not satisfying PR by tumor density decrease
		Appearance of new lesion
		New intratumoral nodule or worsening intratumoral nodule
3D sphere	CR	Disappearance of all lesions. No new lesion
	PR	≥65 % decrease in volume (4/3 πr^3)
	SD	Not satisfying CR, PR or PD
	PD	≥73 % increase in volume (4/3 πr^3)
		Appearance of new lesion
3D ellipsoid	CR	Disappearance of all lesions. No new lesion
	PR	≥30 % decrease in volume (4/3 $\pi\, r_1\, r_2\, r_3$)
	SD	Not satisfying CR, PR, or PD
	PD	≥20 % increase in volume (4/3 $\pi\, r_1\, r_2\, r_3$)
		Appearance of new lesion

RECIST = Response Evaluation Criteria in Solid Tumors
CR = Complete Response
PR = Partial Response
SD = Stable Disease
PD = Progressive disease

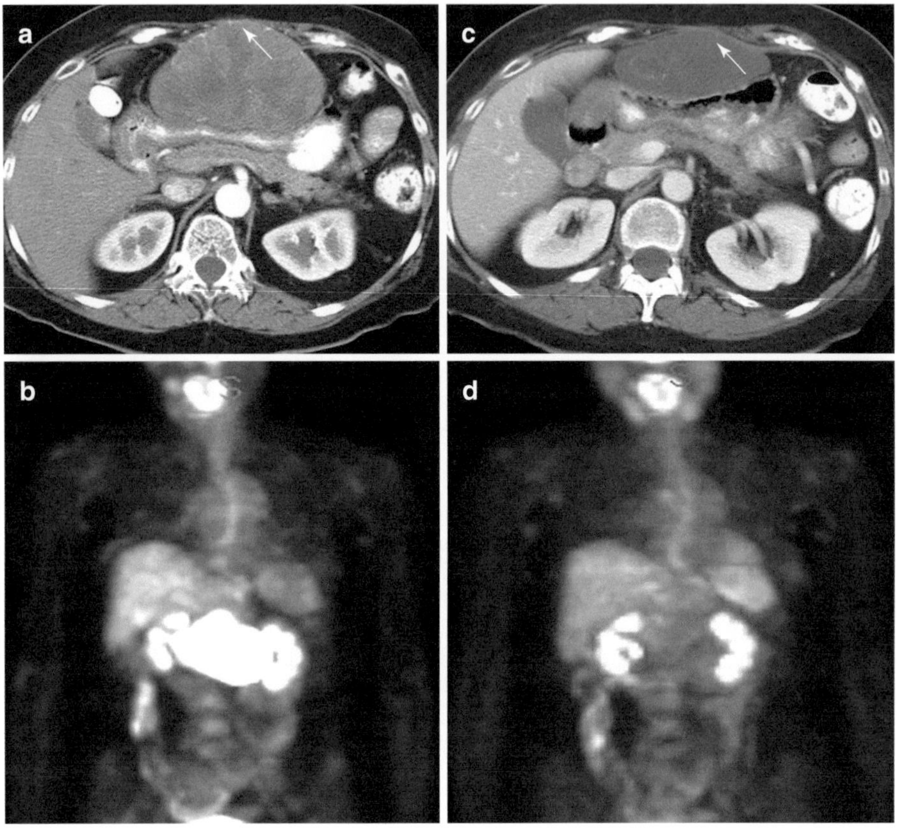

Fig. 2 GIST responding to tyrosine kiviqse inhibitor therapy in a 59-year-old woman with recurrent gastric GIST in the omentum. (**a**, **b**) Pretreatment contrast-enhanced CT scan, (**a**) shows a large, enhancing omental mass abutting the anterior surface of the stomach corresponding to the mass (*arrow*) with markedly increased glucose update shown on pretreatment FDG-PET (**b**). (**c**, **d**) Contrast-enhanced CT scan (**c**) obtained 2 months after treatment showed that the mass (*arrow*) has decreased in size and become homogeneous, with a marked decrease in CT density and no appreciable glucose uptake shown on FDG-PET (**d**) obtained at the same time

cyst formation [28]. These changes can be observed 1 or 2 months after starting treatment. GIST do decrease in size, but the median tumor shrinkage required to satisfy the partial response (PR) criteria by RECIST can take 3–4 months or longer [28]. Moreover, intratumoral hemorrhage or myxoid degenerative change in responding tumors can result in an increase in tumor size (Fig. 3). This paradoxical response can be mistaken for progression of disease (pseudoprogression) if only tumor size is considered when evaluating the treatment response. Similarly, GIST can progress with the development of new intratumoral nodules within the responding tumor without changing the overall tumor size [29]. This nodule-within-a-mass pattern can result in underestimation of disease progression while the tumor size remains stable (Fig. 4).

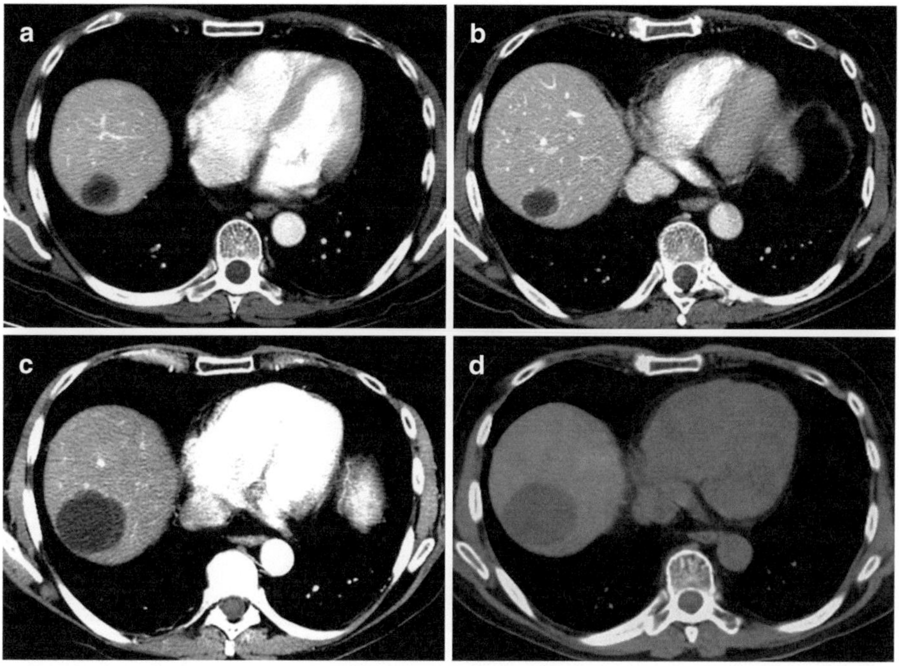

Fig. 3 Responding hepatic metastasis with pseudoprogression in a 56-year-old male with duodenal GIST. (**a**) Pretreatment contrast-enhanced CT shows an enhancing hepatic metastasis in segment 7 with the tumor density measured at 40 HU. Note the peripheral enhancing component. (**b**) Contrast-enhanced CT image obtained 2 months after treatment demonstrates a minimal decrease in size of the hepatic metastasis but with a significant decrease in CT density (27 HU). The peripheral enhancement is no longer evident. This is typical of responding GIST. (**c**, **d**) Contrast-enhanced CT image (**c**) obtained 7 months after treatment shows a homogenously hypoattenuating tumor with a continuous decrease in tumor density (18 HU). Notice the significant increase in tumor size with no appreciable glucose uptake on FDG-PET (**d**). The enlarging homogenous tumor with a continuous decrease in tumor density should not be confused with a progressing tumor. (HU = Hounsfield Unit)

New CT response evaluation criteria were proposed by Choi et al. to address the issues arising from the use of traditional size-based criteria in GIST [30] (Table 1). The Choi criteria incorporate changes in tumor size as well as in CT density, reflecting the morphologic changes in CT characteristics, to evaluate treatment response. These changes include a 10 % decrease in the sum of tumor size of the unidimensional tumor size or a 15 % decrease in tumor density, as determined by the CT attenuation coefficient in Hounsfield units (HUs), at the first follow-up (2 months) (Table 1). The Choi criteria have been shown to correlate well with the responses noted by positron emission tomography (PET) and can best categorize patients into good responders and poor responders, and the category of response is an excellent predictor of progression-free survival [31].

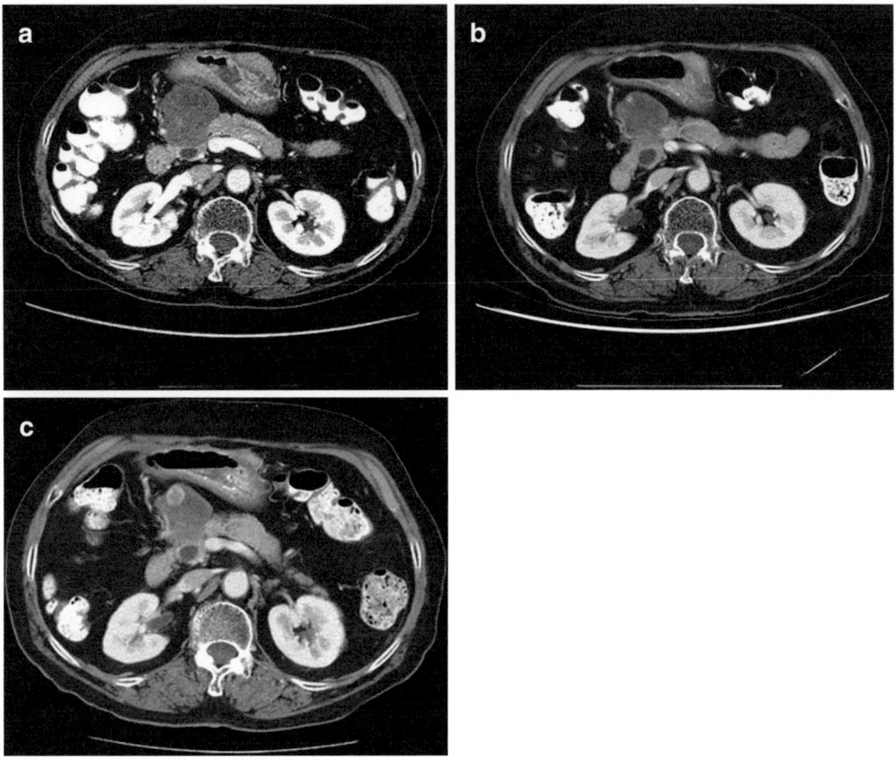

Fig. 4 Recurrence with enlarging intratumoral nodules in a patient with recurrent GIST. (**a**) The recurrent GIST has responded well at 10 months after treatment. (**b**, **c**) Note a tiny enhancing nodule within the responding recurrent tumor at 9 months after treatment (**b**), with an increase in size at 21 months after treatment (**c**)

Caution is needed if intratumoral hemorrhage or calcification occurs in responding tumors following treatment, as these developments could increase tumor density. Unenhanced images may be helpful in overcoming misinterpretation of the findings in this setting (Fig. 5).

Following imatinib treatment, fluid overload can occur as a side effect of the treatment. On imaging, fluid overload can present as ascites, pleural effusion, pericardial effusion, or edema. Such fluid overload should not be mistaken for progression of peritoneal disease [21].

3.3 Surveillance

Once the tumors respond to treatment, the role of imaging is to identify disease recurrence and progression in a timely manner. The tumor's development of resistance to the treatment is believed to be responsible for the recurrence [32].

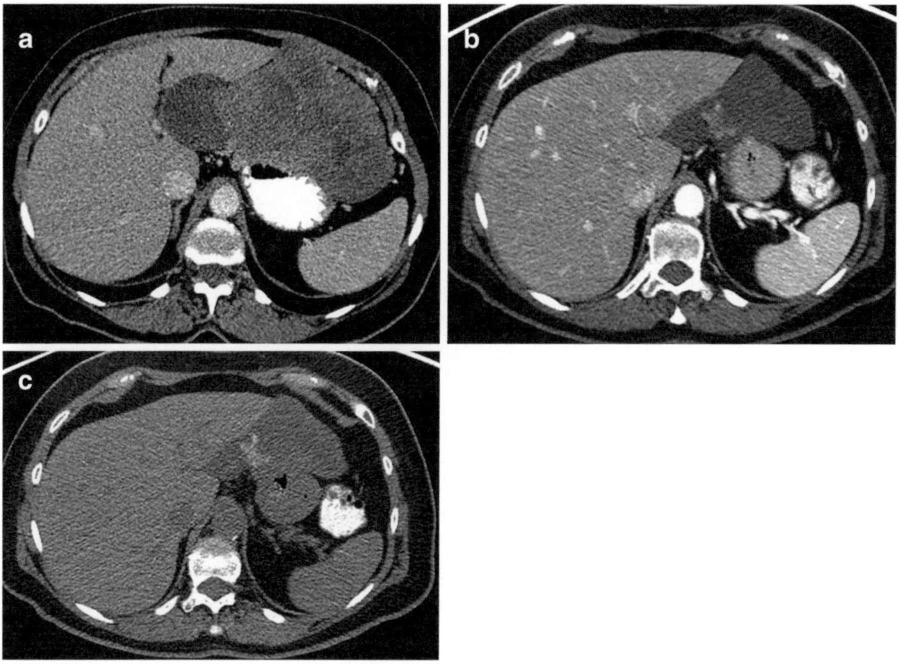

Fig. 5 Pseudoprogression with development of intratumoral calcification in a 66-year-old woman with gastric GIST. (**a**) The pretreatment CT shows an exophytic gastric GIST. (**b**, **c**) At 12 months after treatment, the tumor has responded well, with a significant decrease in size and tumor attenuation. Note that the intratumoral hyperattenuating nodular densities (**b**) are calcifications without enhancement, confirmed on unenhanced imaging (**c**)

Disease progression/recurrence in GIST can be detected by an increase in tumor size, increase in tumor density (enhancement on imaging), appearance of new lesions, presence of distant metastasis, or emergence of a new, intratumoral enhancing nodule.

GIST can recur following margin-free resection, particularly within the first 5 years after treatment [33]. For GIST patients with a high risk of recurrence (e.g., tumor size larger than 5 cm, high mitotic count of more than 5/50 high-power fields), close follow-up with CT imaging is recommended at a 3- to 4-month interval for the first 3 years, twice yearly for up to 5 years, and then annually thereafter.

For GIST patients at low risk for recurrence, CT follow-up twice a year for 5 years is recommended [34], although no standard surveillance protocol has been established in this group.

In cases of inconclusive CT findings, or if imaging findings cannot support the clinical findings, PET imaging can be useful.

3.4 New Techniques

The use of volumetric measurement on CT images has been explored (Table 1). Schiavon et al. reported that the three-dimensional (3D) ellipsoidal model was more sensitive for identifying PR than RECIST was, and 3D criteria were also useful for predicting overall survival [35].

The effect of a new antivascular agent can be monitored using CT perfusion, a fast imaging technique after administration of the iodinated contrast agent that provides quantitative tissue perfusion information such as blood flow, blood volume, and permeability [36]. In GIST, imatinib was postulated to have antivascular activity and to induce tumor apoptosis, which was correlated with a decrease in perfusion CT parameters such as blood volume and blood flow in PET responders [37]. Schlemmer et al. studied the value of perfusion CT on metastatic GIST patients treated with sunitinib or imatinib. Good responders based on Choi criteria were compared with poor responders and showed decreased perfusion parameters such as volume of distribution, blood flow, blood volume, and permeability. This distinct tendency between good responders and poor responders was also observed in hepatic lesions [38]. Although further validation of these findings is needed in a large group of patients, perfusion CT appears to have potential as a functional imaging modality to assist in more accurate assessment of treatment response.

Recently, the role of dual-energy CT (DECT) has been explored in GIST [39, 40]. The use of iodine-related attenuation has shown good correlation with the Choi criteria [39], and new response criteria have been proposed as a potential novel predictor of clinical outcome [40]. Moreover, DECT has a benefit in the possible elimination of unenhanced CT in protocol, reducing radiation exposure to the patient. However, one should keep in mind that this new technique does have technical limitations, especially in obese patients or patients with a large abdomen, and DECT is still in its developmental stage [41].

4 Positron Emission Tomography

PET is a metabolic imaging tool, measuring glucose metabolism using fludeoxyglucose (FDG). Once transported into the intracellular space, the FDG is trapped within the cell without being used as a cellular energy source like glucose is.

Malignant cells usually have increased glycolysis, which presents as increased FDG uptake on imaging. FDG uptake can be evaluated subjectively by visual analysis, semiquantitatively by measuring the standardized uptake value (SUV), and quantitatively by calculating the absolute rate of cellular metabolism using a kinetic model on dynamic sequence [42]. Currently, maximum SUV (SUVmax) is the most used due to its universal availability and semi-quantitative nature.

Combining PET with contrast-enhanced CT (PET-CT) and taking advantage of the features of contrast-enhanced CT can improve the accuracy of tumor detection, tumor characterization, and tumor localization [43]. Combining contrast-enhanced CT with PET can be technically challenging and is not yet universally available, but its use has been increasing.

4.1 *Initial Presentation*

PET offers a relatively high sensitivity for tumor detection and improves staging workup by imaging the whole body. However, PET is limited in its ability to detect small tumors (less than 1 cm in diameter) [44] and is rather nonspecific [45, 46]. Therefore, PET is not routinely used as an initial imaging modality in GIST, but PET is recommended on initial presentation when the tumor has borderline resectability and when PET is the imaging modality used for follow-up and treatment response evaluation [47].

4.2 *Treatment Response Evaluation and Surveillance*

PET is highly sensitive and specific in response evaluation, especially when early response evaluation (e.g., within a month) is needed to plan a further treatment strategy. Quantitative evaluation is possible by calculating the percent change in SUVmax between the baseline and follow-up studies. The changes on PET can be detected as early as 24 hours after the beginning of treatment, well before physical tumor shrinkage [48, 49]. A good correlation was observed between the changes in SUVmax on PET imaging and the changes in enhancement on CT following imatinib treatment [45] (Figs. 2, 3 and 6).

PET is indicated when CT or magnetic resonance imaging findings are equivocal for disease progression or recurrence. In the same context, PET can be useful to delineate the treatment plan when clinical features are inconsistent with imaging features on CT or MRI [17].

4.3 *Limitations*

Despite the great potential of PET as a problem solver and as a reliable tool for early response evaluation in GIST, a standardized image acquisition protocol has not been established yet, and there is no consensus on response evaluation criteria for PET.

European Organization for Research and Treatment of Cancer (EORTC) criteria were proposed in 1999. These criteria were based on multiple small clinical studies of various different tumor types, and GIST was not included [50], and the value of these criteria as a prognostic indicator has not been studied.

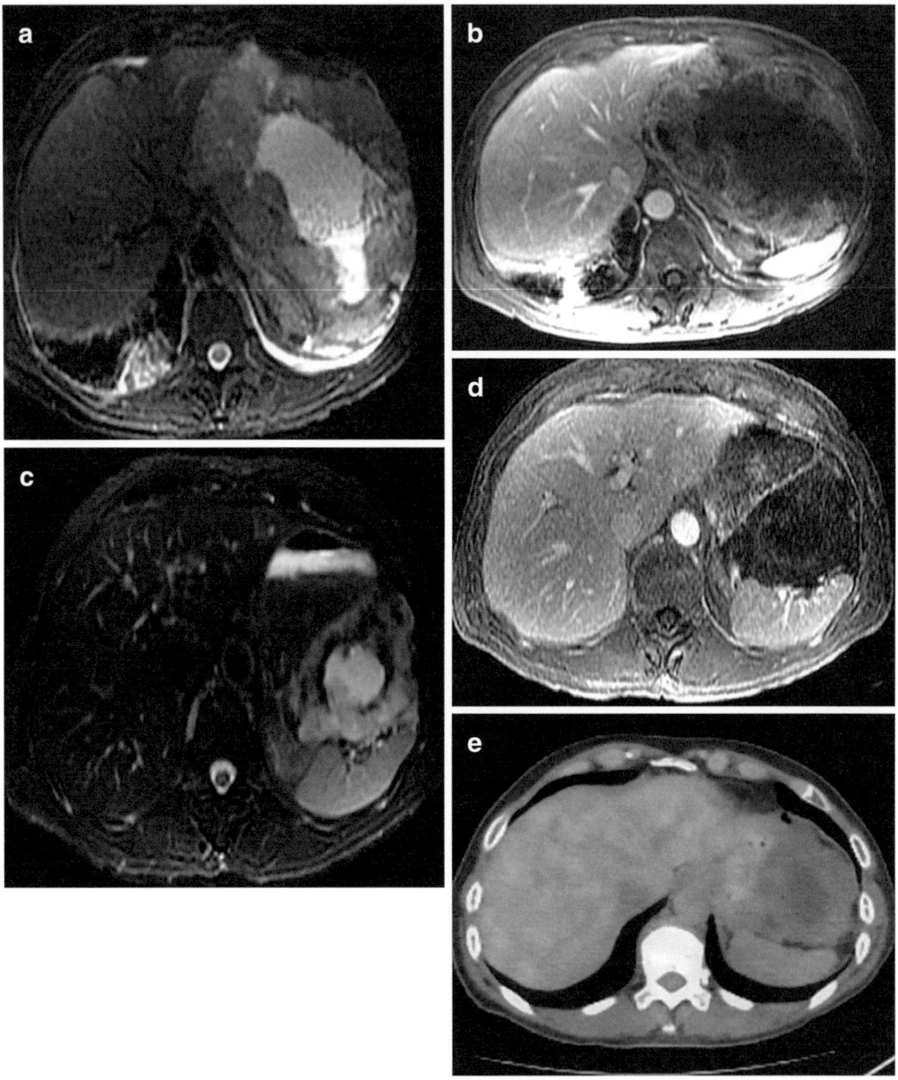

Fig. 6 Gastric GIST responding to therapy on MRI. (**a**, **b**) The centrally necrotic mass in the left upper quadrant demonstrates central T2 hyperintensity due to necrosis (**a**) and relative T2 hyperintense rim of solid enhancing component on a contrast-enhanced T1-weighted image (**b**). (**c**–**e**) At 6 months after treatment, the tumor has shrunk, with a decreasing rim of solid tumor on T2-weighted image (**c**). Note no significant enhancement of the rim on contrast-enhanced T-weighted image (**d**) and no significant FDG update on PET (**e**).

Various cutoff values for SUVmax decrease, ranging from 40 to 70 %, were proposed as a good prognostic indicator for GIST [30, 51, 52]. In 2009, PET Response Criteria in Solid Tumors (PERCIST) were proposed with stricter cutoff values than those of EORTC criteria [53] (Table 2).

Table 2. PET treatment response criteria

Criteria	Response	Description
EORTC	Complete metabolic response (CMR)	Complete resolution of FDG uptake within the entire tumor
	Partial metabolic response (PMR)	≥15–25 % decrease in FDG uptake (SUV) after one cycle of chemotherapy
		≥25 % decrease in FDG uptake (SUV) after ≥2 cycles of chemotherapy
	Stable metabolic disease (SMD)	<25 % increase in FDG uptake (SUV) or <15 % decrease in FDG uptake (SUV)
		and
		No visible increase in size of FDG uptake (≤20 % increase in the longest dimension)
	Progressive metabolic disease (PMD)	≥25 % increase in FDG uptake (SUV) compared with baseline
		or
		Visible increase in size of FDG uptake (>20 % increase in the longest dimension)
		or
		New FDG uptake in metastatic lesion
PERCIST	Complete metabolic response (CMR)	Complete resolution of FDG uptake within the entire target lesions
	Partial metabolic response (PMR)	≥30 % decrease in FDG uptake (SUL) in target lesions & ≥0.8 absolute decrease of SUL
	Stable metabolic disease (SMD)	Not satisfying CMR, PMR, or PMD
	Progressive metabolic disease (PMD)	>30 % increase in FDG uptake (SUL) in target lesions & >0.8 absolute increase of SUL
		or
		Visible increase in size of FDG uptake (75 % in TLG without SUL decrease)
		or
		New FDG uptake

SUL: SUV Lean, *TLG*: total lesion glycolysis

5 Magnetic Resonance Imaging

MRI can be used as an alternative imaging tool for patients with contraindications for contrast-enhanced CT, such as allergy to iodinated contrast. Hepatic metastasis can be better depicted on MRI than on CT, which is primarily used in problem solving. MRI is indicated in rectal GIST for presurgical planning, local tumor staging, and liver metastasis [17]. Depending on the availability of experts within the institution, MRI can be used as a primary imaging modality, but it is technically limited in evaluating peritoneal disease.

5.1 Imaging Presentation

Presentation of GIST on MRI is similar to that on CT. Contrast plays an important role in characterizing the intratumoral structures. GIST shows low signal intensity on T1-weighted images and presents as a heterogeneous mass on T2-weighted images with variably high signal intensity depending on the amount of solid tissue, necrotic tissue, and internal hemorrhage. Intratumoral hemorrhage can be better depicted on MRI than on CT [54, 55] (Fig. 6).

Dynamic contrast-enhanced MRI (DCE-MRI) can aid in assessing tumor viability and vascularity. When the tumor responds to treatment, tumor vascularity and viable tumor components decrease. This change can be quantitated by means of transfer constant (Ktrans), plasma volume, and extravascular leakage space (V_e) [56].

Recently, a diffusion-weighted image (DWI) has been applied as a comparable tool to PET-CT for the assessment of GIST. DWI provides both anatomical and functional image information. By visualizing tissue diffusion characteristics, DWI allows neoplastic tissue to be differentiated from normal tissue by high cell density in neoplastic tissue, resulting in reduced diffusion capability. The diffusion capability can be quantitated by apparent diffusion confident (ADC) values. It has been reported that the changes in ADC values following targeted treatment correlated well with the SUVmax on PET [57, 58]. The utility of DWI requires further validation.

These functional imaging techniques are technically challenging and are undergoing continuous refinement. The use of these techniques in GIST requires further validation.

References

1. Mazur MT, Clark HB. Gastric stromal tumors. Reappraisal of histogenesis. Am J Surg Pathol. 1983;7(6):507–19.
2. Hirota S, Isozaki K, Moriyama Y, Hashimoto K, Nishida T, Ishiguro S, et al. Gain-of-function mutations of c-kit in human gastrointestinal stromal tumors. Science. 1998;279(5350):577–80.
3. Heinrich MC, Corless CL, Duensing A, McGreevey L, Chen CJ, Joseph N, et al. PDGFRA activating mutations in gastrointestinal stromal tumors. Science. 2003;299(5607):708–10.
4. Hirota S, Ohashi A, Nishida T, Isozaki K, Kinoshita K, Shinomura Y, et al. Gain-of-function mutations of platelet-derived growth factor receptor alpha gene in gastrointestinal stromal tumors. Gastroenterology. 2003;125(3):660–7.
5. Rodriguez SA, Faigel DO. Endoscopic diagnosis of gastrointestinal stromal cell tumors. Curr Opin Gastroenterol. 2007;23(5):539–43.
6. Okai T, Minamoto T, Ohtsubo K, Minato H, Kurumaya H, Oda Y, et al. Endosonographic evaluation of c-kit-positive gastrointestinal stromal tumor. Abdom Imaging. 2003;28(3):301–7.
7. Chak A, Canto MI, Rosch T, Dittler HJ, Hawes RH, Tio TL, et al. Endosonographic differentiation of benign and malignant stromal cell tumors. Gastrointest Endosc. 1997;45(6):468–73.

8. Palazzo L, Landi B, Cellier C, Cuillerier E, Roseau G, Barbier JP. Endosonographic features predictive of benign and malignant gastrointestinal stromal cell tumours. Gut. 2000;46(1):88–92.
9. Sepe PS, Moparty B, Pitman MB, Saltzman JR, Brugge WR. EUS-guided FNA for the diagnosis of GI stromal cell tumors: sensitivity and cytologic yield. Gastrointest Endosc. 2009;70(2):254–61.
10. Watson RR, Binmoeller KF, Hamerski CM, Shergill AK, Shaw RE, Jaffee IM, et al. Yield and performance characteristics of endoscopic ultrasound-guided fine needle aspiration for diagnosing upper GI tract stromal tumors. Dig Dis Sci. 2011;56(6):1757–62.
11. Mekky MA, Yamao K, Sawaki A, Mizuno N, Hara K, Nafeh MA, et al. Diagnostic utility of EUS-guided FNA in patients with gastric submucosal tumors. Gastrointest Endosc. 2010;71(6):913–9.
12. Philipper M, Hollerbach S, Gabbert HE, Heikaus S, Bocking A, Pomjanski N, et al. Prospective comparison of endoscopic ultrasound-guided fine-needle aspiration and surgical histology in upper gastrointestinal submucosal tumors. Endoscopy. 2010;42(4):300–5.
13. Hoda KM, Rodriguez SA, Faigel DO. EUS-guided sampling of suspected GI stromal tumors. Gastrointest Endosc. 2009;69(7):1218–23.
14. Fu K, Eloubeidi MA, Jhala NC, Jhala D, Chhieng DC, Eltoum IE. Diagnosis of gastrointestinal stromal tumor by endoscopic ultrasound-guided fine needle aspiration biopsy--a potential pitfall. Ann Diagn Pathol. 2002;6(5):294–301.
15. Kitano M, Sakamoto H, Matsui U, Ito Y, Maekawa K, von Schrenck T, et al. A novel perfusion imaging technique of the pancreas: contrast-enhanced harmonic EUS (with video). Gastrointest Endosc. 2008;67(1):141–50.
16. Sakamoto H, Kitano M, Matsui S, Kamata K, Komaki T, Imai H, et al. Estimation of malignant potential of GI stromal tumors by contrast-enhanced harmonic EUS (with videos). Gastrointest Endosc. 2011;73(2):227–37.
17. Choi H. Imaging modalities of gastrointestinal stromal tumors. J Surg Oncol. 2011;104(8):907–14.
18. Perez EA, Livingstone AS, Franceschi D, Rocha-Lima C, Lee DJ, Hodgson N, et al. Current incidence and outcomes of gastrointestinal mesenchymal tumors including gastrointestinal stromal tumors. J Am Coll Surg. 2006;202(4):623–9.
19. Gold JS, van der Zwan SM, Gonen M, Maki RG, Singer S, Brennan MF, et al. Outcome of metastatic GIST in the era before tyrosine kinase inhibitors. Ann Surg Oncol. 2007;14(1):134–42.
20. Levy AD, Remotti HE, Thompson WM, Sobin LH, Miettinen M. Gastrointestinal stromal tumors: radiologic features with pathologic correlation. Radiographics Rev Publ Radiol Soc N Am Inc. 2003;23(2):283–304, 456; quiz 532.
21. Hong X, Choi H, Loyer EM, Benjamin RS, Trent JC, Charnsangavej C. Gastrointestinal stromal tumor: role of CT in diagnosis and in response evaluation and surveillance after treatment with imatinib. Radiographics Rev Publ Radiol Soc N Am Inc. 2006;26(2):481–95.
22. Lee SH, Ha HK, Byun JY, Kim AY, Cho KS, Lee YR, et al. Radiological features of leiomyomatous tumors of the colon and rectum. J Comput Assist Tomogr. 2000;24(3):407–12.
23. Sandrasegaran K, Rajesh A, Rushing DA, Rydberg J, Akisik FM, Henley JD. Gastrointestinal stromal tumors: CT and MRI findings. Eur Radiol. 2005;15(7):1407–14.
24. Nilsson B, Bumming P, Meis-Kindblom JM, Oden A, Dortok A, Gustavsson B, et al. Gastrointestinal stromal tumors: the incidence, prevalence, clinical course, and prognostication in the preimatinib mesylate era--a population-based study in western Sweden. Cancer. 2005;103(4):821–9.
25. DeMatteo RP, Lewis JJ, Leung D, Mudan SS, Woodruff JM, Brennan MF. Two hundred gastrointestinal stromal tumors: recurrence patterns and prognostic factors for survival. Ann Surg. 2000;231(1):51–8.
26. Therasse P, Arbuck SG, Eisenhauer EA, Wanders J, Kaplan RS, Rubinstein L, et al. New guidelines to evaluate the response to treatment in solid tumors. European Organization for

Research and Treatment of Cancer, National Cancer Institute of the United States, National Cancer Institute of Canada. J Natl Cancer Inst. 2000;92(3):205–16.
27. Eisenhauer EA, Therasse P, Bogaerts J, Schwartz LH, Sargent D, Ford R, et al. New response evaluation criteria in solid tumours: revised RECIST guideline (version 1.1). Eur J Cancer. 2009;45(2):228–47.
28. Demetri GD, von Mehren M, Blanke CD, Van den Abbeele AD, Eisenberg B, Roberts PJ, et al. Efficacy and safety of imatinib mesylate in advanced gastrointestinal stromal tumors. N Engl J Med. 2002;347(7):472–80.
29. Shankar S, vanSonnenberg E, Desai J, Dipiro PJ, Van Den Abbeele A, Demetri GD. Gastrointestinal stromal tumor: new nodule-within-a-mass pattern of recurrence after partial response to imatinib mesylate. Radiology. 2005;235(3):892–8.
30. Choi H, Charnsangavej C, Faria SC, Macapinlac HA, Burgess MA, Patel SR, et al. Correlation of computed tomography and positron emission tomography in patients with metastatic gastrointestinal stromal tumor treated at a single institution with imatinib mesylate: proposal of new computed tomography response criteria. J Clin Oncol Off J Am Soc Clin Oncol. 2007;25(13):1753–9.
31. Benjamin RS, Choi H, Macapinlac HA, Burgess MA, Patel SR, Chen LL, et al. We should desist using RECIST, at least in GIST. J Clin Oncol Off J Am Soc Clin Oncol. 2007;25(13):1760–4.
32. Chen LL, Trent JC, Wu EF, Fuller GN, Ramdas L, Zhang W, et al. A missense mutation in KIT kinase domain 1 correlates with imatinib resistance in gastrointestinal stromal tumors. Cancer Res. 2004;64(17):5913–9.
33. Joensuu H, Vehtari A, Riihimaki J, Nishida T, Steigen SE, Brabec P, et al. Risk of recurrence of gastrointestinal stromal tumour after surgery: an analysis of pooled population-based cohorts. Lancet Oncol. 2012;13(3):265–74.
34. Blay JY, Bonvalot S, Casali P, Choi H, Debiec-Richter M, Dei Tos AP, et al. Consensus meeting for the management of gastrointestinal stromal tumors. Report of the GIST Consensus Conference of 20–21 March 2004, under the auspices of ESMO. Ann Oncol Off J Eur Soc Med Oncol/ESMO. 2005;16(4):566–78.
35. Schiavon G, Ruggiero A, Schoffski P, van der Holt B, Bekers DJ, Eechoute K, et al. Tumor volume as an alternative response measurement for imatinib treated GIST patients. PLoS One. 2012;7(11):e48372.
36. Garcia-Figueiras R, Goh VJ, Padhani AR, Baleato-Gonzalez S, Garrido M, Leon L, et al. CT perfusion in oncologic imaging: a useful tool? AJR Am J Roentgenol. 2013;200(1):8–19.
37. Trent JC, Choi H, Hunt K, Macapinlac H, McConkey D, Charnsangravej C, et al. Apoptotic and anti-vascular activity of imatinib in GIST patients. J Clin Oncol (Meet Abstr). 2005;23(16_Suppl):9001.
38. Schlemmer M, Sourbron SP, Schinwald N, Nikolaou K, Becker CR, Reiser MF, et al. Perfusion patterns of metastatic gastrointestinal stromal tumor lesions under specific molecular therapy. Eur J Radiol. 2011;77(2):312–8.
39. Apfaltrer P, Meyer M, Meier C, Henzler T, Barraza Jr JM, Dinter DJ, et al. Contrast-enhanced dual-energy CT of gastrointestinal stromal tumors: is iodine-related attenuation a potential indicator of tumor response? Invest Radiol. 2012;47(1):65–70.
40. Meyer M, Hohenberger P, Apfaltrer P, Henzler T, Dinter DJ, Schoenberg SO, et al. CT-based response assessment of advanced gastrointestinal stromal tumor: dual energy CT provides a more predictive imaging biomarker of clinical benefit than RECIST or Choi criteria. Eur J Radiol. 2013;82(6):923–8.
41. Graser A, Johnson TR, Chandarana H, Macari M. Dual energy CT: preliminary observations and potential clinical applications in the abdomen. Eur Radiol. 2009;19(1):13–23.
42. Shankar LK, Hoffman JM, Bacharach S, Graham MM, Karp J, Lammertsma AA, et al. Consensus recommendations for the use of 18F-FDG PET as an indicator of therapeutic response in patients in National Cancer Institute Trials. J Nucl Med Off Publ Soc Nucl Med. 2006;47(6):1059–66.

43. Antoch G, Freudenberg LS, Beyer T, Bockisch A, Debatin JF. To enhance or not to enhance? 18F-FDG and CT contrast agents in dual-modality 18F-FDG PET/CT. J Nucl Med Off Publ Soc Nucl Med. 2004;45 Suppl 1:56S–65.
44. Raylman RR, Kison PV, Wahl RL. Capabilities of two- and three-dimensional FDG-PET for detecting small lesions and lymph nodes in the upper torso: a dynamic phantom study. Eur J Nucl Med. 1999;26(1):39–45.
45. Choi H, Charnsangavej C, de Castro FS, Tamm EP, Benjamin RS, Johnson MM, et al. CT evaluation of the response of gastrointestinal stromal tumors after imatinib mesylate treatment: a quantitative analysis correlated with FDG PET findings. AJR Am J Roentgenol. 2004;183(6):1619–28.
46. Hersh MR, Choi J, Garrett C, Clark R. Imaging gastrointestinal stromal tumors. Cancer Control J Moffitt Cancer Center. 2005;12(2):111–5.
47. Van den Abbeele AD. The lessons of GIST--PET and PET/CT: a new paradigm for imaging. Oncologist. 2008;13 Suppl 2:8–13.
48. Van den Abbeele A, editor; for the GIST Collaborative PET Study Group Dana-Farber Cancer Institute, Boston, Massachusetts, OHSU, Portland, Oregon, Helsinki University Central Hospital, Turku University Central Hospital, Finland, Novartis Oncology 2001: F18-FDG-PET provides early evidence of biological response to STI571 in patients with malignant gastrointestinal stromal tumors (GIST). Proc Am Soc Clin Oncol. 2001.
49. Gayed I, Vu T, Iyer R, Johnson M, Macapinlac H, Swanston N, et al. The role of 18F-FDG PET in staging and early prediction of response to therapy of recurrent gastrointestinal stromal tumors. J Nucl Med Off Publ Soc Nucl Med. 2004;45(1):17–21.
50. Young H, Baum R, Cremerius U, Herholz K, Hoekstra O, Lammertsma AA, et al. Measurement of clinical and subclinical tumour response using [18F]-fluorodeoxyglucose and positron emission tomography: review and 1999 EORTC recommendations. European Organization for Research and Treatment of Cancer (EORTC) PET Study Group. Eur J Cancer. 1999;35(13):1773–82.
51. Jager PL, Gietema JA, van der Graaf WT. Imatinib mesylate for the treatment of gastrointestinal stromal tumours: best monitored with FDG PET. Nucl Med Commun. 2004;25(5):433–8.
52. Holdsworth CH, Badawi RD, Manola JB, Kijewski MF, Israel DA, Demetri GD, et al. CT and PET: early prognostic indicators of response to imatinib mesylate in patients with gastrointestinal stromal tumor. AJR Am J Roentgenol. 2007;189(6):W324–30.
53. Wahl RL, Jacene H, Kasamon Y, Lodge MA. From RECIST to PERCIST: evolving considerations for PET response criteria in solid tumors. J Nucl Med Off Publ Soc Nucl Med. 2009;50 Suppl 1:122S–50.
54. Hasegawa S, Semelka RC, Noone TC, Woosley JT, Marcos HB, Kenney PJ, et al. Gastric stromal sarcomas: correlation of MR imaging and histopathologic findings in nine patients. Radiology. 1998;208(3):591–5.
55. Yu MH, Lee JM, Baek JH, Han JK, Choi BI. MRI features of gastrointestinal stromal tumors. AJR Am J Roentgenol. 2014;203(5):980–91.
56. Figueiras RG, Padhani AR, Goh VJ, Vilanova JC, Gonzalez SB, Martin CV, et al. Novel oncologic drugs: what they do and how they affect images. Radiographics Rev Publ Radiol Soc N Am Inc. 2011;31(7):2059–91.
57. Wong CS, Gong N, Chu YC, Anthony MP, Chan Q, Lee HF, et al. Correlation of measurements from diffusion weighted MR imaging and FDG PET/CT in GIST patients: ADC versus SUV. Eur J Radiol. 2012;81(9):2122–6.
58. Schmidt S, Dunet V, Koehli M, Montemurro M, Meuli R, Prior JO. Diffusion-weighted magnetic resonance imaging in metastatic gastrointestinal stromal tumor (GIST): a pilot study on the assessment of treatment response in comparison with 18F-FDG PET/CT. Acta Radiol. 2013;54(8):837–42.

Endoscopic Evaluation of Gastrointestinal Stromal Tumors

Osman Yuksel and William R. Brugge

Abbreviations

AGA	American Gastroenterological Association
CT	Computed tomography
ESD	Endoscopic submucosal dissection
ESMO	The European Society of Medical Oncology
ESMR	Endoscopic submucosal resection
EUS	Endoscopic ultrasonography
EUS-FNA	Endoscopic ultrasonography guided fine needle aspiration
EUS-FNB	Endoscopic ultrasonography guided fine needle biopsy
GIST	Gastrointestinal stromal tumor
MR	Magnetic resonance
NCCN	National Comprehensive Cancer Network
PDGFRA	Alpha-type platelet-derived growth factor receptor
US	Ultrasonography

1 Introduction

Gastrointestinal stromal tumors (GIST) are the most common mesenchymal tumors arising from the gastrointestinal tract. These tumors originate from the interstitial cells of Cajal that are located in the myenteric plexus of the gastrointestinal tract and regulate gastrointestinal tract motility [1, 2]. Stromal cell tumors

O. Yuksel, MD
Pancreas Biliary Center, Gastrointestinal Unit, Massachusetts General Hospital, Boston, MA, USA

Department of Gastroenterology, University of Hacettepe, Ankara, Turkey
e-mail: oyuksel@mgh.harvard.edu

W.R. Brugge, MD (✉)
Pancreas Biliary Center, Gastrointestinal Unit, Massachusetts General Hospital, Boston, MA, USA
e-mail: wbrugge@partners.org

© Springer International Publishing Switzerland 2017

C.R. Scoggins et al. (eds.), *Gastrointestinal Stromal Tumors*,
DOI 10.1007/978-3-319-42632-7_7

may originate throughout the gastrointestinal tract, from the distal esophagus to the anus, but they are most common in the stomach (50–60 %) and the small intestine (30–35 %) and less frequent in the colon (5 %), esophagus (<1 %), and, rarely, the appendix [3, 4].

2 Epidemiology

Analysis of the Surveillance, Epidemiology, and End Result (SEER) cancer data registry between 1993 and 2002 in the United States showed that the average annual incidence of GIST was 0.32/100,000 and the average annual 15-year prevalence was 1.62/100,000 [5]. In Europe, the annual incidence by clinical diagnosis is about 14.5/1,000,000 [6]. Although the global incidence of GIST is not known, the incidence of GIST may be much higher than these figures suggest. In one surgical pathology study by Agaimy et al., the incidence of small gastric GIST was reported to be nearly 22.5 % [7]. The increased incidence of GIST can be related to recent advances in diagnosis using immunohistochemical markers, cross-sectional radiological methods, and invasive endoscopic techniques. The discovery of a mutation in the c-KIT proto-oncogene by Hirota et al. was a milestone in the diagnosis of GIST [8]. This mutation is present in approximately 75–80 % of GIST, whereas mutations in the platelet-derived growth factor alpha receptor (PDGFRA) are observed in only 8 % of GIST [4, 9, 10].

3 Histology

GIST can be histologically subclassified into three morphological patterns, including spindle cell (70 %), epithelioid (20 %), and mixed (10 %) cell types. The prognostic importance of the histologic type is limited, however, the mitotic threshold for malignancy is higher for spindle cell tumors compared to epithelioid cell tumors [11]. Most GIST are immunohistochemically positive for KIT. CD117 antigen, an epitope of KIT, is expressed in approximately 95 % of GIST, both spindle and epithelioid cell types. The presence of c-KIT staining is a strong and universal marker of GIST. Positive staining of c-KİT, together with classic tumor morphology, is a very useful diagnostic approach in differentiating GIST from other mesenchymal tumors [1, 3, 11]. GIST are grossly smooth, gray-white tumors that originate from the muscularis propria of the gastrointestinal tract. These tumors can be located in the submucosal, subepithelial, or subserosal spaces. A pseudocapsule surrounds most small GIST. GIST are rarely invasive tumors, but they have the potential to invade and metastasize to adjacent structures. Cystic, necrotic, and hemorrhagic degeneration are observed in a significant percentage of GIST [2, 3, 12].

4 Clinical Presentation

Approximately 70% of patients with GIST have some clinical symptoms. The clinical presentation of patients with GIST is contingent upon the tumor size and anatomic location of the tumor as well as the behavior of the tumor. The most common clinical presentation is gastrointestinal bleeding and anemia. Other common clinical symptoms include abdominal pain, gastrointestinal obstruction, palpable mass, perforation, fatigue, and dysphagia. Nearly 20–30% of patients with GIST (especially under 2 cm) are incidentally diagnosed during endoscopic, radiological, or surgical procedures [11, 13, 14].

All GIST are regarded to have some degree of malignant potential, however, approximately 10–30% of them are clinically malignant at presentation. Almost half of small intestinal GIST demonstrate malignant behavior and are, in general, more aggressive than gastric GIST. GIST located in the gastric fundus and at the gastroesophageal junction have a higher frequency of malignant behavior than antral GIST. Nevertheless, the clinical risk of malignancy of GIST can be stratified into very low, low, moderate, and high risk according to tumor size, location, and number of mitoses. Further therapeutic approaches and follow-up are dependent upon this risk stratification [13, 15, 16].

Several disciplines, including gastroenterology, oncology, surgery, radiology, pathology, and molecular biology share interests in GIST and in their management. Gastrointestinal endoscopic interventions are commonly used for the evaluation and the diagnosis of GIST [3, 17].

5 Diagnosis

5.1 Standard Endoscopy

Subepithelial lesions of the gastrointestinal tract are often incidentally detected during endoscopic examinations. Hedenbro et al. reported that the incidence of gastric subepithelial lesions was 0.36% during diagnostic endoscopy [18]. Subepithelial lesions are additionally discovered during enteroscopy and colonoscopy. Subepithelial lesions with endoscopic examination are typically observed as a bulge in the gastrointestinal tract with smooth, intact, normal overlying mucosa (Fig. 1). The differential diagnosis of the lesion is broad and comprises GIST, carcinoid tumors, aberrant pancreas, inflammatory tumors, leiomyomas, lipomas, leiomyosarcomas, liposarcomas, hemangiomas, neuroma, cysts, pseudocysts, varices, aneurysms, polyps, extramural structures, and tumors of adjacent organs [4, 13, 19]. However, some endoscopic findings of the lesion, including location, stiffness, size, color, and appearance of the mucosa help to narrow the differential diagnosis. The endoscopic features suggestive of GIST include an oval or smooth shape with an overlying normal mucosa or with ulceration (Fig. 2). These features are usually insufficient to identify the tissue type of a subepithelial lesion. Thus, tissue sampling from these lesions is necessary in order to achieve a definitive histologic diagnosis. As these tumors often originate in the muscularis propria, standard endoscopic biopsy does not provide sufficient information for the diagnosis of GIST [20]. Sampling with endoscopic mucosal biopsy is successful in only 20–30 % of GIST cases. Thus, tissue for histologic examination is often obtained via more invasive methods. Bite-on-bite biopsies or jumbo forceps biopsies can be used to unroof the epithelial layer in order to obtain tissue from deep layers [3, 21]. In one study using jumbo forceps, the diagnostic yield ratio was 42 % (15/36) [22]. In a retrospective

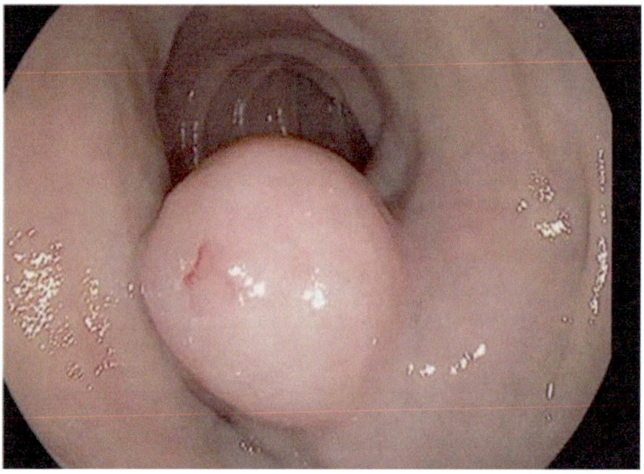

Fig. 1 Duodenal gastrointestinal stromal tumor with overlying normal mucosa

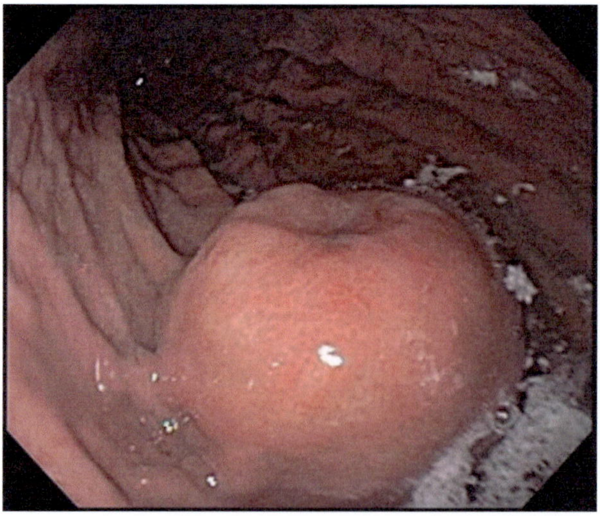

Fig. 2 Gastrointestinal stromal tumor with overlying ulcers in the proximal gastric body

multicenter study, the success rates had a wide range depending on the layer in which the tumor was placed. Jumbo forceps biopsies for third-layer lesions had a yield of 65.1 % (56/86) but was only 40 % (10/25) for fourth-layer lesions. Moreover, 34.9 % patients had significant bleeding after biopsies were obtained with jumbo forceps and required some form of hemostatic treatment [21, 23]. Therefore, a definitive diagnosis of GIST often requires further evaluation with endoscopic ultrasonography (EUS) and cross-sectional imaging methods [13].

5.2 Endoscopic Ultrasonography

Standard endoscopy provides imaging of subepithelial lesions, whereas EUS can reveal the entire tumor and provide information regarding the size and origin of the tumor. EUS has become an important diagnostic tool in the evaluation of subepithelial lesions. High-frequency ultrasound imaging is capable of differentiating between intramural tumors, intramural vascular lesions, and tumors with extramural compression. EUS also provides valuable information about tumor shape, size, layer in which the tumor is situated, tumor border, regional lymphadenopathy, echogenic pattern of the lesion, and local spread of the tumor. With EUS, GIST have classically a round or oval shape and a dark or hypoechoic appearance, but they are comparatively hyperechoic to the muscle layer, and they typically arise in the fourth layer, which represents the muscularis propria (Figs. 3 and 4) [13, 24].

EUS has become a preferable diagnostic method to further evaluate subepithelial lesions discovered by ultrasonography (USG), computed tomography (CT), magnetic resonance (MR), or esophagogastroduodenoscopy. In a prospective study of 150 patients who had a presumptive diagnosis of a submucosal lesion in the gastrointestinal tract, the sensitivity and specificity of EUS to differentiate extramural lesions and submucosal lesions were 92 % and 100 %, respectively [25]. Many

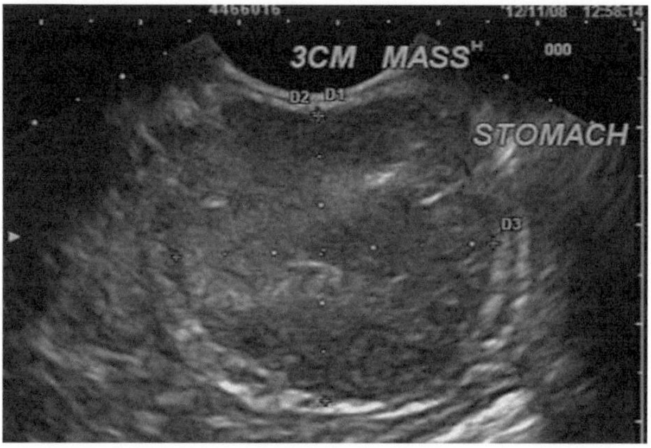

Fig. 3 Linear EUS examination revealing a gastric GIST surrounded by a pseudocapsule

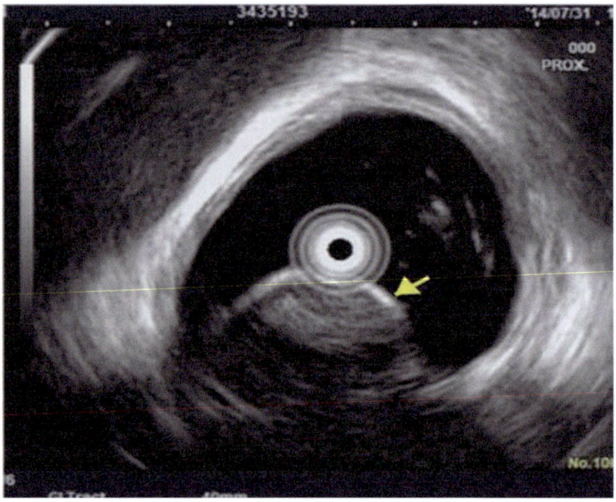

Fig. 4 Radial probe EUS examination demonstrating a small, homogenous subepithelial mass

studies have demonstrated the capability of EUS to differentiate GIST from other subepithelial tumors. Okai et al. attempted to differentiate the various gastric mesenchymal tumors via the imaging of EUS. They reported that a marginal halo and a relatively higher echogenicity suggested a GIST. However, a marginal hypoechoic halo was also detected in patients with schwannomas [26]. In a study of 181 consecutive patients with submucosal lesions in the upper gastrointestinal tract, the authors reported a sensitivity and specificity of 95 % and 72 %, respectively, for the diagnosis of GIST by EUS [27]. Kim et al. reported that four features in particular – relative echogenicity, homogeneity, echogenic foci, and marginal halo – conferred a sensitivity and specificity of 89.1 % and 85.7 %, respectively, for the diagnosis of a GIST [28].

EUS imaging is currently used to differentiate gastrointestinal submucosal lesions and is certainly more effective in this regard than standard endoscopy. Nevertheless, EUS imaging alone is not able to differentiate gastrointestinal subepithelial lesions with sufficient accuracy. EUS is also highly dependent on the skill and experience of the endoscopist and is subject to variation in image interpretation [13, 29].

5.3 EUS Imaging of GIST Malignancy

Most GIST are benign, yet malignant characteristics are observed in approximately 20 % of gastric GIST and 40–50 % of small intestinal GIST. Assessment of the malignant potential of GIST is a challenge to clinicians. EUS features can help to distinguish the malignant potential of GIST. Many studies have sought to define the EUS features that predict the malignant behavior of GIST [16, 28]. Pari et al. reported that the following EUS features could be used to predict the malignant behavior of a GIST: tumor size >5 cm, irregular extraluminal border, local invasion, and a heterogenous appearance. In this study, all lesions were completely removed surgically, and thus a diagnosis of GIST was secured with histology [30]. Kim et al. suggested that except for the tumor size and the irregularity of the tumor border, most of the EUS features were not useful in establishing the malignant risk of a given GIST. In patients with a tumor size ≥35 mm, they showed a sensitivity and specificity of 92.3 % and 78.8 %, respectively, for the diagnosis of GIST [28]. In a French study, the EUS criteria for malignancy were tested in 56 surgically resected gastrointestinal lesions and demonstrated that the presence of an irregular extraluminal margin, cystic spaces, and malignant-appearing lymph nodes were predictive of malignancy. The presence of at least one of these criteria had 91 % sensitivity, 88 % specificity, and an 83 % positive predictive value for malignancy [31]. Okai et al. found that exogastric growth, cystic changes, and echogenic foci within the tumor were not related to malignant behavior; however, lobulation of the lesion surface was often seen by EUS in the malignant GIST [26]. Jeon et al. found that certain EUS findings, including irregular tumor borders, mucosal ulceration, nonoval shape, and tumor size >3 cm, were correlated with a risk of malignancy [32].

In summary, there have been several studies to differentiate benign and malignant GIST based on EUS features. Irregular tumor border and tumor sizes have been associated with a risk of malignancy in the majority of studies. Thus, these parameters should be considered as predictive factors of malignancy for GIST when detected by EUS. Other EUS features, including echogenic foci, heterogeneity, and cystic spaces, have proven less consistent than irregular border and diameter of tumor in their capability to predict the risk of malignancy in a GIST [13]. New EUS techniques for tissue evaluation, including contrast-enhanced EUS, real-time elastography, and digital image analysis may be helpful in the differential diagnosis of GIST. Some studies have reported the capability of digital image analysis in differentiating benign from malignant subepithelial lesions on EUS [21, 33, 34].

5.4 Biopsy

Although EUS features can provide considerable clues to the risk of malignancy for GIST, the accuracy of EUS imaging features is not sufficient. Thus, tissue samples are often used to increase the diagnostic accuracy of EUS. Preoperative tissue sampling may not be necessary for large tumors or symptomatic tumors that need surgery regardless of the pathological diagnosis. The options for tissue sampling from GIST include EUS-guided fine-needle aspiration (FNA), EUS-guided fine-needle biopsy (FNB), EUS-guided Tru-cut biopsy, jumbo forceps or bite-on bite biopsy, surgical excision, endoscopic submucosal resection (ESMR), endoscopic submucosal dissection (ESD), percutaneous biopsy, unroofing, and tunneling techniques. Percutaneous biopsy is not usually recommended due to the risk of tumor rupture and peritoneal spread [13, 21, 35, 36].

5.4.1 EUS-Guided Fine-Needle Aspiration

The American Gastroenterological Association (AGA) and National Comprehensive Cancer Network (NCCN) state that EUS-guided sampling of GIST is the preferred technique for tissue acquisition. Many studies have demonstrated that EUS-guided sampling is an effective and a safe method for GIST. However, these series of studies often include a modest number of patients with GIST [37–40]. Akahoshi et al. reported a diagnostic yield of 82 % with the use of 22 gauge (G) FNA from subepithelial hypoechoic tumors. Major complications were not observed in their study [40]. Watson et al. reported a yield of 80 % for the EUS-FNA (19G or 22G needle) sampling of submucosal lesions in the upper gastrointestinal tract. They found that the diagnostic yield of EUS-FNA was higher for gastric tumors compared to esophageal or duodenal tumors. Diagnostic material was obtained in 79 % with the use of a 19G needle and in 64 % with a 22G needle [41]. In a study of 120 patients with gastrointestinal lesions, the authors reported that adequate samples for histological evaluation were obtained in 116 of the 119 patients. The diagnostic accuracy of EUS-FNA with a 19G needle in this study was 93.2 % [42]. In the study of Sekine et al., the sensitivity was 82.5 % for the diagnosis of GIST and 81.3 % for the diagnosis of small GIST (<20 mm). They suggested that EUS-FNA for both large and small GIST is a valuable modality [43]. Some authors use a stylet for the initial puncture, but there is no convincing data about its effectiveness [44, 45].

Despite providing sufficient cytologic material from subepithelial tumors, the diagnostic success of EUS has been reported to vary from 38 to 82 % [29, 41, 46]. This wide range of success may lead to concerns about the role of EUS-FNA. Up to 33.3 % of FNA samples may be nondiagnostic and/or insufficient for assessing the malignant potential of the lesion. However, the capability of EUS-FNA for biopsy of GIST is better than any other. In summary, the performance of EUS-FNA for the diagnosis of GIST is good, but it is not accepted as an excellent technique [13].

5.4.2 EUS-Guided Core Biopsy

EUS-FNA cannot always provide cytological material for immunohistochemical evaluation and assessment for malignancy. EUS-guided tissue core biopsy with a Tru-cut needle has been tried to improve tissue acquisition of EUS-FNA [29]. EUS-guided Tru-cut core biopsy may have improved accuracy for the diagnosis of mesenchymal tumors, however, the results have been controversial. Fernández-Esparrach et al. found that a histological diagnosis of mesenchymal tumor was achieved in 60 % of patients by EUS-guided Tru-cut core biopsy [47]. DeWitt et al. used EUS-FNA and EUS-guided Tru-cut core biopsy to obtain cytologic material from 38 patients with gastrointestinal tumors. Diagnostic cytology yield was 76 %, and immunochemistry was achieved in 50 % of cases by EUS-FNA. Diagnostic histology yield by EUS-guided Tru-cut core biopsy technique was 79 %, and immunochemistry was successfully employed in 97 % of patients [48]. In 76 patients with GIST and 51 patients with non-GIST subepithelial tumors, An et al. performed Tru-cut biopsy (19 gauge) and EUS-FNA (22 gauge) biopsy. The diagnostic success of Tru-cut biopsy was greater than that of EUS-FNA biopsy (77.8 % versus 38.7 %). The percentage of nondiagnostic materials (suspicious and insufficient) was significantly higher in the EUS-FNA group (22.6 and 38.7 %) than in the Tru-cut biopsy group (6.7 and 15.5 %). The diagnostic yield for GISTs was significantly higher with EUS-guided Tru-cut biopsy than with EUS-FNA biopsy (90.9 % versus 68.8 %) [49].

EUS-guided Tru-cut core biopsy technique provides a grossly visible piece of tissue sample that can permit diagnostic histology and immunochemistry. The device performance is similar in the esophagus, rectum, and stomach. However, its use is limited to tumors located in the fundus and cardia of the stomach and the duodenal bulb due to the echoendoscope angulation interfering with its deployment. EUS-guided Tru-cut core biopsy of smaller subepithelial tumors is more difficult. Additionally, it has been reported to cause sepsis and peritoneal spillage of malignant cells [13, 50, 51].

Due to anatomical limitations, the risk of complications, and conflicting results, EUS-guided Tru-cut core biopsy is usually kept in reserve for obtaining samples from tumors that cannot be sufficiently sampled by EUS-FNA [13]. New core biopsy needles will likely replace Tru-cut needles in the future.

6 EUS Surveillance

There are no published large studies to evaluate the safety of EUS surveillance in patients with GIST. Optimal timing of surveillance with EUS has not been established for GIST. Frequency of EUS evaluation should be adjusted depending on the clinical scenario of patients. There are slight differences between guidelines in patients with GIST. The NCCN recommends that very small gastric GIST should be evaluated by abdominal/pelvic CT with contrast and/or EUS-guided FNA. If the tumor has no high-risk features including irregular border, cystic spaces, ulceration, echogenic foci, and heterogeneity, endoscopic surveillance at 6- to 12-month intervals may be considered. But complete surgical resection patients with very small gastric GIST with high-risk features should be considered [52]. The European Society of Medical Oncology (ESMO) and the NCCN released guidelines about management of GIST. The Guideline of ESMO recommends resection for gastric GISTs with diameter >2 cm. NCCN recommends removal of all GIST with size 2 cm or larger. However, resection is recommended for all GIST of diameter ≥3 and <3 cm with concerning EUS features including heterogeneity, an irregular tumor border, echogenic foci, and presence of cystic appearance by the AGA [13, 35, 52, 53].

EUS is a good diagnostic method for the differential diagnosis of subepithelial tumors. Also it is useful in the choice of the appropriate treatment method for GIST. EUS precisely determines the size of lesion, layer of origin, and growth pattern of tumor (intraluminal or/and extraluminal). All of these features are important features to use in the endoscopic resection techniques. An experienced team should be available before endoscopic resection [13, 20].

References

1. Joensuu H, Hohenberger P, Corless CL. Gastrointestinal stromal tumour. Lancet. 2013;382(9896):973–83.
2. Miettinen M, Lasota J. Histopathology of gastrointestinal stromal tumor. J Surg Oncol. 2011;104:865–73.
3. Miettinen M, Lasota J. Gastrointestinal stromal tumors. Gastroenterol Clin North Am. 2013;42(2):399–415.
4. Poveda A, del Muro XG, López-Guerrero JA, Martínez V, Romero I, Valverde C, Cubedo R, Martín-Broto J. GEIS 2013 guidelines for gastrointestinal sarcomas (GIST). Cancer Chemother Pharmacol. 2014;74(5):883–98.
5. Rubin JL, Sanon M, Taylor DC, Coombs J, Bollu V, Sirulnik L. Epidemiology, survival, and costs of localized gastrointestinal stromal tumors. Int J Gen Med. 2011;4:121–30.
6. Nilsson B, Bümming P, Meis-Kindblom JM, Odén A, Dortok A, Gustavsson B, Sablinska K, Kindblom LG. Gastrointestinal stromal tumors: the incidence, prevalence, clinical course, and prognostication in the preimatinib mesylate era – a population-based study in western Sweden. Cancer. 2005;103(4):821–9.
7. Agaimy A, Wünsch PH. Sporadic Cajal cell hyperplasia is common in resection specimens for distal oesophageal carcinoma. A retrospective review of 77 consecutive surgical resection specimens. Virchows Arch. 2006;448(3):288–94.
8. Hirota S, Isozaki K, Moriyama Y, Hashimoto K, et al. Gain-of-function mutations of c-kit in human gastrointestinal stromal tumors. Science. 1998;279:577–80.
9. Corless CL, Heinrich MC. Molecular pathobiology of gastrointestinal stromal sarcomas. Annu Rev Pathol. 2008;3:557–86.
10. Lasota J, Miettinen M. Clinical significance of oncogenic KIT and PDGFRA mutations in gastrointestinal stromal tumours. Histopathology. 2008;53(3):245–66.
11. Iorio N, Sawaya RA, Friedenberg FK. Review article: the biology, diagnosis and management of gastrointestinal stromal tumours. Aliment Pharmacol Ther. 2014;39(12):1376–86.
12. Chourmouzi D, Sinakos E, Papalavrentios L, Akriviadis E, Drevelegas A. Gastrointestinal stromal tumors: a pictorial review. J Gastrointestin Liver Dis. 2009;18(3):379–83.
13. Sepe PS, Brugge WR. A guide for the diagnosis and management of gastrointestinal stromal cell tumors. Nat Rev Gastroenterol Hepatol. 2009;6(6):363–71.
14. Tryggvason G, Kristmundsson T, Orvar K, Jónasson JG, Magnússon MK, Gíslason HG. Clinical study on gastrointestinal stromal tumors (GIST) in Iceland, 1990–2003. Dig Dis Sci. 2007;52(9):2249–53.
15. Chen TH, Hsu CM, Chu YY, Wu CH, Chen TC, Hsu JT, Yeh TS, Lin CJ, Chiu CT. Association of endoscopic ultrasonographic parameters and gastrointestinal stromal tumors (GISTs): can endoscopic ultrasonography be used to screen gastric GISTs for potential malignancy? Scand J Gastroenterol. 2016;51(3):374–7.
16. Kim MN, Kang SJ, Kim SG, Im JP, Kim JS, Jung HC, Song IS. Prediction of risk of malignancy of gastrointestinal stromal tumors by endoscopic ultrasonography. Gut Liver. 2013;7(6):642–7.
17. Humphris JL, Jones DB. Subepithelial mass lesions in the upper gastrointestinal tract. J Gastroenterol Hepatol. 2008;23(4):556–66.
18. Hedenbro JL, Ekelund M, Wetterberg P. Endoscopic diagnosis of submucosal gastric lesions. The results after routine endoscopy. Surg Endosc. 1991;5(1):20–3.
19. Menon L, Buscaglia JM. Endoscopic approach to subepithelial lesions. Therap Adv Gastroenterol. 2014;7(3):123–30.
20. Schmidt A, Bauder M, Riecken B, Caca K. Endoscopic resection of subepithelial tumors. World J Gastrointest Endosc. 2014;6(12):592–9.
21. Eckardt AJ, Jenssen C. Current endoscopic ultrasound-guided approach to incidental subepithelial lesions: optimal or optional? Ann Gastroenterol. 2015;28(2):160–72.

22. Hunt GC, Smith PP, Faigel DO. Yield of tissue sampling for submucosal lesions evaluated by EUS. Gastrointest Endosc. 2003;57(1):68–72.
23. Buscaglia JM, Nagula S, Jayaraman V, Robbins DH, Vadada D, Gross SA, DiMaio CJ, Pais S, Patel K, Sejpal DV, Kim MK. Diagnostic yield and safety of jumbo biopsy forceps in patients with subepithelial lesions of the upper and lower GI tract. Gastrointest Endosc. 2012;75(6):1147–52.
24. Mullady DK, Tan BR. A multidisciplinary approach to the diagnosis and treatment of gastrointestinal stromal tumor. J Clin Gastroenterol. 2013;47(7):578–85.
25. Rösch T, Kapfer B, Will U, Baronius W, Strobel M, Lorenz R, Ulm K, German EUS Club. Endoscopic ultrasonography. Accuracy of endoscopic ultrasonography in upper gastrointestinal submucosal lesions: a prospective multicenter study. Scand J Gastroenterol. 2002;37(7):856–62.
26. Okai T, Minamoto T, Ohtsubo K, Minato H, Kurumaya H, Oda Y, Mai M, Sawabu N. Endosonographic evaluation of c-kit-positive gastrointestinal stromal tumor. Abdom Imaging. 2003;28(3):301–7.
27. Brand B, Oesterhelweg L, Binmoeller KF, Sriram PV, Bohnacker S, Seewald S, De Weerth A, Soehendra N. Impact of endoscopic ultrasound for evaluation of submucosal lesions in gastrointestinal tract. Dig Liver Dis. 2002;34(4):290–7.
28. Kim GH, Park do Y, Kim S, Kim DH, Kim DH, Choi CW, Heo J, Song GA. Is it possible to differentiate gastric GISTs from gastric leiomyomas by EUS? World J Gastroenterol. 2009;15(27):3376–81.
29. Tae HJ, Lee HL, Lee KN, Jun DW, Lee OY, Han DS, Yoon BC, Choi HS, Hahm JS. Deep biopsy via endoscopic submucosal dissection in upper gastrointestinal subepithelial tumors: a prospective study. Endoscopy. 2014;46(10):845–50.
30. Shah P, Gao F, Edmundowicz SA, Azar RR, Early DS. Predicting malignant potential of gastrointestinal stromal tumors using endoscopic ultrasound. Dig Dis Sci. 2009;54(6):1265–9.
31. Palazzo L, Landi B, Cellier C, Cuillerier E, Roseau G, Barbier JP. Endosonographic features predictive of benign and malignant gastrointestinal stromal cell tumours. Gut. 2000;46(1):88–92.
32. Jeon SW, Park YD, Chung YJ, Cho CM, Tak WY, Kweon YO, Kim SK, Choi YH. Gastrointestinal stromal tumors of the stomach: endosonographic differentiation in relation to histological risk. J Gastroenterol Hepatol. 2007;22(12):2069–75.
33. Nguyen VX, Nguyen CC, Li B, Das A. Digital image analysis is a useful adjunct to endoscopic ultrasonographic diagnosis of subepithelial lesions of the gastrointestinal tract. J Ultrasound Med. 2010;29(9):1345–51.
34. Kim GH, Kim KB, Lee SH, Jeon HK, Park do Y, Jeon TY, Kim DH, Song GA. Digital image analysis of endoscopic ultrasonography is helpful in diagnosing gastric mesenchymal tumors. BMC Gastroenterol. 2014;14:7.
35. Hwang JH, Rulyak SD, Kimmey MB, American Gastroenterological Association Institute. American Gastroenterological Association Institute technical review on the management of gastric subepithelial masses. Gastroenterology. 2006;130(7):2217–28.
36. Karaca C, Turner BG, Cizginer S, Forcione D, Brugge W. Accuracy of EUS in the evaluation of small gastric subepithelial lesions. Gastrointest Endosc. 2010;71(4):722–7.
37. Ando N, Goto H, Niwa Y, Hirooka Y, Ohmiya N, Nagasaka T, Hayakawa T. The diagnosis of GI stromal tumors with EUS-guided fine needle aspiration with immunohistochemical analysis. Gastrointest Endosc. 2002;55(1):37–43.
38. Vander Noot 3rd MR, Eloubeidi MA, Chen VK, Eltoum I, Jhala D, Jhala N, Syed S, Chhieng DC. Diagnosis of gastrointestinal tract lesions by endoscopic ultrasound-guided fine-needle aspiration biopsy. Cancer. 2004;102(3):157–63.
39. Sepe PS, Moparty B, Pitman MB, Saltzman JR, Brugge WR. EUS-guided FNA for the diagnosis of GI stromal cell tumors: sensitivity and cytologic yield. Gastrointest Endosc. 2009;70(2):254–61.

40. Akahoshi K, Sumida Y, Matsui N, Oya M, Akinaga R, Kubokawa M, Motomura Y, Honda K, Watanabe M, Nagaie T. Preoperative diagnosis of gastrointestinal stromal tumor by endoscopic ultrasound-guided fine needle aspiration. World J Gastroenterol. 2007;13(14):2077–82.
41. Watson RR, Binmoeller KF, Hamerski CM, Shergill AK, Shaw RE, Jaffee IM, Stewart L, Shah JN. Yield and performance characteristics of endoscopic ultrasound-guided fine needle aspiration for diagnosing upper GI tract stromal tumors. Dig Dis Sci. 2011;56(6):1757–62.
42. Larghi A, Verna EC, Ricci R, Seerden TC, Galasso D, Carnuccio A, Uchida N, Rindi G, Costamagna G. EUS-guided fine-needle tissue acquisition by using a 19-gauge needle in a selected patient population: a prospective study. Gastrointest Endosc. 2011;74(3):504–10.
43. Sekine M, Imaoka H, Mizuno N, Hara K, Hijioka S, Niwa Y, Tajika M, Tanaka T, Ishihara M, Ito S, Misawa K, Ito Y, Shimizu Y, Yatabe Y, Ohnishi H, Yamao K. Clinical course of gastrointestinal stromal tumor diagnosed by endoscopic ultrasound-guided fine-needle aspiration. Dig Endosc. 2015;27(1):44–52.
44. Salah W, Faigel DO. When to puncture, when not to puncture: submucosal tumors. Endosc Ultrasound. 2014;3(2):98–108.
45. Wani S, Early D, Kunkel J, Leathersich A, Hovis CE, Hollander TG, Kohlmeier C, Zelenka C, Azar R, Edmundowicz S, Collins B, Liu J, Hall M, Mullady D. Diagnostic yield of malignancy during EUS-guided FNA of solid lesions with and without a stylet: a prospective, single blind, randomized, controlled trial. Gastrointest Endosc. 2012;76(2):328–35.
46. Williams DB, Sahai AV, Aabakken L, Penman ID, van Velse A, Webb J, Wilson M, Hoffman BJ, Hawes RH. Endoscopic ultrasound guided fine needle aspiration biopsy: a large single centre experience. Gut. 1999;44(5):720–6.
47. Fernández-Esparrach G, Sendino O, Solé M, Pellisé M, Colomo L, Pardo A, Martínez-Pallí G, Argüello L, Bordas JM, Llach J, Ginès A. Endoscopic ultrasound-guided fine-needle aspiration and trucut biopsy in the diagnosis of gastric stromal tumors: a randomized crossover study. Endoscopy. 2010;42(4):292–9.
48. DeWitt J, Emerson RE, Sherman S, Al-Haddad M, McHenry L, Cote GA, Leblanc JK. Endoscopic ultrasound-guided Trucut biopsy of gastrointestinal mesenchymal tumor. Surg Endosc. 2011;25(7):2192–202.
49. Na HK, Lee JH, Park YS, Ahn JY, Choi KS, Kim do H, Choi KD, Song HJ, Lee GH, Jung HY, Kim JH. Yields and utility of endoscopic ultrasonography-guided 19-gaugeTrucut biopsy versus 22-gauge fine needle aspiration for diagnosing gastric subepithelial tumors. Clin Endosc. 2015;48(2):152–7.
50. Polkowski M, Gerke W, Jarosz D, Nasierowska-Guttmejer A, Rutkowski P, Nowecki ZI, Ruka W, Regula J, Butruk E. Diagnostic yield and safety of endoscopic ultrasound-guided trucut [corrected] biopsy in patients with gastric submucosal tumors: a prospective study. Endoscopy. 2009;41(4):329–34.
51. Kim MY, Jung HY, Choi KD, Song HJ, Lee JH, Kim do H, Choi KS, Lee GH, Kim JH. Natural history of asymptomatic small gastric subepithelial tumors. J Clin Gastroenterol. 2011;45(4):330–6.
52. Demetri GD, von Mehren M, Antonescu CR, DeMatteo RP, Ganjoo KN, Maki RG, Pisters PW, Raut CP, Riedel RF, Schuetze S, Sundar HM, Trent JC, Wayne JD. NCCN Task Force report: update on the management of patients with gastrointestinal stromal tumors. J Natl Compr Canc Netw. 2010;8 Suppl 2:S1–41; quiz S42-4.
53. ESMO/European Sarcoma Network Working Group. Gastrointestinal stromal tumours: ESMO Clinical Practice Guidelines for diagnosis, treatment and follow-up. Ann Oncol. 2014;25 Suppl 3:iii21–6.

Endoscopic Management of Small GIST

Kavitha M. Nair and Field F. Willingham

1 Introduction

Gastrointestinal stromal tumors (GISTs) comprise approximately 60–70 % of all masses identified in the GI tract. Approximately 5,000–6,000 new cases of GISTs arise in the United States each year, and of these, an estimated 30 % will become malignant. GISTs are diagnosed via biopsy or resection and are stained for the KIT protein, also referred to as CD117. If the cells do not contain KIT, then they can be checked for the PDGFRA gene, which is found in approximately 5–10 % of GISTs [1]. They are often discovered incidentally during esophagogastroduodenoscopy (EGD) [2]. The National Institutes of Health (NIH) classifies low-risk and high-risk GISTs based on the size of the lesion, mitotic count, and proliferating cell nuclear antigen (PCNA) proliferative index (<10 % vs. >10 %). In order to completely assess the mitotic count, complete resection of the entire lesion may be required [3]. Some data suggest a higher incidence of subclinical GISTs than had been previously thought. In one study, 100 whole stomachs were resected from patients with gastric cancer and examined for microscopic GISTs. They found 50 microscopic GISTs, all of which were positive for KIT and/or CD34 and negative for desmin. Most microscopic GISTs (90 %) were located in the upper stomach [1, 4]. Another study found that microscopic gastric GISTs were present in 22.5 % of consecutive autopsies performed on patients aged 50 years or older [5] and a retrospective study

K.M. Nair, MD
Department of Medicine, Emory University School of Medicine, Atlanta, GA, USA

F.F. Willingham, MD, MPH (✉)
Division of Digestive Diseases, Department of Medicine, Emory University School of Medicine, Atlanta, GA, USA

Department of Medicine, Emory University Hospital,
1364 Clifton Road, NE, Atlanta, GA 30322, USA
e-mail: field.willingham@emoryhealthcare.org

© Springer International Publishing Switzerland 2017

C.R. Scoggins et al. (eds.), *Gastrointestinal Stromal Tumors*,
DOI 10.1007/978-3-319-42632-7_8

reported a prevalence of subepithelial gastric masses of 0.36 % during routine endoscopy [6]. Given the low reported annual incidence of clinical GISTs, presumably few microscopic GISTs are significant clinically.

While GISTs are the most common tumor type, there are other submucosal tumors (SMTs) in the upper GI tract. Endoscopic ultrasound (EUS) plays a key role in the evaluation of submucosal tumors in the upper GI tract. EUS has the ability to assess the layer of origin, the depth of invasion, and via fine needle aspirates, can often provide a tissue diagnosis. Standard endoscopic techniques such as forceps biopsy often sample the overlying mucosal layer and are frequently unsuccessful in establishing a tissue diagnosis for submucosal tumors. Percutaneous biopsy is rarely appropriate as most smaller submucosal tumors are not well visualized by cross-sectional imaging. In addition, there could be a small risk of tumor dissemination or rupture. Studies report the accuracy of EUS fine-needle aspiration (EUS-FNA) to be in the range of 80–85 % [7]. EUS is considered to be the procedure of choice for tissue diagnosis. In addition, certain tumor characteristics observed by endoscopy and EUS (ulceration, tumor size >5 cm, extraluminal growth, local invasion, and heterogeneity) are thought to be associated with more aggressive behavior [2].

Small GISTs are defined as tumors less than 2 cm in the widest dimension. They are often discovered incidentally on EGD. Some guidelines suggest that GISTs 2 cm or larger in size should be surgically resected, and recent data suggest that this is reasonable [8]. For example, a large study of 1,765 cases of small gastric GISTs (defined as less than 2 cm in size) demonstrated no metastasis with tumors in this size range [9]. The management of incidentally encountered GISTs smaller than 2 cm is debated. Some guidelines suggest that small asymptomatic gastric GISTs (less than 2 cm) with no high-risk features by EUS can be managed conservatively with endoscopic surveillance [10]. Others recommend endoscopic resection given that the natural history of these small tumors has not been clearly established [1].

Unlike more superficial submucosal tumors, GISTs typically arise from the muscularis propria layer or the fourth endosonographic layer. While mucosal cancers and more superficial tumors can often be resected endoscopically, leaving the deep muscle layer intact, GISTs arising from the muscularis propria layer create a unique challenge. Resecting across the base of a fourth-layer tumor may leave a positive deep muscle margin [11]. However, it is not clear that such an R1 resection has a clinical significance. Multiple studies have examined endoscopic techniques for the resection of smaller GIST-type tumors [11]. These have included endoscopic mucosal resection (EMR), endoscopic band ligation, endoscopic submucosal dissection (ESD), and endoscopic enucleation using an insulated-tip electrosurgical knife [6] (Figs. 1 and 2).

2 Endoscopic Mucosal Resection

Cap-assisted endoscopic mucosal resection uses a cap affixed to the tip of the endoscope that is then positioned immediately over the target lesion. Suction is used to retract the lesion into the cap. A standard snare excision technique is then used to resect the banded lesion [12]. Resecting these lesions via EMR is often safe;

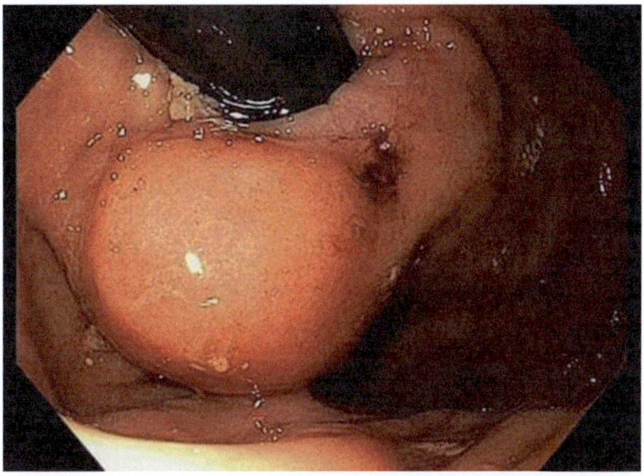

Fig. 1 Submucosal mass (1.5 cm) in the cardia viewed on retroflexion

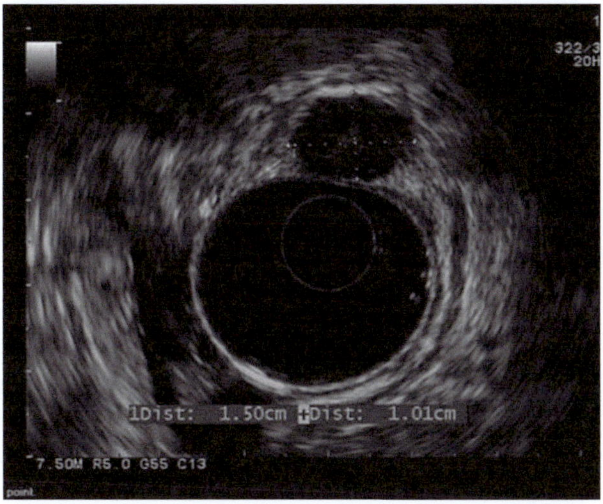

Fig. 2 Echoendosonographic image of a hypoechoic 1.5 cm submucosal mass lesion arising from the muscularis propria layer

however, complications may include bleeding and perforation. EMR is better suited for lesions which are superficial to the muscularis propria layer. The deep muscle layer does not suction easily into the cap, and, due to the origination of most GIST tumors in the muscularis propria layer, the EMR system may be unable to constrain the lesion. Very small tumors or GISTs originating from the muscularis mucosa layer might be approachable in this manner.

3 Endoscopic Band Ligation

Another case series examined the efficacy of endoscopic band ligation as a method of resection of GIST. In this study, 29 patients were diagnosed with GIST by EUS and deep endoscopic biopsies. A standard endoscope with a transparent cap attached to the tip was used. The cap was placed over the lesion, suction was applied, and an elastic band was released around the base. All patients then underwent EUS every 2–3 months on schedule to visualize progression of the banding. They found that 28 GISTs sloughed completely with a mean of 4.8 weeks for complete healing. One lesion did not slough due to incomplete ligation, and when the procedure was repeated, it sloughed completely. There was one episode of bleeding that required intervention with metallic clips and no perforation events. They noted one episode of recurrence that was documented 4 months postprocedure. Of note, this approach does not allow for tumor sampling, which is a limitation given the prognostic importance of the number of mitoses [13].

4 Endoscopic Submucosal Dissection

A case series evaluated the efficacy and safety of endoscopic submucosal dissection (ESD) for the removal of small GISTs. GISTs were diagnosed by endoscopic ultrasonography (EUS) and managed by ESD with incision of the surrounding mucosa followed by dissection of the submucosal tissue to display the GIST, and followed finally by resection of the lesion in its entirety. Of the 20 GISTs with a mean size 1.6 cm, 19 were resected with ESD completely and 1 required additional surgery because of tumor residual in the wound after the ESD resulting in a success rate of 95 %. Of note, the mean ESD procedure time was 87.5 min. Complications included perforation in three cases after the dissection of the GIST and no delayed bleeding events [14]. The utility of ESD was also evaluated for the removal of subepithelial tumors (SETs) from the muscularis propria layer in 12 patients. An insulated-tip knife was used to remove tumor from the muscularis propria primarily. A suction and cap method (EMR-c) was used to obtain a tissue diagnosis if complete resection by ESD was not possible. A total of nine tumors were resected completely by ESD with a mean tumor size of 20.7 mm. GIST was the histological diagnosis for eight lesions and leiomyoma for four tumors. The mean procedure time was 60.9 min. There were no (?) reported perforations, bleeding or other post-procedural complications [15]. Endoscopic enucleation has also been examined in a case series of 15 patients. It is a technically difficult procedure and may lead to perforation and/or bleeding. The method utilizes an insulated-tip electrosurgical knife. Four of these patients were found to have GIST and 11 of these cases had a tumor that arose from the muscularis propria. Enucleation was successful in 14 cases with a mean procedure time of 35 min. One episode of perforation was documented in the anterior wall of the proximal gastric body and required management by endoscopic clip application [16].

5 Hybrid Endoscopic and Laparoscopic Resection

A laparoscopic approach was reported in 1999 describing a gastric wedge resection for the management of GIST [17]. One major challenge with this type of resection is the determination of the appropriate resection line. Particularly for endoluminal lesions, laparoscopic visualization may not be possible. Additionally, while some gastric lesions are very accessible, tumors in areas such as the GE junction and pyloric channel pose significant challenges. For example, postoperative transformation of the stomach is a complication of excessive gastric resection with implications for long-term quality of life. From these concepts, the idea of laparoscopic and endoscopic cooperative surgery (LECS) was developed [18]. The hybrid approach to resection of GISTs merges minimally invasive laparoscopic and interventional endoscopic techniques. It is an approach that has shown to be beneficial in a highly selected subset of patients with tumors of the foregut [19]. Combined endoscopic and laparoscopic hybrid local resection was originally performed only with the intragastric resection of posterior lesions [20–22]. A larger study analyzed 52 cases of confirmed GIST within the gastric posterior wall. All patients underwent LECS without procedural complications and a median hospital stay of 5 days. There was no incidence of tumor rupture intraoperatively. One postoperative complication of anastomatic bleeding was reported. These studies suggested that a minimally invasive hybrid approach may be effective for curative treatment, with negative surgical margins and a short time to recovery.

Another study conducted reviewed seven patients who underwent LECS for the resection of gastric submucosal tumors. The purpose was to investigate the utility of hybrid laparoscopic and endoscopic techniques in the resection of gastric submucosal tumors independent of tumor location such as at the gastroesophageal junction or pyloric ring. Endoscopic submucosal dissection was used to dissect around the mucosal and submucosal layers. The seromuscular layer was then laparoscopically dissected and the tumor was removed via the abdominal cavity. All tumors were successfully removed using this approach. Of the seven tumors, two were greater than 5 cm in size and one was a confirmed GIST. The mean operation time was 169 min with negligible blood loss. There were no reported postoperative complications (Table 1).

Another series employed a hybrid approach to manage foregut mass lesions endoluminally using laparoscopic assistance. All of the lesions had been deemed to be problematic for a straightforward surgical resection. The lesions were approached endoscopically and laparoscopically. Endoscopic transection at the base of the lesions was performed with the aid of laparoscopic assistance via the serosal surface of the gastric wall. A total of seven patients underwent the hybrid approach in this study and of these patients, five underwent successful hybrid endoscopic and laparoscopic resections. There were two cases that required conversion to a larger laparoscopic resection but no conversions to open resection were required. The mean procedural time was 119 min and there were no complications [19].

The same researchers also investigated GISTs with a predominantly endophytic component. Endophytic tumors may be difficult to locate laparoscopically and as a result, a large portion of the gastric wall is often excised in order to achieve a negative margin. A push-pull technique was developed to enable resection of fourth layer tumors endoscopically followed by laparoscopic resection of the resection site to obtain a negative margin. In this series, four patients in two institutions underwent the push-pull hybrid procedure where an endoscopic resection of the tumor was

Table 1 Summary of techniques

Author	*N*	Method	Mean operation time (min)	Mean tumor diameter (mm)	Complete resection rate (%)	Complications
Zhou et al. [14]	20	ESD	87.5	16	95	Three cases of perforation
Lee et al. [15]	12	ESD	60.9	20.7	100	None
Sun et al. [13]	29	Endoscopic band ligation	Not reported	Not clearly reported but all less than 12 mm	96 (28 of 29)	One episode of recurrence that was documented 4 months postprocedure. One lesion did not slough because it was not completely ligated. Bleeding in one patient because the lesion sloughed early
Park et al. [16]	15	Endoscopic enucleation	35	20	93 (14 of 15)	One episode of perforation was documented in the anterior wall of proximal gastric body and required management by endoscopic clip application
Ding et al. [22]	52	Hybrid	80	25	100	None
Hiki et al. [18]	7	Hybrid	169	2 were greater than 5 cm	100	None
Willingham et al. [11]	7	Hybrid	119	35	70 (5 of 7)	None
Willingham et al. [19]	4	Hybrid	162	33	100	None
Daiko et al. [23]	4	Hybrid	137.7	51	100	None
Mori et al. [24]	6	Hybrid	288	41	100	None
Xu et al. [25]	15	STER	78.7	19	100	One case of pneumothorax and subcutaneous emphysema requiring chest tube placement and pneumoperitoneum that required needle aspiration for resolution

(continued)

Table 1 (continued)

Author	*N*	Method	Mean operation time (min)	Mean tumor diameter (mm)	Complete resection rate (%)	Complications
Ye et al. [29]	85	STER	57.2	19.2	100	Eight patients with pneumothorax, subcutaneous emphysema, and/or pneumoperitoneum, 26.3 % complication rate for GISTs
Gong et al. [26]	12	STER	48.3	19.5	100 (10 patients with en bloc resection and two patients in two pieces)	Two patients had both pneumothorax and subcutaneous emphysema
Inoue et al. [28]	9	STER	152	18.5	78 (7 of 9); two had tumors that were too large (60 mm and 75 mm, respectively)	None
Zhou et al. [34]	26	EFTR	105	28	100	None
Feng et al. [27]	48	EFTR	60	16	100	None
Ye et al. [35]	51	EFTR	52	24	98 (50 of 52)	One case of failure and conversion to laparoscopy

performed with laparoscopic assistance (push) followed by full-thickness laparoscopic resection of the base with endoscopic assistance (pull). While the endoscopic resection alone was associated with a positive deep margin, the push-pull hybrid technique allowed for complete R0 resections. In this study, endophytic GISTs in anatomically challenging locations could be safely and effectively managed using an oncologically sound, minimally invasive approach [11].

Another hybrid technique utilizing EGD and thorascopy for the management of GISTs originating in the thoracic esophagus has been described. Whereas the conventional transthoracic approach is highly invasive, the hybrid approach provided a minimally invasive alternative. They identified four tumors, one of which was confirmed to be GIST. The resection plane between the tumor and the mucosal layer of the esophagus was first identified. This was accomplished using a sodium hyaluronate solution stained with indigo carmine. Using EGD, it was injected into the submucosa. Following this, using three-port thorascopy, the tumor was enucleated using the dyed submucosa as a guide, thus minimizing the risk of full-thickness perforation of the esophagus. The muscle layer was then sutured and the tumor was removed. The mean surgical time was 137.7 min and mean blood loss was 21.2 ml. No perioperative complications were reported. This procedure was performed using three access ports, and was felt to reduce postoperative pain and hasten early postoperative recovery [23].

A case series of six patients with GISTs was reported utilizing a hybrid natural orifice transluminal endoscopic surgery (NOTES) approach. The procedure involved conventional flexible endoscopic devices and conventional flexible endoscopes without special functions. There was minimal supportive use of a laparoscope, which was primarily employed to observe the endoscopic resection of the GIST and visualize appropriate gastric closure. Two oral endoscopes and one nasal endoscope were used to remove the excised tumor under laparoscopic observation. Any perforations were closed using loop clip three-point circumferential suturing followed by full-thickness suturing under laparoscopy. All patients were discharged from the hospital within 10 days and without any reported complications. The time to discharge was shorter than patients who underwent laparoscopic surgery for gastric GISTs. Because of insufflation during laparoscopy, it can be difficult to obtain a good visualization of endoscopic resection. They found that blocking gas flow to the duodenum and subsequently downstream parts of the intestine prevented distension of the intestine, which allowed for a clearer laparoscopic view [24].

6 Submucosal Tunneling Endoscopic Resection (STER)

Submucosal tunneling has been extensively utilized in peroral endoscopic myotomy (POEM) for the treatment of achalasia [28]. In POEM, a submucosal tunnel is created to allow for circular muscle layer dissection. The same approach can also be used to access lesions located in the muscle layer [29]. This technique enabled the development of submucosal tunneling endoscopic resection (STER) for the treatment of upper GI submucosal tumors (SMTs) originating from the muscularis propria layer [25]. This therapeutic approach was reported initially in 15 patients [25]. In STER procedures, a submucosal tunnel is created endoscopically starting approximately 5 cm proximal to the lesion. A tunnel is created to reach the lesion which is then resected. The lesion is withdrawn through the tunnel and the mucosal entry site is then closed [30]. In this series, of the 15 SMTs, nine were located in the esophagus, three in the stomach, and three in the cardia. All originated from the muscularis propria layer, and they had an average size of 1.9 cm. A total of five tumors were confirmed GISTs. Estimated blood loss was minimal. Complications included one case of pneumothorax and subcutaneous emphysema requiring chest tube placement and pneumoperitoneum requiring needle aspiration. This study eased initial concerns regarding the risk of bleeding and the formation of hematoma as well as infection risk within the submucosal tunnel. There were no reported cases of delayed bleeding or infectious complications. There appeared to be lower rates of postoperative GI tract leakage and secondary infection when compared to endoscopic submucosal dissection (ESD) [25].

This was followed by a larger prospective study evaluating submucosal tunneling endoscopic resection (STER) for small (≤3 cm) upper gastrointestinal subepithelial tumors (SETs) originating from the muscularis propria layer. In this study, 85 patients with upper GI SETs originating from the muscularis propria were treated with STER. The tumors were identified and marked. A tunnel was created between the submucosal and muscular layers 5 cm above the tumor. The tumors were resected and retrieved via the tunnel. The mucosal entry site was then closed with endoclips. Of these 85 tumors, 60 were located in the esophagus, 16 in the cardia, and 9 in the stomach, and 19 of the 85 were confirmed to be GISTs. They reported a total of eight patients developing pneumothorax, subcutaneous emphysema, and/or pneumoperitoneum that required conservative management [29].

In another study, a similar complication rate was reported with submucosal tunnel dissection for upper gastrointestinal submucosal tumors. In a study of 12 patients, two patients had both pneumothorax and subcutaneous emphysema requiring conservative management [26]. The total complication rate varied by the tumor subtype (26.3 % for GISTs, 4.6 % for leiomyomas, 0 % for calcifying fibrous tumors). Both studies identified the same limitations. Because of the submucosal tunnel capacity, it was only possible to remove tumors ≤3.0 cm in diameter. They found that tumors greater than 3 cm were challenging to remove endoscopically [29].

Another study focused on this limitation evaluating endoscopic submucosal tumor resection in nine patients with tumors of size >2 cm located in either the esophagus or cardia. No upper size limit was established. As with the previous studies, the mucosal entry incision was made approximately 5 cm proximally to the tumor. The tumors were resected with electrocautery and extracted by suctioning the tumor into a cap device. The entry site was closed with endoclips. Two patients required conversion to surgery for removal as the tumors were too large (75 and 60 mm). Large tumors compromised adequate endoscopic visualization because of the tumor mass effect in the small submucosal space. They proposed a slightly larger tumor size limitation of 4 cm. Of the nine tumors, one was histologically confirmed GIST. There were no reported postprocedural complications of hematoma, infection, or perforation [31].

7 Endoscopic Full-Thickness Resection (EFTR)

EFTR was developed to enable complete resection of tumors from the luminal aspect. With the intact tumor and all layers represented, the specimen may allow a more complete histologic examination, providing histology more similar to surgical specimens. A feasibility and safety study was performed in an animal model addressing several concerns. First, bleeding complications, because large vessels are common in the submucosa or the serosal surface. Also, as part of the procedure, the formation of a large defect might result in intragastric air leakage into the peritoneal cavity with subsequent collapse of the stomach. Additionally, this procedure requires significant operator experience with endoscopic suturing of large full-thickness defects in the stomach. Studies were completed on a total of 12 pigs. Feasibility was first confirmed in four pigs via laparoscopy. This animal study confirmed that it was possible to take full-thickness specimens from the gastric wall in all the pigs (100 %, 8/8) and to adequately close the defect after resection with this method (100 %, 8/8) [32, 33].

In humans, another study evaluated 26 patients with gastric submucosal tumors originating from the muscularis propria to evaluate the efficacy, safety, and feasibility of EFTR. Endoscopic submucosal dissection was used to incise around the tumor. Incision into the serosal layer surrounding the lesion was made using a Hook knife. All aspects of the procedure were completed without the aid of laparoscopy. EFTR was successful in all 26 patients with a mean operation time of 105 min and an average lesion size of 2.8 cm. Of the 26 tumors, 16 were histologically confirmed GISTs. No complications of bleeding, peritonitis, or abdominal abscess were reported [34]. This study addressed potential infectious complications, closure of the gastric wall incision, and limited visualization following the gastrotomy. In order to avoid infectious complications, they prevented the escape of gastric fluid into the peritoneal cavity through careful hemostasis, a semireclining position, administration of antibiotics and proton-pump inhibitors, nasogastric decompression, and use of suction of fluid and gas in the stomach during incisions. Closure of the gastric wall incision was achieved through the use of suction, clip, and suture whereby the incision site was reduced by air suction prior to the application of metallic clips. A 20-gauge needle was inserted at the right lower costal margin to decompress the abdomen until the gastric closure was achieved and gas release from the needle ceased [34]. Other researchers also succeeded in EFTR for resection of GISTs without laparoscopic assistance. In this study, 48 patients having undergone EFTR were analyzed retrospectively. GISTs were histologically confirmed in 43 cases. The mean tumor size was 1.59 cm (range, 0.50–4.80 cm; standard deviation, 1.01 cm). No postoperative complications were reported [27].

In a larger retrospective study, EFTR was evaluated in 51 patients with SETs arising from the muscularis propria. The patients underwent EFTR and closure with metallic clips and an endoloop to fix and tighten the clips together. Of these tumors, 30 were histologically confirmed GISTs. There was one reported case of failure and subsequent conversion to laparoscopy because tumor was lost to the peritoneal cavity during resection. The mean procedure time was 52 min and no other complications were reported [35].

8 Conclusions

GISTs represent a unique challenge due to their origination in the fourth, muscular layer. This layer provides the barrier when more superficial lesions are resected endoscopically. For lesions arising from this layer, additional considerations related to the likelihood of a positive deep margin have led to varying approaches. However, the significance of a positive microscopic margin is uncertain with GISTs and the management of a positive deep margin is not well defined. A study analyzed the outcomes in 200 patients with GISTs over a 16-year time period. The patient characteristics, tumor features, and type of treatment were examined to identify factors that might predict tumor recurrence and survival. Researchers identified a subgroup of 80 patients who presented without metastasis and underwent complete gross resection of the tumor. They found size of tumor to be an important predictor of survival; however, the status of the microscopic margin of the resection did not affect survival. It was suggested that the microscopic margin of resection of the organ from which they arise may not be as important a predictor of survival as the potential for tumor shedding [36, 37, 38]. Minimally invasive approaches are predicated on the low rates of lymph node metastasis and malignant progression with small GISTs.

EMR, endoscopic encucleation, and ESD may enable minimally invasive resection of small GISTs from the luminal side; however, the deep margin can be a concern. More invasive techniques such as STER and EFTR aim to provide an endoluminal approach with the benefits of an R0 resection; however, there are concerns raised regarding seeding. These techniques also require highly advanced endoscopic skills, and there is no coding model for long endoscopic surgeries in countries such as the US. The hybrid approach marries endoscopy and laparoscopy with the advantage of a minimally invasive procedure, improved visualization, and higher complete resection rate; however, it requires two separate teams and still necessitates a laparoscopic surgery and hospital stay. The operative risks and anticipated postoperative recovery must be weighed against the oncologic benefit of the tumor resection taking into account the patient's age, comorbidities, and performance status. While it may be reasonable to resect a small tumor along the greater curvature of the stomach in an elderly patient with several comorbidities, a similar tumor at the GE junction in a young patient may require an entirely different approach. A multidisciplinary care team is vital in reviewing the potential risks and benefits of each approach and developing a consensus plan for management [1]. The ultimate goal is to offer the best procedure for the specific patient based on their specific tumor and performance status. As the armamentarium broadens, patients may benefit from more targeted approaches to their particular presentation.

References

1. Demetri G, Mehren M, Antonescu C, DeMatteo R, Ganjoo K, Maki R, Pisters P, Raut C, Riedel R, Schuetze S, Sundar H, Trent J, Wayne J. NCCN Task Force report: update on the management of patients with gastrointestinal stromal tumors. J Natl Compr Canc Netw. 2010;8 Suppl 2:S1–44.
2. Shah P, Gao F, Edmundowicz S, Azar R, Early D. Predicting malignant potential of gastrointestinal stromal tumors using endoscopic ultrasound. Dig Dis Sci. 2009;54(6):1265–9.
3. Joensuu H. Risk stratification of patients diagnosed with gastrointestinal stromal tumor. Hum Pathol. 2008;39(10):1411–9.
4. Kawanowa K, Sakuma Y, Sakurai S, Hishima T, Iwasaki Y, Saito K, Hosoya Y, Nakajima T, Funata N. High incidence of microscopic gastrointestinal stromal tumors in the stomach. Hum Pathol. 2006;37(12):1527–35.
5. Agaimy A, et al. Minute gastric sclerosing stromal tumors (GIST tumorlets) are common in adults and frequently show c-KIT mutations. Am J Surg Pathol. 2007;31:113–20.
6. Hedenbro JL, Ekelund M, Wetterberg P. Endoscopic diagnosis of submucosal gastric lesions. The results after routine endoscopy. Surg Endosc. 1991;5:20–3.
7. Rammohan A, Sathyanesan J, Rajendran K, Pitchaimuthu A, Perumal S, Srinivasan UP, Ramasamy R, Palaniappan R, Govindan M. A gist of gastrointestinal stromal tumors: a review. World J Gastrointest Oncol. 2013;5(6):102–12.
8. Miettinen M, Lasota J. Gastrointestinal stromal tumors: pathology and prognosis at different sites. Semin Diagn Pathol. 2006;23(2):70–83.
9. Miettinen M, Sobin LH, Lasota J. Gastrointestinal stromal tumors of the stomach: a clinicopathologic, immunohistochemical, and molecular genetic study of 1765 cases with long-term follow-up. Am J Surg Pathol. 2005;29(1):52–68.
10. American Gastroenterological Association Institute. American Gastroenterological Association Institute medical position statement on the management of gastric subepithelial masses. Gastroenterology. 2006;130:2215–6.
11. Willingham F, Reynolds P, Lewis M, Ross A, Maithel S, Rocha F. Hybrid push-pull endoscopic and laparoscopic full thickness resection for the minimally invasive management of gastrointestinal stromal tumors (GIST). Gastroenterol Res Pract. 2015;2015:618756.
12. Kantsevoy SV, et al. Endoscopic mucosal resection and endoscopic submucosal dissection. Gastrointest Endosc. 2008;68(1):11–8.
13. Sun S, Ge N, Wang C, Wang M, Lü Q. Endoscopic band ligation of small gastric stromal tumors and follow-up by endoscopic ultrasonography. Surg Endosc. 2007;21:574–8.
14. Zhou P, Yao L, Qin X. Endoscopic submucosal dissection for gastrointestinal stromal tumors: a report of 20 cases. Zhonghua Wei Chang Wai Ke Za Zhi. 2008;11:219–22.
15. Lee IL, et al. Endoscopic submucosal dissection for the treatment of intraluminal gastric subepithelial tumors originating from the muscularis propria layer. Endoscopy. 2006;38:1024–8.
16. Park YS, et al. Endoscopic enucleation of upper-GI submucosal tumors by using an insulated-tip electrosurgical knife. Gastrointest Endosc. 2004;59:409–15.
17. Ohgami M, Otani Y, Kumai K, Kubota T, Kim YI, Kitajima M. Curative laparoscopic surgery for early gastric cancer: five years experience. World J Surg. 1999;23:187–92.
18. Hiki N, Yamamoto Y, Fukunaga T, et al. Laparoscopic and endoscopic cooperative surgery for gastrointestinal stromal tumor dissection. Surg Endosc. 2008;22:1729–35.

19. Willingham F, Garud S, Davis S, Lewis M, Maithel S, Kooby D. Human hybrid endoscopic and laparoscopic management of mass lesions of the foregut (with video). Gastrointest Endosc. 2012;75(4):905–12.
20. Ludwig K, Wilhelm L, Scharlau U, Amtsberg G, Bernhardt J. Laparoscopic-endoscopic rendezvous resection of gastric tumors. Surg Endosc. 2002;16:1561–5.
21. Ridwelski K, Pross M, Schubert S, Wolff S, Gunther T, Kahl S, Lippert H. Combined endoscopic intragastral resection of a posterior stromal gastric tumor using an original technique. Surg Endosc. 2002;16:537.
22. Ding P, Zhao Y. Endo-laparoscopic rendezvous approach for pericardia with gastric posterior wall of gastrointestinal stromal tumor: analysis of 52 consecutive cases. J Cancer Res Ther. 2014;10:259–62.
23. Daiko H, Fujita T, Ohgara T, Yamazaki N, Fujii S, Ohno Y, Yano T. Minimally invasive hybrid surgery combined with endoscopic and thoracoscopic approaches for submucosal tumor originating from thoracic esophagus. World J Surg Oncol. 2015;13:40.
24. Mori H, Kobara H, Kobayashi M, Muramatsu A, Nomura T, Hagiike M, Izuishi K, Suzuki Y, Masaki T. Establishment of pure NOTES procedure using a conventional flexible endoscope: review of six cases of gastric gastrointestinal stromal tumors. Endoscopy. 2011;43(7):631–4.
25. Xu MD, et al. Submucosal tunneling endoscopic resection: a new technique for treating upper GI submucosal tumors originating from the muscularis propria layer (with videos). Gastrointest Endosc. 2012;75:195–9.
26. Gong W, Xiong Y, Zhi F, Liu S, Wang A, Jiang B. Preliminary experience of endoscopic submucosal tunnel dissection for upper gastrointestinal submucosal tumors. Endoscopy. 2012;44(3):231–5.
27. Feng Y, Yu L, Yang S, Li X, Ding J, Chen L, Xu Y, Shi R. Endolumenal endoscopic full-thickness resection of muscularis propria-originating gastric submucosal tumors. J Laparoendosc Adv Surg Tech A. 2014;24:171–6.
28. Inoue H, Kobayashi M. Peroral endoscopic myotomy (POEM) for esophageal achalasia. Endoscopy. 2010;42:265–71.
29. Ye LP, Zhang Y, Mao XL, Zhu LH, Zhou X, Chen JY. Submucosal tunneling endoscopic resection for small upper gastrointestinal sub- epithelial tumors originating from the muscularis propria layer. Surg Endosc. 2014;28(2):524–30.
30. Kobara H, Mori H, Rafiq K, Fujihara S, Nishiyama N, Ayaki M, Yachida T, Matsunaga T, Tani J, Miyoshi H, Yoneyama H, Morishita A, Oryu M, Iwama H, Masaki T. Submucosal tunneling techniques: current perspectives. Clin Exp Gastroenterol. 2014;7:67–74.
31. Inoue H, Ikeda H, Hosoya T, et al. Submucosal endoscopic tumor resection for subepithelial tumors in the esophagus and cardia. Endoscopy. 2012;44(3):225–30.
32. Ikeda K, Mosse A, Park P. Endoscopic full-thickness resection: circumferential cutting method. Gastrointest Endosc. 2006;64:82–9.
33. Kantsevoy S. Endoscopic full-thickness resection: new minimally invasive therapeutic alternative for GI-tract lesions. Gastrointest Endosc. 2006;64(1):90–1.
34. Zhou PH, Yao LQ, Qin XY, Cai MY, Xu MD, Zhong YS, Chen WF, Zhang YQ, Qin WZ, Hu JW, Liu JZ. Endoscopic full-thickness resection without laparoscopic assistance for gastric submucosal tumors originated from the muscularis propria. Surg Endosc. 2011;25(9):2926–31.
35. Ye L, Yu Z, Mao X, Zhu L, Zhou X. Endoscopic full-thickness resection with defect closure using clips and an endoloop for gastric subepithelial tumors arising from the muscularis propria. Surg Endosc. 2014;28(6):1978–83.
36. DeMatteo RP, Lewis JJ, Leung D, et al. Two hundred gastrointestinal stromal tumors: recurrence patterns and prognostic factors for survival. Ann Surg. 2000;231:51–8.
37. Sepe P, Brugge W. A guide for the diagnosis and management of gastrointestinal stromal cell tumors. Nat Rev Gastroenterol Hepatol. 2009;6:363–71. doi:10.1038/nrgastro.2009.43.
38. Kim H. Endoscopic treatment for gastrointestinal stromal tumor: advantages and hurdles. World J Gastrointest Endosc. 2015;7(3):192–205.

Operative Management of Gastrointestinal Stromal Tumors

Jack W. Rostas and Prejesh Philips

1 Introduction

The definitive management of gastrointestinal stromal tumors (GIST) is a complete (R0) resection. While this goal is shared with the majority of gastrointestinal malignancies, such as a gastric or colon adenocarcinoma, the major similarities end there. The unique growth characteristics of GIST dictate a divergent operative approach. While an R0 resection for GIST is ideal, microscopically involved margins do not mandate repeat resection [1]. Furthermore, the need for formal organ resection with en bloc lymphadenectomy is uncommon due to the rarity of lymph node metastasis and availability of effective and well-tolerated adjuvant therapy in the form of tyrosine kinase inhibitors [2]. Broadened clinical experience in the management of GIST has led to more tailored resections and an expanded role of minimally invasive approaches. This chapter will focus on the open surgical approaches and apply these concepts in the operative management of primary GIST.

2 Fundamentals of Operative Management

2.1 General Concepts

Tumor location and biology are the most important factors in the selection of operative candidates. Favorable locations happen to be the most common (i.e., the body of the stomach, Table 1) and yield the most therapeutic choices. Surgical

J.W. Rostas, MD • P. Philips, MD (✉)
Division of Surgical Oncology, Department of Surgery, University of Louisville, Louisville, KY, USA
e-mail: prejesh.philips@louisville.edu

© Springer International Publishing Switzerland 2017

C.R. Scoggins et al. (eds.), *Gastrointestinal Stromal Tumors*,
DOI 10.1007/978-3-319-42632-7_9

Table 1 Frequency of GIST location per abdominal site

Site	%
Gastric	60–70
Small intestine	25–33
Jejunum/ileum	27
Duodenum	5
Rectum	3–10
Large intestine	3–5
Esophagus	<1
Other intra-abdominal	8
Extra-abdominal	<5

exploration should proceed for localized disease amenable to primary resection with minimal morbidity. Locations such as the duodenum, near the gastroesophageal junction, or the rectum present a more complicated management algorithm. These sites should be managed with a conservative, organ-sparing approach whenever possible. There should be a low threshold for the use of neoadjuvant therapy to facilitate a difficult resection or to reduce the morbidity of a potentially extensive resection. All decisions for (neo)adjuvant therapy should be performed in the multidisciplinary setting [2–4].

GIST tends to be quite friable and great care must be taken during operative manipulation. Rupture, no matter the clinical circumstances, significantly increases the risk for local recurrence and decreases survival [5–7]. It is therefore imperative to avoid violating the tumor pseudocapsule during extirpative surgery. In this regard, it is often prudent to pack off surrounding structures before attempting resection or mobilization of friable GIST. Preoperative imaging can provide some clues regarding tumor texture, as some GIST have areas that are partially cystic and prone to rupture with operative traction (Fig. 1).

2.2 Selection Criteria

Clear indications for resection include isolated lesions that are amenable to complete resection with expected negative margins [3]. Symptoms that represent traditional indications for intervention, such as hemorrhage refractory to endoscopic management, bowel perforation, and obstruction, also clearly mandate exploration [8]. Localized lesions larger than 5 cm in anatomically difficult locations may benefit from preoperative therapy, with each clinical scenario being assessed individually (see below regarding neoadjuvant therapy).

The management of small (<2 cm) incidentally discovered, asymptomatic GIST is less clear. These lesions are often found incidentally during upper endoscopy. Some are potentially resectable by endoscopic means, however, this approach requires specialized skills. The endoscopic management of GIST is covered in detail in a separate chapter in this book. Endoscopic ultrasound (EUS)

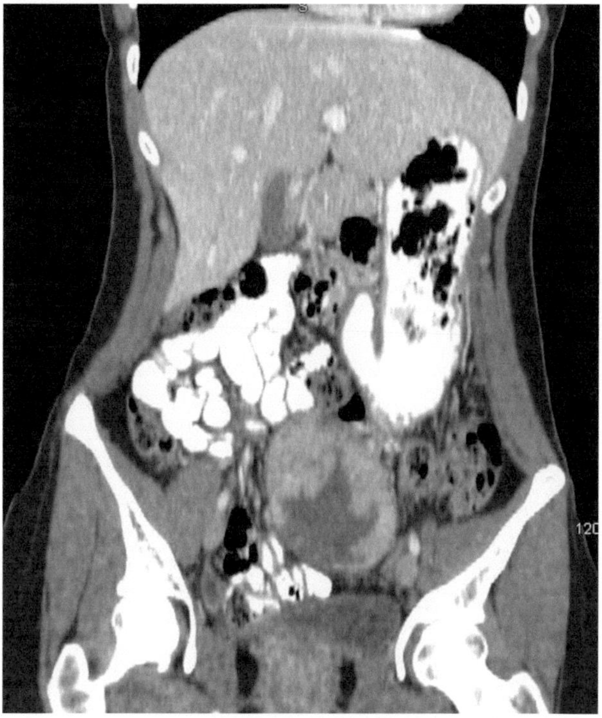

Fig. 1 CT demonstrating partially cystic GIST arising from the stomach

is an excellent diagnostic adjunct to assess the size as well as the depth of the lesions. Formal resection is indicated in the presence of high-risk features on EUS (echogenic foci, ulceration, or irregular margins). Otherwise, serial (every 6–12 months) endoscopic surveillance may be recommended for small, low-risk lesions, especially in a patient whose comorbid conditions might be otherwise prohibitive [3, 4].

2.3 Margin of Resection

Complete resection is the treatment of choice for GIST, either as primary therapy or after a favorable response to neoadjuvant therapy. While the optimal margin of resection is controversial, the decided trend is toward less aggressive resections. This approach is grounded in a tumor physiology lacking significant intramural spread or areas of skip metastasis, as well as favorable outcome data for these more limited resections. In addition, focal, microscopically involved margins (focal R1 resections) do not adversely impact survival on long-term follow-up [1]. Furthermore, the resection of GIST does not mandate the routine removal of large lymph node basins, similar to most soft tissue sarcomas lacking a predilection for lymph node invasion. Lymph nodes should only be removed if involvement is noted on preoperative imaging or during intraoperative exploration [2].

2.4 Neoadjuvant Therapy

Patients with early disease who are clearly amenable to resection are best served by resection. However, for patients deemed unresectable, the use of imatinib (Gleevac®, tyrosine kinase inhibitor) may be indicated as first-line therapy. A favorable response to therapy can lead to downsizing and subsequent resection. For those patients with unfavorable (large, difficult locations) yet clearly resectable tumors, the decision to use neoadjuvant imatinib is less clear. The key issue, yet to be determined, is the threshold at which the benefit of the therapy outweighs its risks (albeit minor) and costs. Specific biology can be critical; for example, tumors harboring exon 9 mutations appear to require higher doses of imatinib to attain a clinical response [9]. Of course, patients not harboring the c-kit mutation have no clear response to imatinib and should not be considered for neoadjuvant therapy with the available drugs. Indications for the preoperative use of imatinib are listed in Table 2. Although not a strict requirement if primary resection is chosen, a biopsy will be necessary if the decision is made to institute neoadjuvant therapy. In addition to reducing surgical morbidity, a response to therapy has also been shown to yield a reduced rate of tumor rupture during subsequent resection [10, 11].

When instituting targeted therapy in advance of a planned resection, there are two traditional approaches to determine the timing of operative intervention. The first strategy is to allow a set time after the institution of chemotherapy, typically 8–12 weeks based on the original RTOG 0132 protocol, before proceeding with surgical intervention [12]. This allows a reasonable period for therapy based on early phase II trials in advanced disease [13]. The second, more contemporary option is intervention based on assessing for a maximal response to therapy by serial imaging. For the majority of tumors that respond to imatinib, resection can be performed with maximal benefit of preoperative therapy, but well before the development of resistant clones [14]. The median interval to maximal tumor response has been shown at 28 weeks, with a plateau at 34 weeks [15]. The NCCN recommends treatment until a plateau response is reached, as evidenced by two consecutive stable imaging studies [3]. Our preference is to obtain baseline cross-sectional imaging

Table 2 Indications for neoadjuvant (first-line) imatinib

Disease stage	Anticipated goals of therapy
Locally advanced	
Unresectable	Convert to resectable
Extensive disease	Reduce extent or expected morbidity of resection
Localized in an anatomically challenging organ/location	Facilitate a minimally invasive approach to resection

(CT or MRI) before institution of neoadjuvant therapy, and serial repeat imaging until a plateau response is reached, at which time an operative intervention is performed.

Early observation and regular imaging are critical, as disease progression requires prompt reassessment [4]. Repeated PET, although highly accurate, is not always available or feasible for surveillance in advance of operative intervention [3, 16]. While CT is the workhorse for perioperative imaging, interpretation can be difficult. For example, an initial response pattern of GIST can manifest as swelling and be misinterpreted as tumor progression. Many criteria have been described to objectively quantify tumor response by imaging. RECIST criteria, while widely used and accurate in many tumors, can underestimate GIST response to therapy. The criteria by Choi et al. (>10 % decrease in tumor size and >15 % decrease in tumor density) more reliably predict therapeutic response by CT [17, 18].

The perioperative scheduling of neoadjuvant therapy varies significantly between imatinib and the newer targeted therapies. Imatinib can be stopped immediately prior to surgery and reinstituted as soon as oral medications are tolerated. Newer agents such as sunitinib and regorafenib are more systemically caustic and should be stopped a week prior to operative intervention. These second-line agents should be restarted more judiciously based on individual patient recovery [3].

2.5 Technical Considerations

Potential approaches for resection of GIST include endoscopic, open, laparoscopic, hand-assisted laparoscopic, robot-assisted, or a combination of these techniques. In achieving an R0 resection, application of these techniques can vary widely according to tumor size, location, and extent of local invasion. Traditional dogma has relegated the laparoscopic approach to small, easily accessible tumors over the fear of violating margins and tumor spillage. This concern is valid, such that great care and gentle handing of the specimen should be taken with any approach. A specimen retrieval bag should be utilized during every minimally invasive approach [3].

Contemporary evidence demonstrates equivalent oncological outcomes, along with the expected reduced morbidity conferred by the minimally invasive approach [7, 19–21]. One caveat of early data is short follow-up, small studies, and a significant selection bias toward smaller and generally more favorable tumors in the minimally invasive approach. Hand-assisted surgery can provide many of the advantages of open and minimally invasive techniques and until recently was explicitly recommended by the NCCN for tumors over 5 cm to help ensure safe specimen handling [3, 22]. Robot-assisted surgery can be particularly effective for resections in difficult locations, such as the pelvis. The only contraindication to the minimally invasive approach is the inability to safely conduct an oncologically sound procedure. The operative approach chosen should be tailored to the tumor characteristics as well as the level of comfort and experience of the surgeon.

3 Location and Management

3.1 Esophagus

GIST of the esophagus are quite rare and difficult to manage given the lack of serosa to help confine the tumor. As can be expected, these lesions display higher risk features compared to gastric GIST. Surveillance can be considered for small (<2 cm) GIST. For a symptomatic submucosal tumor, or one that is larger than 2 cm, an endoscopic biopsy should be performed. If the biopsy confirms that the tumor is a GIST, then preoperative imatinib should be considered given the anatomic difficulty with resection and the overall biologic aggressiveness of GIST arising in the esophagus [22–25].

The goals of resection are to impart minimal morbidity while achieving an R0 resection. Enucleation via a thoracic approach is recommended for small lesions (2–5 cm), as this approach can decrease morbidity rates by half relative to esophagectomy [26]. The long-term results of enucleation are unclear given the limited data and follow-up, however, small GIST with low mitotic rates might be adequately treated with this organ-preserving approach. In general, there should be a low threshold for preoperative imatinib due to the high-risk nature of these tumors. Furthermore, imatinib may facilitate downsizing and esophagus preservation for larger lesions in which an esophagectomy is considered necessary for cure [23–25, 27, 28]. Esophagectomy should be performed in the appropriate candidate for large, persistent, lesions in which organ preservation is not considered oncologically feasible.

3.2 Stomach

The stomach represents the most common location for primary GIST and yields the most therapeutic options. Negative margins can typically be accomplished with a wedge resection for the majority of lesions [2]. Even large gastric GIST often have a narrow pedicle arising from a relatively small area of the stomach, such that a local wedge resection suffices for a margin negative resection (Fig. 2). Extensive resections (subtotal or total gastrectomy) are rarely indicated. As in other tumor locations, great care must be taken to avoid tumor spillage and capsular rupture. Rarely, large gastric GIST may involve adjacent organs such as spleen, mesocolon, or pancreas. In most cases, local structures can be separated with careful dissection; in the instance of dense adhesions, en bloc resection of adjacent organs should be performed to reduce the risk of involved margins or capsular rupture.

In general, proximal or distal lesions, especially those abutting the gastroesophageal junction, pose the greatest difficulty (Fig. 3). Robotic-assisted resections can facilitate resections in the narrow hiatal confines. As stated above, imatinib is indicated to facilitate organ preservation. Tumors involving the pylorus will frequently require distal gastrectomy [22].

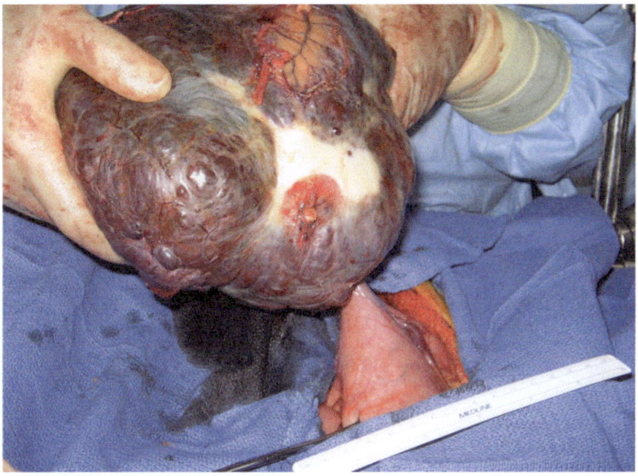

Fig. 2 Massive gastric GIST arising from a narrow portion of the stomach

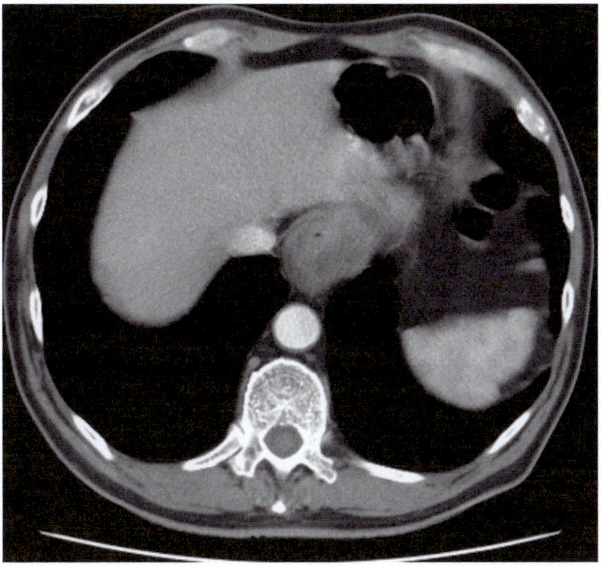

Fig. 3 Distal esophageal GIST

3.3 Duodenum

The approach to duodenal GIST varies greatly depending on the specific location and extent of the tumor. Locations in proximity to the ampulla require particular attention. Organ-sparing, segmental resection is preferable when feasible, with the goal of preserving bowel caliber and function. As stated previously, there should be a low threshold to administer neoadjuvant therapy to facilitate organ preservation. Pancreaticoduodenectomy may be required in tumors refractory to neoadjuvant therapy, and in those in which segmental resection is not feasible [29]. After

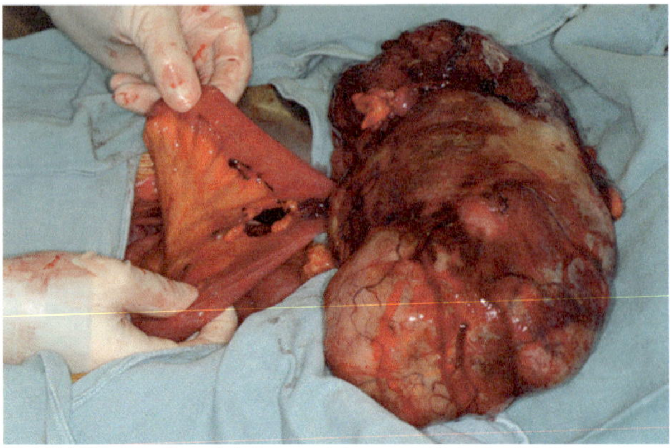

Fig. 4 Jejunal GIST. Note the two feeding blood vessels that have been ligated

appropriate downsizing therapy, most duodenal GIST can be resected in a segmental fashion. For large GIST located in the first part of duodenum, a distal gastrectomy is often needed [22]. For GIST that involve the antipancreatic wall of the descending duodenum without the involvement of the duodenal wall that touches the pancreas (including near the ampulla), a partial duodenectomy may be feasible and the resultant defect closed with a roux-Y-duodenojejunostomy.

3.4 Jejunum and Ileum

Small intestinal GIST of similar size and grade display a more aggressive clinical course than those from a gastric source [30, 31]. Segmental resection is the favored treatment of jejunal and ileal lesions; extensive en bloc resections are usually unnecessary, unless adjacent organs are involved with the GIST [2]. Once again, these small bowel GIST often arise from a narrow stalk and a segmental resection is often sufficient to achieve an R0 resection (Fig. 4). In the rare event of nodal extension, mesenteric resection should include any concerning lymphadenopathy. Lesions in proximity to the ileocecal junction should be resected with a right hemicolectomy if there is a concern over stenosis at the ileocecal junction from a more limited segmental resection.

3.5 Large Intestine

As with small bowel lesions, primary resection is the management of choice for lesions of the intra-abdominal colon. Ensuring preservation of adequate vascular inflow is critical to segmental resection of the colon. Unlike the management of colon adenocarcinoma, large vascular pedicles can be preserved to facilitate reconstruction. However, formal segmental resections including the attendant vascular pedicle are not unreasonable.

3.6 Rectum

Rectal GIST appear to display unique characteristics as they tend be higher risk than more common locations in general [31, 32]. Furthermore, these lesions can be subclassified as low or high risk based on tumor size (low: <5 cm) and mitotic rate (low: <5 mitosis per HPF) [30, 32]. A critical focus of intervention for rectal GIST is sphincter and functional preservation. As with other tumors proximate to critical structures, there should be a low threshold to administer neoadjuvant therapy. Extensive multivisceral excisions should be performed only if absolutely necessary [22, 32].

The bony confines of the pelvis make the approach to resection of rectal lesions complex. Management of proximal rectal lesions is segmental resection, with more distal lesions often requiring low anterior resection for adequate margins. Mesorectal excision is unnecessary without evidence of nodal involvement, although most surgeons are comfortable with rectal mobilization in this dissection plane. For distal lesions, local excision is preferred when appropriate and can be performed via trans-anal, trans-sacral, or trans-vaginal approaches. For extensive lesions, abdomino-perineal resection or exenteration may be necessary for local control, only as a last resort in those tumors refractory to a judicious administration of targeted therapy.

3.7 Recurrent or Metastatic Disease

The relief of significant symptoms, as with primary disease, represents a clear indication for operative intervention for recurrent or metastatic disease. However, many factors must be taken into account before embarking on the elective resection of such lesions. In no other clinical scenario does tumor biology dictate the clinical course of GIST more than in the management of recurrent or metastatic disease. For those patients not currently on therapy, imatinib is the first-line treatment for recurrent disease or the development of metastasis. A surgery-only approach is associated with poor outcomes. Furthermore, preoperative CT imaging can underestimate tumor burden, especially with regards to peritoneal disease. Should the disease burden be deemed resectable with minimal morbidity, surgery can follow the administration of imatinib [33].

For patients with an extensive tumor burden, only those harboring disease that is stable or responsive to imatinib have been shown to benefit from surgical resection. This may reflect tumor cytoreduction, in which the potential for developing therapy-resistant mutations is physically reduced, or simply be a consequence of favorable tumor biology in general [33]. Patients harboring disseminated but stable disease can develop a new focus of progression while on adjuvant therapy. For the appropriate candidate, resection can be considered to eliminate the clones that have presumably developed resistance. In any scenario, the decision to proceed with operative intervention should be made with multidisciplinary support [3, 4, 33].

Second-line therapy (sunitinib and regorafenib) is currently available for those who progress on imatinib. Outcomes for operative intervention for those patients on second-line therapy are uncertain, with little correlation to preoperative response (as opposed to first-line therapy), lower survival, and higher morbidity. Careful patient selection is critical in this cohort [33].

Recurrent and metastatic GIST display unique characteristics based on location. Two-thirds of patients with metastatic GIST harbor disease in the liver, with over 50 % of these patients having liver-only metastasis. Metastatic liver involvement is typically diffuse and often precludes resection. Ablative techniques or hepatic arterial therapies are an option for liver lesions not amenable to resection [2, 33]. These techniques may be especially useful for focal yet unresectable recurrences, such as in the scenario of CT progression in a single hepatic lesion in a patient with other significant (but stable) disease burden. In patients with extensive bilobar liver-dominant metastatic GIST, intra-arterial therapy in the form of bland or radioactive beads can be used to delay tumor progression.

Peritoneal recurrence is the next most common manifestation of disease progression and is found in 20 % of patients [34] (Fig. 5). As stated previously, peritoneal disease if difficult to detect and is often underrepresented on surveillance CT. Gastric primaries tend to recur in the lesser sac, and rectal primaries tend to recur in the recto-vesicular or recto-vaginal spaces [33]. True local-only recurrences are uncommon after an R0 resection. Cytoreduction and hyerthermic intraperitoneal chemotherapy (HIPEC) has a limited role in peritoneal sarcomatosis from GIST, although experience and data are limited [35]. HIPEC for GIST should be considered experimental and performed within the confines of a clinical trial or protocol. Lung metastasis is uncommon and if deemed resectable should be treated with an organ-sparing approach in highly selected patients.

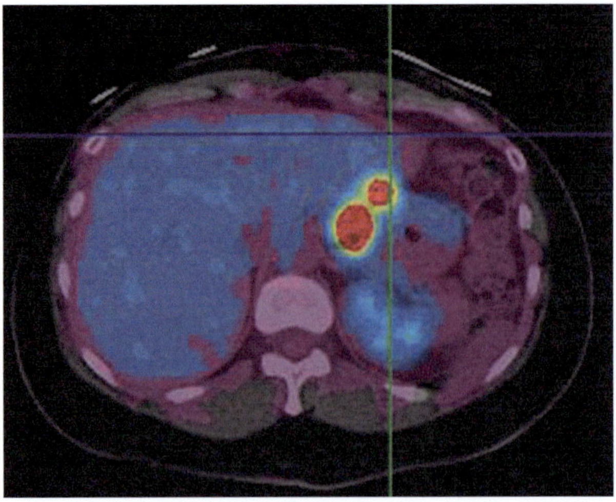

Fig. 5 PET demonstrating peritoneal metastases along the lesser omentum

4 Conclusion

Definitive management of GIST involves resection with clear margins. The anatomical location and tumor characteristics dictate the need for neoadjuvant therapy, extent of resection, capacity for negative margins (anatomical constraints), and operative approach (open or minimally invasive). The availability of excellent adjuvant and neoadjuvant therapy has diminished the need for heroic resections for curative intent. While advances in operative techniques have allowed the minimally invasive approach to reduce the morbidity of resection, the focus should be on a complete resection without tumor spillage in order to achieve optimal oncological outcomes.

References

1. McCarter MD, Antonescu CR, et al. Microscopically positive margins for primary gastrointestinal stromal tumors: analysis of risk factors and tumor recurrence. J Am Coll Surg. 2012;215(1):53–9.
2. Bamboat ZM, DeMatteo RP. Updates on the management of gastrointestinal stromal tumors (GIST). Surg Oncol Clin N Am. 2012;21(2):301–16.
3. von Mehren M, Randall RL, Benjamin RS, et al. Soft tissue sarcoma version 1.2015 NCCN Clinical Practice Guidelines in Oncology. Web 10.2015.
4. Casali PG, Blay JY, ESMO/CONTICANET/EUROBONET Consensus Panel of Experts. Gastrointestinal stromal tumors: ESMO clinical practice guidelines for diagnosis, treatment, and follow-up. Ann Oncol. 2012;23(7):vii49–57.
5. Joensuu H. Risk stratification of patients diagnosed with gastrointestinal stromal tumor. Hum Pathol. 2008;39:1411–9.
6. Rutkowski P, Bylina E, Wozniak A, et al. Validation of the Joensuu risk criteria for primary resectable gastrointestinal stromal tumor, impact of tumour rupture on outcomes. Eur J Surg Oncol. 2011;37:890–6.
7. Bischof DA, Kim Y, Dodson R, et al. Open versus minimally invasive resection of gastric GIST: a multi-institutional analysis of short- and long-term outcomes. Ann Surg Oncol. 2014;21:2941–8.
8. Rutkowski P, Ruka W. Emergency surgery in the era of molecular treatment of solid tumors. Lancet Oncol. 2009;10:157–63.
9. Debiec-Rychter M, Sciot R, Cesne AL, et al. KIT mutations and dose selection for imatinib in patients with advanced gastrointestinal stromal tumors. Eur J Cancer. 2006;42:1093–103.
10. Rutkowski P, Gronchi A, Hohenberger P, et al. Neoadjuvant imatinib in locally advanced gastrointestinal stromal tumors (GIST): the EORTC STBSG experience. Ann Surg Oncol. 2013;20:2937–43.
11. Koontz MZ, Visser BM, Kunz PL. Neoadjuvant imatinib for borderline resectable GIST. J Natl Compr Canc Netw. 2012;10(12):1477–82.
12. Eisenberg BL, Harris J, Blanke CD, et al. Phase II trial of neoadjuvant/adjuvant imatinib mesylate (IM) for advanced primary and metastatic/recurrent operable gastrointestinal stromal tumor (GIST): early results of RTOG 0132/ACRIN 6665. J Surg Oncol. 2009;99:42–7.
13. Demetri GD, von Mehren M, Blanke CD, et al. Efficacy and safety of imatinib mesylate in advanced gastrointestinal stromal tumors. N Engl J Med. 2002;347:472–80.
14. Wang D, Zhang Q, Blanke CD, et al. Phase II trial of neoadjuvant/adjuvant imatinib mesylate for advanced primary and metastatic/recurrent operable gastrointestinal stromal tumors: long-term follow-up results of radiation therapy oncology group 0132. Ann Surg Oncol. 2012;19:1074–80.

15. Tirumani SH, Shinagare AB, Jagannathan JP, et al. Radiological assessment of earliest, best, and plateau response of gastrointestinal stromal tumors to neoadjuvant imatinib prior to successful surgical resection. Eur J Surg Oncol. 2014;40:420–8.
16. Van den Abbeele AD, Gatsonis C, de Vries DJ, et al. ACRIN 6665/RTOG 0132 phase II trial of neoadjuvant imatinib mesylate for operable malignant gastrointestinal stromal tumor: monitoring with 18F-FDG PET and correlation with genotype and GLUT4 expression. J Nucl Med. 2012;53:567–74.
17. Benjamin RS, Choi H, Macapinlac HA, et al. We should desist using RECIST, at least in GIST. J Clin Oncol. 2007;25:1760–4.
18. Choi H, Charnsangavej C, Faria SC, et al. Correlation of CT and PET in patients with metastatic GIST with imatinib, new CT response criteria. J Clin Oncol. 2007;25:1753–9.
19. Chen QL, Pan Y, Cai JQ, et al. Laparoscopic versus open resection for gastric gastrointestinal stromal tumors: an updated systematic review and meta-analysis. World J Surg Oncol. 2014;12:206.
20. Pucci MJ, Berger AC, Lim PW, et al. Laparoscopic approaches to gastric gastrointestinal stromal tumors: an institutional review of 57 cases. Surg Endosc. 2012;26:3509–14.
21. Karakousis GC, Singer S, Zheng J, et al. Laparoscopic versus open gastric resections for primary gastrointestinal stromal tumors (GISTs): a size-matched comparison. Ann Surg Oncol. 2011;18:1599–605.
22. Demetri GD, von Mehren M, Antonescu CR, et al. NCCN Task Force report: update on the management of patients with gastrointestinal stromal tumors. J Natl Compr Canc Netw. 2010;8(2):S1–44.
23. Lott S, Schmieder M, Mayer B, et al. Gastrointestinal stromal tumors of the esophagus: evaluation of a pooled case series regarding clinicopathological features and clinical outcome. Am J Cancer Res. 2015;5(1):333–43.
24. Lee HJ, Park SI, Kim DK, et al. Surgical resection of esophageal gastrointestinal stromal tumors. Ann Thorac Surg. 2009;87:1569–72.
25. Blum MG, Bilimoria KY, Wayne JD, et al. Surgical considerations for the management and resection of esophageal gastrointestinal stromal tumors. Ann Thorac Surg. 2007;84:1717–23.
26. Robb WB, Bruyere E, Amielh D, et al. Esophageal gastrointestinal stromal tumor: is tumoral enucleation a viable therapeutic option? Ann Surg. 2015;261:117–24.
27. Jiang P, Jiao Z, Han B, et al. Clinical characteristics and surgical treatment of oesophageal gastrointestinal stromal tumors. Eur J Cardiothorac Surg. 2010;38:223–7.
28. Coccolini F, Catena F, Ansaloni L, et al. Esophagogastric junction gastrointestinal stromal tumor: resection vs enucleation. World J Gastroenterol. 2010;16(35):4374–6.
29. Liang X, Yu H, Zhu LH, et al. Gastrointestinal stromal tumors of the duodenum: surgical management and survival results. World J Gastroenterol. 2013;19(36):6000–10.
30. Miettinen M, Lasota J. Gastrointestinal stromal tumors review on morphology, molecular pathology, prognosis, and differential diagnosis. Arch Pathol Lab Med. 2006;130:1466–78.
31. DeMatteo RP, Gold JS, Saran L, et al. Tumor mitotic rate, size, and location independently predict recurrence after resection of primary gastrointestinal stromal tumor (GIST). Cancer. 2008;112:608–15.
32. Jakob J, Mussi C, Ronellenfitsch U, et al. Gastrointestinal stromal tumor of the rectum: results of surgical and multimodality therapy in the era of imatinib. Ann Surg Oncol. 2013;20:586–92.
33. Bamboat ZM, DeMatteo RP. Metastatecomy for gastrointestinal stromal tumors. J Surg Oncol. 2014;109(1):23–7.
34. DeMatteo RP, Lewis JJ, Leung D, et al. Two hundred gastrointestinal stromal tumors, recurrence patterns and prognostic factors for survival. Ann Surg. 2000;231(1):51–8.
35. Bryan ML, Fitzgerald NC, Levine EA, et al. Cytoreductive surgery with hyperthermic intraperitoneal chemotherapy in sarcomatosis from gastrointestinal stromal tumor. Am Surg. 2014;80(9):890–5.

Minimally Invasive Approaches to Gastrointestinal Stromal Tumors (GISTs)

Tiffany C. Cox, Vedra A. Augenstein, Sam Schell, and B. Todd Heniford

1 Introduction

The concept and proof of concept of minimally invasive surgical techniques began with the introduction of laparoscopic cholecystectomy in 1987. Since then, laparoscopy has improved patient outcomes and transitioned through all surgical specialties, including general surgery thoracic, vascular, gynecology, and urology. Minimally invasive surgery has evolved since its creation due to improvements in instruments, visualization, hemostatsis, robotics, the ability to combine laparoscopy with intraoperative endoscopy, and the wide availability of these technologies to maximize favorable outcomes. The application of minimally invasive surgical techniques to the treatment of gastrointestinal stromal tumors (GISTs) has been extensively studied, and the general conclusion is that laparoscopic removal of GIST in most patients is associated with a shorter hospital stay and comparable long-term oncologic outcomes compared to open resection [1–8]. However, as with any operation for GIST, the adherence to oncologic surgical practices, including prevention of tumor spillage and appropriate resection, must be considered before deciding on a minimally invasive resection [1].

GISTs are an uncommon yet important type of gastric neoplasm, representing 1–3 % of surgically resected gastric tumors [9]. These tumors comprise a spectrum of variable malignant potential that ranges from benign to aggressive. In fact, the metastatic potential is difficult to predict due to a lack of signs of malig-

T.C. Cox, MD • V.A. Augenstein, MD, FACS • S. Schell • B.T. Heniford, MD, FACS (✉)
Division of Gastrointestinal and Minimally Invasive Surgery, Carolinas Laparoscopic and Advanced Surgery Program, Carolinas Medical Center,
1025 Morehead Medical Drive, Suite 300, Charlotte, NC 28204, USA
e-mail: todd.heniford@carolinashealthcare.org

© Springer International Publishing Switzerland 2017

C.R. Scoggins et al. (eds.), *Gastrointestinal Stromal Tumors*,
DOI 10.1007/978-3-319-42632-7_10

nancy beyond histologic mitotic rate or metastasis at the time of surgery. Historically, GISTs were labeled as leiomyomas, leiomyoblastomas, and leiomyosarcomas due to the belief that they originated from smooth muscle cells. However, more recently, the interstitial cells of Cajal, a pleuro-potential intestinal pacemaker cell, have been identified as the origin of GISTs [10]. Further research into their origin has revealed that gain of function mutation in the c-KIT or PDGFRa genes is a hallmark of GISTs, which has allowed further delineation of the cellular characteristics of these neoplasms [11]. This genetic understanding is utilized to predict the use of adjuvant therapy as well as its potential aggressive nature.

GISTs are often found during routine endoscopy for other reasons, but they can also be discovered due to upper gastrointestinal bleeding, pain, or obstruction. Surgical resection is currently the only curative procedure and, thereby, is the preferred treatment when such lesions are encountered. Previously, smaller GISTs might have undergone surveillance, but due to their indeterminate natural history, resection is recommended whenever possible [9]. When GIST resection was first discussed, traditional open surgery was all that was available. With the advent of laparoscopy, case reports and isolated series began to describe the feasibility of using a minimally invasive approach to resect GISTs [12–20]. However, the size criteria for tumors amenable to minimally invasive surgery have been disputed. With little evidence, it was originally proposed that laparoscopic resection only be attempted for lesions less than 2 cm [21, 22]. This cutoff was subsequently challenged, and numerous articles reported favorable results performing minimally invasive resection of GISTs larger than 2 cm [10, 23–25]. The National Comprehensive Cancer Network (NCCN) guidelines published in 2010 recommend that all GISTs, 2 cm or larger, should be resected. GISTs smaller than 5 cm are amenable to laparoscopic wedge resection, and those larger than 5 cm can be resected laparoscopically or using laparoscopic-assisted hand port [26]. Currently, a strict size criterion does not exist to guide surgeons as the NCCN guidelines admit that the 2 cm cutoff for resection is somewhat arbitrary, and the decision to perform a minimally invasive or open surgery is dependent upon factors such as tumor size, mitotic index, as well as surgeon preference, skill, and confidence with laparoscopic surgery. Similarly, 2-cm margins were proposed to be necessary for adequate surgical resection, but more recently it has been demonstrated that tumor size and not negative microscopic surgical margins determine survival [17, 27, 28]. Given this, the lymph node resection is not required due to the lack of spread to lymph nodes, the long history of technical success of laparoscopic gastric procedures for reflux and weight loss, the availability and reliability of laparoscopic staplers, and the capability of easily and quickly reaching the stomach with an endoscope, GIST tumors appear to be uniquely approachable via minimally invasive surgery. Due to improved short-term outcomes, laparoscopy is recommended whenever deemed appropriate, although it should be performed by those surgeons with advanced laparoscopic skills.

2 Operative Techniques

2.1 General Laparoscopic Technique

The operative approach can depend on tumor location, size, and characteristics of its growth. For laparoscopic, laparoendoscopic (intragastric), or laparoscopic hand-assisted resection, patient positioning and trocar placement are often similar to most foregut procedures (Fig. 1) [10]. The technique described previously [10] begins with the patient placed in a supine position with abduction of both arms. A split leg table or stirrups should be used to allow the surgeon the option of standing between the patient's legs for optimum triangulation of the trocars. Video monitors are typically placed laterally to each of the patient's shoulders or one can be positioned above the patient's head depending on surgeon preference. The initial trocar is typically placed in the midline, about one-third of the distance between the umbilicus and the xiphoid. A liver retractor is most often placed through a right subcostal, midclavicular line trocar. The surgeon operates through two working ports, one placed in the epigastrium and the second in the left subcostal, midclavicular line. An additional trocar is placed in the left upper-quadrant trocar for the assistant. After insertion of the initial ports, a formal abdominal exploration should be performed to rule out peritoneal seeding or hepatic metastasis. If necessary, an intraoperative ultrasound can be used to evaluate the liver for metastases, especially in the case of suspicious lesions found on preoperative imaging. Intraoperative flexible endoscopy often facilitates determining the best approach for resection by localization of the lesion from proximal to distal and whether it is anterior, posterior, or along the greater of lesser curve while also looking at the stomach with the laparoscope. It also can aid in the delineation of resection margins during the operation. At the end of surgery, endoscopy is utilized to evaluate the integrity of the staple/suture lines after resection. Importantly,

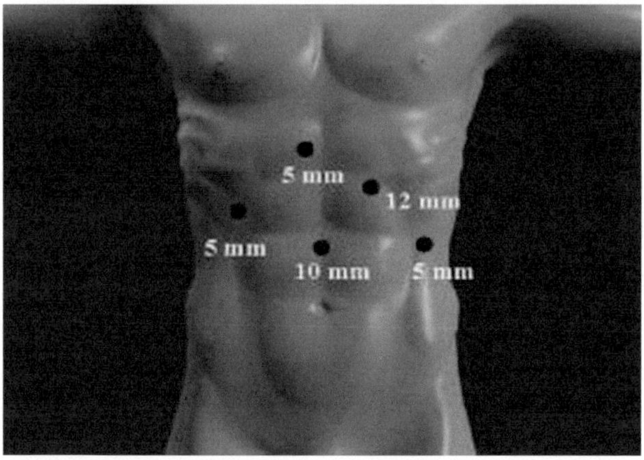

Fig. 1 Port placement and patient positioning for laparoscopic wedge resection [10]

while evaluating the tumor and during resection, surgeons should attempt to avoid directly handling the lesions with the laparoscopic instruments to reduce the risk of tumor rupture.

2.2 Laparoendoscopic Technique

This technique, as previously described [19], is for patients with predominantly intraluminal masses. Positioning is similar to the laparoscopic approach in that the patient is positioned on a split-leg operating table, and the operating surgeon stands between the legs. One assistant is required for the laparoscopic procedure, and a surgical endoscopist is positioned at the head of the operating table and the endoscopic screen is positioned next to the laparoscopic monitor. The resection can be performed with either 2- or 5-mm laparoscopic instruments depending on their availability, size of the patient, size of the lesion, and its location. The advantage of using 2-mm instruments is that it can eliminate the need for closure of the gastric wall port sites and improve cosmesis.

An initial diagnostic laparoscopy is performed to exclude metastatic disease and unsuspected transmural extension of the stromal tumor. Typically, the peritoneal cavity is accessed at the umbilicus or just above it by an open or closed technique. With the laparoscope looking from the intraperitoneal location, diagnostic endoscopy is performed to visualize the lesion and plan trocar placement. This allows for the appropriate planning for triangulation of the trocars as they come through the abdominal wall and into the stomach. This can allow the surgeon to have sufficient intertrocar distance, make sure that there is adequate distance from the trocars to the lesion, and also make sure that the trocars penetrate the stomach perpendicularly instead of tangentially or through the greater omentum. This can be achieved by the combination of digital palpation of the abdominal wall or penetration with a spinal needle, perspective from the endoscopic view, all the while under laparoscopic visualization with reduced pneumoperitoneum. Indeed, the spinal needle can be very helpful to simulate trocar position and direction prior to placement. Maximal gastric distension and further release of the pneumoperitoneum will then allow trocar placement into the stomach with endoscopic guidance (Fig. 2). Intragastric stabilization of the trocars is then secured by a balloon (5-mm trocars, Entec Corp., Madison, CT, USA), flanges (2-mm trocars, Imagyn Surgical, Newport Beach, CA, USA), or simply suturing the stomach to the abdominal wall. This can be performed by adding an additional intraperitoneal port and then introducing a suture with a needle (such as a 2–0 silk on a straightened SH needle) using a suture passer next to the proposed intragastric port site. Placement of two intragastric trocars is needed if the endoscopic visualization alone is used, and three trocars for laparoscopic visualization. Use of the intragastric laparoscope is certainly easier; endoscopic vision can result in an image inversion (left is right, up is down, etc.) and a masterful endoscopist is absolutely needed.

A hemostatic dissection and demarcation of the mass from the submucosa and normal muscle fibers is achieved with the submucosal and intramuscular injection of dilute epinephrine (1:100,000) performed by endoscopic sclerotherapy needle or a transabdominal spinal needle (Fig. 3). Circumferential incision of the mucosa just beyond the base of the lesion is then accomplished with hook cautery with meticulous dissection to not disrupt the lesion which is typically well circumscribed. Appropriate retraction of the mass can be gained by grasping the overlying mucosa or endolooping the lesion. If necessary for complete resection a transmural defect may result which is closed with intragastric suturing and knot-tying (Fig. 4). Once excised, the lesion is delivered through the mouth after placing it in a bag (Catch purse, Hakko Trading Co., Japan) or with the use of an endoscopic snare. An endoscopic overtube may be utilized. Adequate closure of the stomach is verified with gastric distension under laparoscopic inspection. Closure of gastric port sites is done with the same trocars after pulling them from the stomach and into the peritoneal cavity (Fig. 5).

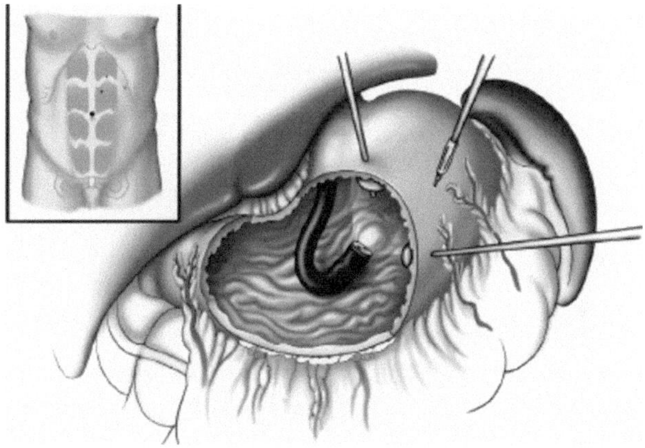

Fig. 2 Endoscopically guided intragastric placement of trocars [19]

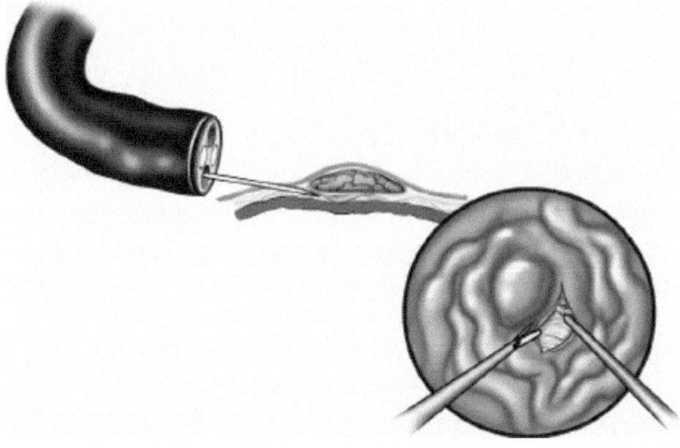

Fig. 3 Submucosal epinephrine injection endoscopically for hemostatic dissection [19]

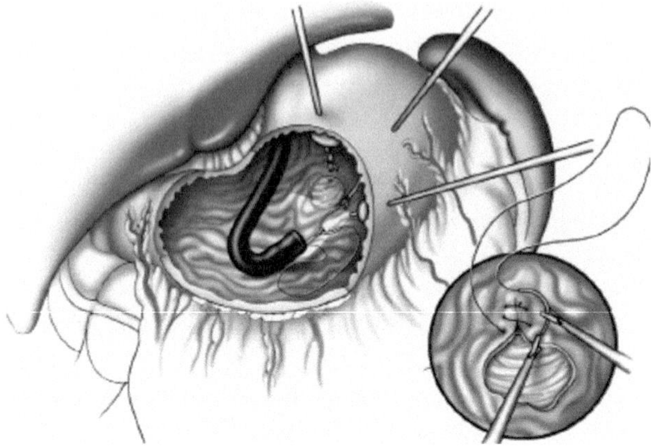

Fig. 4 Closure of mucosal-mural defect laparoscopically with endoscopic passage of suture and visualization [19]

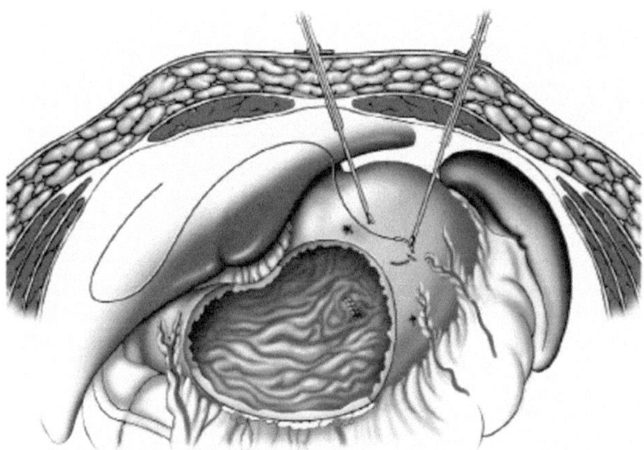

Fig. 5 Closure of intragastric port sites utilizing same ports pulled from the stomach and into the intra-abdominal cavity [19]

2.3 Needlescopic Technique

The surgical treatment for stromal tumors of the gastroesophageal junction is potentially resected percutaneous, transgastric needlescopic approach as previously described [16]. A 2-mm needlescopic umbilical port (Imagyn Medical Technologies, Irvine, CA, USA) is inserted using a Veress technique and the abdomen is insufflated to a 12-mmHg pneumoperitoneum. The abdomen is explored with a 2-mm endoscope (Karl Storz, Inc., Culver City, CA, USA). If necessary, two additional 2-mm ports are inserted under needlescopic guidance in the left midclavicular and left midaxillary positions. After exploration, a flexible endoscope is passed into the stomach and the tumor is localized. A video mixer can provide simultaneous endoscopic and needlescopic visualization.

The stomach is distended by the endoscope, and the 2-mm ports are passed through the gastric wall under combined visualization. The abdominal cavity is desufflated, and the remainder of the procedure is performed under endoscopic guidance. As described with the laparoendoscopic approach, circumferential injection of the tumor submucosally with 1:100,000 epinephrine solution is accomplished with a spinal needle. A 2-mm grasper and hook cautery are used to incise the mucosa around the tumor. An endoloop is placed around the tumor to accomplish retraction without manipulating the tumor directly, and the tumor is enucleated from the underlying muscularis and encircled with an endoscopic snare for final removal transorally.

2.4 Hand-Assisted Laparoscopic Technique

Similar patient positioning and trocar placement are used on occasion when a hand-assisted port is needed [10]. Selective use is recommended for larger tumors, such as those greater than 7 cm, or lesions in difficult locations. The incision is typically 6–7 cm in length and placed in the midline for possible conversion to an open procedure if necessary. The benefits of the hand-assisted technique for the larger tumors can allow for gentle handling, assist in appropriate positioning of endoscopic staplers, and allow retraction for optimal visualization when in difficult locations or in cases involving bulky tumors.

3 Technique Based on Location

3.1 Anterior Gastric Wall Tumors

Masses within the anterior wall of the stomach are frequently amenable to wedge resection with a linear endoscopic GI anastomotic stapler as described previously [10, 16, 17]. If the tumor is extraluminal, it is usually visualized on initial inspection with the laparoscope. Those lesions that are intraluminal are often identified by a characteristic dimpling of the gastric serosal surface or by bimanual palpation of the stomach with laparoscopic instruments. As mentioned previously, intraluminal visualization by a flexible endoscope assists with tumor localization and may guide resection to ensure adequate margins and to safeguard against comprising the gastric inlet or outlet. After identifying the lesion itself, the short gastric vessels are divided with ultrasonic coagulating shears. By elevating the gastric wall with two seromuscular sutures placed opposite each other within 1 cm of the mass to accomplish a no-touch technique laparoscopic gastric wedge resection and to ensure that the stitches do not penetrate or perforate the tumor. The sutures are elevated simultaneously and the stapler is placed just under the sutures to resect the tumor and a small margin of the normal stomach.

Another technique is to circumferentially excise the gastric tumor and a surrounding margin of the normal tissue using ultrasonic coagulating shears [19]. This technique is simplified by insufflating the stomach with a flexible endoscope, allowing the site where the stomach is to be opened to be determined by observing the tumor both endoscopically and laparoscopically. Typically, the incision into the stomach is made 2 cm from the lesion to make certain that the tumor is not lacerated. This technique allows for a more precise excision of the normal tissue at the margins of the tumor compared to the technique utilizing an endoscopic GIA stapler. The gastrotomy can be closed by laparoscopic intracorporeal suturing or by placing two to four full-thickness traction sutures along the cut edge of the gastrotomy and using an endoscopic linear stapler to reapproximate ("close") the gastrotomy.

3.2 Posterior Gastric Wall Lesions

Posterior wall lesions are commonly approached through the lesser sac [10, 16, 17]. Exposure of the posterior surface of the stomach is achieved following division of the gastrocolic omentum and short gastric vessels allowing the greater curvature to be elevated and rotated cephalad. The lesion can then be resected similar to the technique described for anterior lesions [19]. An alternative approach to the posterior gastric wall tumor entails creating an anterior gastrotomy over the lesion after it is endoscopically localized. As described previously, the location of the gastrotomy is determined by visual cues from the gastroscope and laparoscope while simultaneously palpating the gastric wall with laparoscopic graspers. Through the anterior gastrostomy, normal gastric tissue adjacent to the tumor is grasped with laparoscopic bowel grasper or, alternatively, traction sutures can be placed on each side of the tumor much as described for anterior gastric tumors. The tumor and the surrounding margin of normal stomach are elevated through the gastrotomy and resected by an endoscopic linear stapler. The staple line is examined for bleeding and any bleeding points are oversewn. The anterior gastrotomy is closed with the GIA stapler or sutures.

Intraluminal posterior wall lesions such as those near the gastroesophageal junction not amenable to the above treatment are approached via a percutaneous, laparoscopic, intragastric resection. Laparoscopic intragastric or "endoluminal" surgery, as described previously in this chapter, involves the placement of balloon or mushroom-tipped laparoscopic trocars (2–10 mm) percutaneously into the stomach (insufflated by a flexible endoscope) similar to the placement of a percutaneous endoscopic gastrostomy tube [29]. The pylorus may be occluded with a balloon-tipped nasogastric tube but is infrequently needed. An angled laparoscope, positioned through one of the percutaneous gastric trocars, is preferred for visualization of the operative field, but a flexible endoscope can be used in combination with two working trocars. A dilute epinephrine solution (1:100,000) is injected circumferentially around the tumor as a tumescent to aid in the dissection of the submucosal plane surrounding the tumor and to limit bleeding. The lesion is enucleated from the submucosal-muscular junction using an electrocautery hook as needed. The mucosal defect is left open to heal or can be closed with laparoscopic intragastric suturing. The tumor is placed in a retrieval bag and removed trans-orally.

3.3 Greater and Lesser Curvature Lesions

Simple wedge resection with an endoscopic linear stapler is commonly the preferred approach for lesions near the greater and lesser curvatures [10, 16, 17]. For all lesions located on the greater curve, the greater omentum needs to be divided and similarly for the lesser omentum/gastrohepatic ligament for those tumors located on the lesser curve. Ultrasonic coagulation shears or Ligasure allows for a hemostatic division of the short gastric vessels on the greater curvature and likewise the branches of the left gastric artery and coronary vein on the lesser curvature. Appropriate positioning during laparoscopy such as rotating the stomach so that the stromal tumor faces anteriorly can facilitate the ease of the resection. The tumor is resected using an endoscopic linear stapler and then removed through an extraction bag via an enlarged 12-mm trocar site.

3.4 Gastroesophageal Junction Tumors

Masses in the proximity of the gastroesophageal (GE) junction can be managed similar to tumors near the pylorus. The goals remain, if possible, to achieve an adequate surgical margin while maintaining the normal function of the lower esophageal sphincter mechanism. Lesions found more than 2–3 cm from the GE junction are approached according to their location, as an anterior, posterior, or greater/lesser curve mass, as previously described. The resection of a tumor at the GE junction is more difficult. If it is a mucosal or submucosal lesion, enucleation is a viable option and is one that we have used effectively on multiple occasions. Endoscopic ultrasound (EUS) verification of the tumors' depth of penetration is invaluable in determining the tactics of resection for these masses. Posterior lesions at the gastroesophageal junction are easier to approach in this fashion because the instrument angle coming down from the abdominal wall is naturally pointing toward the posterior GE junction.

In this technique, the vessels around the fundus and cardia of the stomach are usually not transected, but they can be if needed. If the upper portion of the greater curve needs to be mobilized, the assistant on the left gently retracts the gastrosplenic ligament toward the lateral abdominal wall with a laparoscopic bowel grasper placed through the left lateral port. The surgeon uses the upper mid-line port to pull the stomach medially and inferiorly and the mid-right subcostal port to coagulate and transect the short gastric vessels using the ultrasonic coagulating shears. The anterior gastrotomy can be made linearly or horizontally, but one needs to remember that the gastrostomy closure must not constrict the upper stomach. Enucleation proceeds with an electrocautery hook after submucosal, peritumoral injection with dilute epinephrine. After removal of the lesion within an entrapment sac, we typically close the mucosa of the GE junction, but, on occasion, we have left it open to heal on its own.

A novel technique we described for small gastroesophageal junction stromal tumors is a laparoscopic or minilaparoscopic intragastric resection [18], which has been somewhat described in this chapter. The technique is similar to the endoluminal technique, although the minilaparoscopic or laparoscopic intragastric resection utilizes the flexible endoscope as the "camera" and insufflator nearly always. We again perform a local injection with dilute epinephrine via a 7-in., 22-gauge spinal needle placed through one of the 2-mm ports or by injection needle though the endoscope. An electrocautery hook is used to enucleate the gastroesophageal junction tumor and the mass is removed transorally with the flexible endoscope.

If the gastric stromal tumor is located in the cardia or at the gastroesophageal junction, it may not be amenable to a wedge resection technique [16, 17]. An esophagogastrectomy can be performed, although this is a technically demanding procedure to perform laparoscopically. In short, following division of the short gastric vessels and the lesser curve attachments, the mobilization of the proximal esophagus is necessary well into the mediastinum with meticulous dissection utilizing the visible plane between the pleura and the esophagus with a combination of blunt and electrosurgical dissection. Once complete, the distal esophagus is transected proximal to the gastrointestinal stromal tumor with an endoscopic linear stapler. The vasculature of the stomach is taken circumferentially using the Ligasure or other vascular sealing device. The duodenum is transected distal to the pylorus using a GIA stapler. For reconstruction, a Roux-en-Y esophagojejunostomy. This portion of the operation is initiated by taking the patient out of Trendelenberg's position and maintaining them in a more neutral orientation. The omentum is rolled upward and over the colon and a colonic epiploica is grasped and pulled upward to expose the full undersurface of the transverse colon mesentery and to identify the ligament of Treitz. We measure approximately 30–45 cm distal to the ligament of Treitz and roll this portion of the jejunum upward to the distal esophagus. If the intestine easily reaches the distal esophagus, an anticolic route will be chosen. To facilitate the anticolic positioning of the jejunal limb, one can split the omentum midline in a caudal-cranial fashion using the ultrasonic coagulating shears. Otherwise, a small window can be made in the avascular area of the transverse mesocolon just above and lateral to the ligament of Treitz. The loop of the jejunum can be brought through the mesocolon easily in a retrocolic, retrogastric fashion. The anastomosis is performed in an isoperistaltic manner. We then complete the esophagojejunostomy with a 25 mm EEA stapler with facilitation of the anvil to the distal esophagus by way of securing it to the end of a 16-French orogastric tube and initial passage of the proximal end of the tube which is then pulled through an enterotomy made in the distal esophagus and brought out through the abdomen via a trocar site. An existing trocar site is enlarged to allow access of the EEA stapler trasnabdominally and advanced through an enterotomy on the antimesenteric border of the jejunum antegrade through the Roux limb. After the stapler and anvil are fastened, tightened, and fired, the Roux limb enterotomy can be closed with sutures or an endoscopic linear stapler. This anastomosis can also be performed using laparoscopic linear staplers alone with anastomosis of the Roux limb to the posterior esophagus. Again, the common enterotomy is closed with either sutures or an endoscopic linear stapler. The mesenteric defects are closed using 2–0 suture.

3.5 Distal Stomach/Pylorus Tumors

Small tumors in the prepyloric region may be excised by wedge resection with an endoscopic linear stapler as previously described [17]. Tumors near the pylorus, but not truly involving the pylorus, are approached using methods to achieve negative margins while not obstructing the pylorus. Posterior lesions that lie 1½–2 cm from the pylorus and whose depth of penetration is limited to the mucosa or submucosa can usually be removed without compromising the pylorus. We have found EUS confirmation of the tumors' depth of penetration invaluable in planning our approach to pyloric masses. Our usual approach is through a horizontal, anterior gastrotomy, which can be effectively performed with the ultrasonic shears. The position of the gastrotomy is again localized with the aid of an endoscope, but the gastric opening is made no closer than 3–4 cm from the pylorus. Traction sutures are then placed proximally and distally within a centimeter or so of the tumor, and it is pulled through the anterior gastrotomy out into the abdominal cavity. The mass can then be enucleated with an electrocautery hook or it can be elevated and removed with an endoscopic linear stapler. The enucleation site is closed with a running suture. If the tumor is to be enucleated, we frequently we inject a dilute epinephrine solution (1:100,000) circumferentially around the tumor as described for the endoluminal technique. As a rule, the horizontal, distal, anterior gastrotomy is closed vertically so as to not compromise the luminal diameter of the distal stomach. Two to four full-thickness traction sutures are used to approximate the gastric wall and a thick-tissue (4.8 mm) GIA cartridge(s) is used to close the stomach. The endoscope, which is usually pulled back into the proximal stomach during the resection, is used to insufflate the stomach in order to evaluate the resection site and gastrostomy closure for bleeding, check the patency of the distal stomach, and to assess the integrity of the gastrostomy closure.

Large or full-thickness tumors in close proximity to the pylorus or those tumors causing gastric outlet obstruction often require a more formal resection (antrectomy and gastrojejunostomy) due to the high probability that a wedge resection will result in the narrowing of the distal stomach causing iatrogenic gastric outlet obstruction [30, 31]. An endoscopic linear stapler is utilized to accomplish the proximal and distal resection. To perform the anastomosis, the ligament of Treitz is located and the jejunal limb is selected approximately 30–40 cm distally. A window in the transverse mesocolon is created to perform a retrocolic anastomosis. Enterotomies are created on the posterior aspect of the stomach and antimesenteric border of the jejunum and the final anastomosis is created with multiple firings of an endoscopic linear stapler. The anastomosis is closed with either an endoscopic stapler or laparoscopic intracorporeal suturing depending on the common enterotomy size and surgeon preference.

3.6 Duodenum

This resection approach as previously described [32] starts with similar abdominal access via the infraumbilical position using an open Hasson technique. The abdomen is insufflated to 15 mmHg with CO_2, and two 5-mm ports are placed, one each in the right upper quadrant and left lateral rectus sheath, with an additional port 12 mm in the right paramedian position in a triangulated fashion. The liver is retracted cephalad and laterally, allowing for the visualization of the first and second portions of the duodenum.

A flexible endoscope is introduced through the oropharynx into the stomach and passage into the pylorus to appropriately visualize the duodenal mass. Endoscopic transillumination with a concomitant injection of methylene blue into the duodenal wall aids in laparoscopic localization of this nonpalpable lesion. Electrosurgical dissection is used to create a duodenotomy at the site of the dye-stained portion. The lesion is elevated through this duodenotomy with similarly described suture elevation alongside the mass to retract the lesion out of its intraluminal location for transected at its base using the Endo-GIA stapler (USSC, Norwalk, Connecticut). The mass is then placed in an extraction bag and removed via the 12-mm trocar site. After excision, the duodenotomy is closed using interrupted 3–0 silk sutures. The endoscope is then passed beyond the duodenotomy closure to perform a leak test at the closure with the assist of the intraluminal insufflation and overlying irrigation intra-abdominally to identify any bubbles demonstrating areas of potential leak. As a final buttress, the omentum is placed over the suture line.

4 Postoperative Care and Follow-Up

Postoperatively, nasogastric tubes can be used and intraoperatively confirmed of appropriate placement. A gastrograffin swallow is performed in the morning of the first postoperative day for selective patients. Diets are advanced as patient tolerates and patients should be discharged home after the resumption of a regular diet. In regards outpatient follow-up, in addition to routine visits at approximately 10 and 30 days after surgery, postoperative follow-up includes physical examination every 3–4 months for the first 3 years, every 6 months for 2 years, and then yearly. For those lesions 3 cm or greater or with higher mitotic indices, a chest radiograph, abdominal computed tomography (CT) scan, and serum chemistries should be obtained at 6 months, 1 year, and then annually for 5 years. Upper endoscopy is performed at approximately 6 months and subsequently 1 year postoperatively with surveillance annually for at least 2 years after resection. A PET scan, MR imaging, and chest CT scan are obtained if abnormalities are found on any of the surveillance studies. All patients should be evaluated with a multidisciplinary approach to be considered by oncology for eligibility in a clinical trial or adjuvant therapy [10].

5 Outcomes

5.1 Laparoscopic

Laparoscopic surgery to resect GISTs has grown in popularity since it was first introduced with published data demonstrating better short-term results and similar long-term outcomes compared to open resection in properly selected patients. Matthews et al. reported that laparoscopic resection was associated with a shorter hospital stay (3.8 days vs. 6.2 days, $P<0.05$) and similar long-term oncologic outcomes for the open and laparoscopic approach [16]. This finding has been corroborated by numerous subsequent studies [5, 8, 33–36], with reports of quicker time to return of bowel function [33, 34], less of a delay for resumption of oral intake [33, 34], lower estimated blood loss [5, 33, 35], and lower overall morbidity for patients undergoing the laparoscopic approach [5, 34, 36]. While there has been tumor sized-matched comparison of the open and laparoscopic technique demonstrating favorability to the laparoscopic approach [35], there is no prospective randomized trial comparing the outcomes of laparoscopic and open resection, which is necessary to strengthen the evidence supporting the use of the laparoscopic technique instead of open resection.

5.2 *Laparoendoscopic*

In 1998, an intraluminal resection of gastric stromal tumors was performed using a laparoendoscopic technique with favorable initial results as the patient was asymptomatic at the 9-month follow-up visit [18]. A follow-up study performed by Walsh et al. reported on 14 gastric stromal tumors excised from 13 patients, with a mean length of stay of 3.8 days and no recurrences at a mean follow-up of 16.2 months [19]. Beyond this series, only single smaller series case reports using the laparoendoscopic technique demonstrate feasibility for GIST tumors located in the duodenum [37], cardia [38], or gastric GIST lesions utilizing laparoendoscopic resection [39, 40].

5.3 *Endoscopic Full-Thickness Resection*

The major concern of complete endoscopic resection is full-thickness mucosal injury causing perforation, thus the use of endoscopic resection is generally restricted to the mucosal and submucosal layers. Recently, submucosal tumors (SMTs) that are closely related to the serosa or reach the muscularis propria have been resected using endoscopic full-thickness resection (EFR). In a study of 26 patients with SMTs of which 16 were stromal tumors, no short-term complications and no recurrence were observed after a mean follow-up time of 8 months [41]. A comparison of 32 patients who underwent EFR with 30 treated laparoscopically observed similar operative time and complication rate as well as no recurrences in either group, demonstrating the potential usefulness of EFR in treating stromal tumors arising from the muscularis propria [42]. Even nonintracavitary stromal tumors have demonstrated feasibility of EFR [43].

5.4 *Robotic-Assisted Resection*

Robotic-assisted resections of GIST lesions, although lacking high-level evidence, have been tried [44–46]. In a case series consisting of five patients, successful resection of tumors in the distal antrum ($n=3$) and in the cardia/gastroesophageal junction ($n=2$) has been demonstrated with one conversion to open and disease-free survival at 18-month postoperatively [44]. Even for tumors >3 cm, GIST lesions have successfully been resected and disease free 1-year postoperatively [45]. Preliminary reports of robotically assisted resection of GISTs are promising, however, only case reports and case series currently exist; thus, more research is required to understand its utility and long-term outcomes.

6 Conclusion

Minimally invasive approaches to GIST compared to open in selective patients have been shown to result in better short-term outcomes and demonstrated of long-term outcomes equivalent to the open approach. The proper technique to use depends on location, size, and preference of the surgeon to perform the technique with which they are most confident. Resection of GIST lesions with a turn toward laparoscopic and laparoendoscopic technique is growing, and current literature is supporting the feasibility and optimistic outcomes for the minimally invasive approach.

References

1. Nishimura J, Nakajima K, Omori T, Takahashi T, Nishitani A, Ito T, Nishida T. Surgical strategy for gastric gastrointestinal stromal tumors: laparoscopic vs. open resection. Surg Endosc. 2007;21(6):875–8. doi:10.1007/s00464-006-9065-z.
2. Pelletier JS, Gill RS, Gazala S, Karmali S. A systematic review and meta-analysis of open vs. Laparoscopic resection of gastric gastrointestinal stromal tumors. J Clin Med Res. 2015;7(5):289–96. doi:10.14740/jocmr1547w.
3. Liao CH, Yeh CN, Wang SY, Fu CY, Tsai CY, Liu YY, Cheng CT, Yeh TS. Surgical option for intestinal gastrointestinal stromal tumors--perioperative and oncological outcomes of laparoscopic surgery. Anticancer Res. 2015;35(2):1033–40.
4. Chen QL, Pan Y, Cai JQ, Wu D, Chen K, Mou YP. Laparoscopic versus open resection for gastric gastrointestinal stromal tumors: an updated systematic review and meta-analysis. World J Surg Oncol. 2014;12:206. doi:10.1186/1477-7819-12-206.
5. Bischof DA, Kim Y, Dodson R, Carolina Jimenez M, Behman R, Cocieru A, Blazer 3rd DG, Fisher SB, Squires 3rd MH, Kooby DA, Maithel SK, Groeschl RT, Clark Gamblin T, Bauer TW, Karanicolas PJ, Law C, Quereshy FA, Pawlik TM. Open versus minimally invasive resection of gastric GIST: a multi-institutional analysis of short- and long-term outcomes. Ann Surg Oncol. 2014;21(9):2941–8. doi:10.1245/s10434-014-3733-3.
6. Fisher SB, Kim SC, Kooby DA, Cardona K, Russell MC, Delman KA, Staley 3rd CA, Maithel SK. Gastrointestinal stromal tumors: a single institution experience of 176 surgical patients. Am Surg. 2013;79(7):657–65.
7. Tabrizian P, Nguyen SQ, Divino CM. Laparoscopic management and longterm outcomes of gastrointestinal stromal tumors. J Am Coll Surg. 2009;208(1):80–6. doi:10.1016/j.jamcollsurg.2008.08.028.

8. Melstrom LG, Phillips JD, Bentrem DJ, Wayne JD. Laparoscopic versus open resection of gastric gastrointestinal stromal tumors. Am J Clin Oncol. 2012;35(5):451–4. doi:10.1097/COC.0b013e31821954a7.
9. Walsh RM, Heniford BT. Laparoendoscopic treatment of gastric stromal tumors. Semin Laparosc Surg. 2001;8(3):189–94.
10. Novitsky YW, Kercher KW, Sing RF, Heniford BT. Long-term outcomes of laparoscopic resection of gastric gastrointestinal stromal tumors. Ann Surg. 2006;243(6):738–45. doi:10.1097/01.sla.0000219739.11758.27; discussion 745–37.
11. Kim HH. Endoscopic treatment for gastrointestinal stromal tumor: advantages and hurdles. World J Gastroint Endoscopy. 2015;7(3):192–205. doi:10.4253/wjge.v7.i3.192.
12. Cheng HL, Lee WJ, Lai IR, Yuan RH, Yu SC. Laparoscopic wedge resection of benign gastric tumor. Hepatogastroenterology. 1999;46(27):2100–4.
13. Kimata M, Kubota T, Otani Y, Ohgami M, Ishikawa Y, Yokoyama T, Issiki S, Abe S, Egawa T, Tokuyama J, Wada N, Kumai K, Kitajima M, Mukai M. Gastrointestinal stromal tumors treated by laparoscopic surgery: report of three cases. Surg Today. 2000;30(2):177–80.
14. Matsui H, Uyama I, Fujita J, Komori Y, Sugioka A, Hasumi A. Gastrointestinal stromal tumor of the stomach successfully treated by laparoscopic proximal gastrectomy with jejunal interposition. Surg Laparosc Endosc Percutan Tech. 2000;10(4):239–42.
15. Tagaya N, Mikami H, Kogure H, Kubota K, Hosoya Y, Nagai H. Laparoscopic intragastric stapled resection of gastric submucosal tumors located near the esophagogastric junction. Surg Endosc. 2002;16(1):177–9. doi:10.1007/s004640080158.
16. Matthews BD, Walsh RM, Kercher KW, Sing RF, Pratt BL, Answini GA, Heniford BT. Laparoscopic vs open resection of gastric stromal tumors. Surg Endosc. 2002;16(5):803–7. doi:10.1007/s00464-001-8319-z.
17. Matthews BD, Joels CS, Kercher KW, Heniford BT. Gastrointestinal stromal tumors of the stomach. Minerva Chir. 2004;59(3):219–31.
18. Heniford BT, Arca MJ, Walsh RM. The mini-laparoscopic intragastric resection of a gastroesophageal stromal tumor: a novel approach. Surg Laparosc Endosc Percutan Tech. 2000; 10(2):82–5.
19. Walsh RM, Ponsky J, Brody F, Matthews BD, Heniford BT. Combined endoscopic/laparoscopic intragastric resection of gastric stromal tumors. J Gastroint Surg Off J Soc Surg Alimentary Tract. 2003;7(3):386–92.
20. Nguyen NT, Jim J, Nguyen A, Lee J, Chang K. Laparoscopic resection of gastric stromal tumor: a tailored approach. Am Surg. 2003;69(11):946–50.
21. Heinrich MC, Corless CL. Gastric GI stromal tumors (GISTs): the role of surgery in the era of targeted therapy. J Surg Oncol. 2005;90(3):195–207. doi:10.1002/jso.20230; discussion 207.
22. Demetri GD, Benjamin R, Blanke CD, Choi H, Corless C, DeMatteo RP, Eisenberg BL, Fletcher CD, Maki RG, Rubin BP, Van den Abbeele AD, von Mehren M, Force NGT. NCCN Task Force report: optimal management of patients with gastrointestinal stromal tumor (GIST)–expansion and update of NCCN clinical practice guidelines. J Natl Compr Cancer Network JNCCN. 2004;2 Suppl 1:S1–26; quiz 27–30.
23. De Vogelaere K, Van Loo I, Peters O, Hoorens A, Haentjens P, Delvaux G. Laparoscopic resection of gastric gastrointestinal stromal tumors (GIST) is safe and effective, irrespective of tumor size. Surg Endosc. 2012;26(8):2339–45. doi:10.1007/s00464-012-2186-7.
24. Mochizuki Y, Kodera Y, Fujiwara M, Ito S, Yamamura Y, Sawaki A, Yamao K, Kato T. Laparoscopic wedge resection for gastrointestinal stromal tumors of the stomach: initial experience. Surg Today. 2006;36(4):341–7. doi:10.1007/s00595-005-3164-7.
25. Nakamori M, Iwahashi M, Nakamura M, Tabuse K, Mori K, Taniguchi K, Aoki Y, Yamaue H. Laparoscopic resection for gastrointestinal stromal tumors of the stomach. Am J Surg. 2008;196(3):425–9. doi:10.1016/j.amjsurg.2007.10.012.
26. Demetri GD, von Mehren M, Antonescu CR, DeMatteo RP, Ganjoo KN, Maki RG, Pisters PW, Raut CP, Riedel RF, Schuetze S, Sundar HM, Trent JC, Wayne JD. NCCN Task Force report: update on the management of patients with gastrointestinal stromal tumors. J Natl Compr Cancer Network JNCCN. 2010;8 Suppl 2:S1–41; quiz S42–44.
27. Appleman HD, Helwig EB. Gastric epithelioid leiomyoma and leiomyosarcoma (leiomyoblastoma). Cancer. 1976;38(2):708–28.

28. DeMatteo RP, Lewis JJ, Leung D, Mudan SS, Woodruff JM, Brennan MF. Two hundred gastrointestinal stromal tumors: recurrence patterns and prognostic factors for survival. Ann Surg. 2000;231(1):51–8.
29. Ohashi S. Laparoscopic intraluminal (intragastric) surgery for early gastric cancer. A new concept in laparoscopic surgery. Surg Endosc. 1995;9(2):169–71.
30. Cuschieri A. Laparoscopic gastric resection. Surg Clin North Am. 2000;80(4):1269–84. viii.
31. Goh PM, Alponat A, Mak K, Kum CK. Early international results of laparoscopic gastrectomies. Surg Endosc. 1997;11(6):650–2.
32. Gersin KS, Heniford BT, Baradi H, Ponsky JL. Laparoendoscopic excision of a duodenal mass. Endoscopy. 1999;31(5):398–400. doi:10.1055/s-1999-25.
33. Zheng L, Ding W, Zhou D, Lu L, Yao L. Laparoscopic versus open resection for gastric gastrointestinal stromal tumors: a meta-analysis. Am Surg. 2014;80(1):48–56.
34. Koh YX, Chok AY, Zheng HL, Tan CS, Chow PK, Wong WK, Goh BK. A systematic review and meta-analysis comparing laparoscopic versus open gastric resections for gastrointestinal stromal tumors of the stomach. Ann Surg Oncol. 2013;20(11):3549–60. doi:10.1245/s10434-013-3051-1.
35. Karakousis GC, Singer S, Zheng J, Gonen M, Coit D, DeMatteo RP, Strong VE. Laparoscopic versus open gastric resections for primary gastrointestinal stromal tumors (GISTs): a size-matched comparison. Ann Surg Oncol. 2011;18(6):1599–605. doi:10.1245/s10434-010-1517-y.
36. Schwameis K, Fochtmann A, Schwameis M, Asari R, Schur S, Kostler W, Birner P, Ba-Ssalamah A, Zacherl J, Wrba F, Brodowicz T, Schoppmann SF. Surgical treatment of GIST–an institutional experience of a high-volume center. Int J Surg (London, England). 2013;11(9):801–6. doi:10.1016/j.ijsu.2013.08.016.
37. Kato M, Nakajima K, Nishida T, Yamasaki M, Nishida T, Tsutsui S, Ogiyama H, Yamamoto S, Yamada T, Mori M, Doki Y, Hayashi N. Local resection by combined laparoendoscopic surgery for duodenal gastrointestinal stromal tumor. Diagn Therap Endosc. 2011;2011:645609. doi:10.1155/2011/645609.
38. Singaporewalla RM, Baladas GH, Lee TD. Laparoendoscopic removal of a benign gastric stromal tumor at the cardia. JSLS J Soc Laparoendosc Surg Soc Laparoendosc Surg. 2006;10(1):117–21.
39. Hirano Y, Watanabe T, Uchida T, Yoshida S, Kato H, Hosokawa O. Laparoendoscopic single site partial resection of the stomach for gastrointestinal stromal tumor. Surg Laparosc Endosc Percutan Tech. 2010;20(4):262–4. doi:10.1097/SLE.0b013e3181e36a5b.
40. Henckens T, Van de Putte D, Van Renterghem K, Ceelen W, Pattyn P, Van Nieuwenhove Y. Laparoendoscopic single-site gastrectomy for a gastric GIST using double-bended instruments. J Laparoendosc Adv Surg Tech A. 2010;20(5):469–71. doi:10.1089/lap.2009.0391.
41. Zhou PH, Yao LQ, Qin XY, Cai MY, Xu MD, Zhong YS, Chen WF, Zhang YQ, Qin WZ, Hu JW, Liu JZ. Endoscopic full-thickness resection without laparoscopic assistance for gastric submucosal tumors originated from the muscularis propria. Surg Endosc. 2011;25(9):2926–31. doi:10.1007/s00464-011-1644-y.
42. Huang LY, Cui J, Wu CR, Zhang B, Jiang LX, Xian XS, Lin SJ, Xu N, Cao XL, Wang ZH. Endoscopic full-thickness resection and laparoscopic surgery for treatment of gastric stromal tumors. World J Gastroenterol WJG. 2014;20(25):8253–9. doi:10.3748/wjg.v20.i25.8253.
43. Wang L, Ren W, Fan CQ, Li YH, Zhang X, Yu J, Zhao GC, Zhao XY. Full-thickness endoscopic resection of nonintracavitary gastric stromal tumors: a novel approach. Surg Endosc. 2011;25(2):641–7. doi:10.1007/s00464-010-1189-5.
44. Buchs NC, Bucher P, Pugin F, Hagen ME, Morel P. Robot-assisted oncologic resection for large gastric gastrointestinal stromal tumor: a preliminary case series. J Laparoendosc Adv Surg Tech A. 2010;20(5):411–5. doi:10.1089/lap.2009.0385.
45. Moriyama H, Ishikawa N, Kawaguchi M, Hirose K, Watanabe G. Robot-assisted laparoscopic resection for gastric gastrointestinal stromal tumor. Surg Laparosc Endosc Percutan Tech. 2012;22(3):e155–6. doi:10.1097/SLE.0b013e3182491ff6.
46. Ortiz-Oshiro E, Exposito PB, Sierra JM, Gonzalez JD, Barbosa DS, Fernandez-Represa JA. Laparoscopic and robotic distal gastrectomy for gastrointestinal stromal tumour: case report. Int J Med Robot Computer Aassist Surg MRCAS. 2012;8(4):491–5. doi:10.1002/rcs.1456.

Neoadjuvant Therapy and Surgical Consolidation for Localized Gastrointestinal Stromal Tumors

W.W. Tseng, S. Chopra, E. Jung, and B.L. Eisenberg

1 Introduction

The standard treatment for localized gastrointestinal stromal tumor (GIST) is the complete surgical resection with histologically negative margins [1]. In fact, patients in whom complete resection is achieved have up to a threefold improvement in survival compared to those with unresectable disease. Overall, at initial presentation, the majority of patients (70–80 %) have disease that is amenable to resection; however, a substantial subset of patients will have disease that is locally advanced and either borderline resectable, often with substantial morbidity, or unresectable.

GISTs are characterized by the expression of KIT, a transmembrane receptor tyrosine kinase encoded by the c-kit proto-oncogene and recognized by an immunohistochemical stain for CD117.

Approximately 75 % of GISTs harbor a KIT gene mutation, and these mutations lead to constitutive activation of the kinase. Two-thirds of GISTs harbor mutations in exon 11 while approximately 10 % of GISTs have a mutation in an extracellular domain encoded by exon 9. Other mutations (exon 17, 13, and PDGFR-alpha) are also known to exist and are discussed in more detail elsewhere.

W.W. Tseng • B.L. Eisenberg (✉)
Department of Surgery, Keck School of Medicine, University of Southern California, Los Angeles, CA, USA

Hoag Family Cancer Institute, Hoag Memorial Presbyterian Hospital, Newport Beach, CA, USA
e-mail: Burton.eisenberg@hoag.org

S. Chopra
Department of Pathology, Keck School of Medicine, University of Southern California, Los Angeles, CA, USA

E. Jung
Department of Surgery, Keck School of Medicine, University of Southern California, Los Angeles, CA, USA

© Springer International Publishing Switzerland 2017

C.R. Scoggins et al. (eds.), *Gastrointestinal Stromal Tumors*,
DOI 10.1007/978-3-319-42632-7_11

KIT inhibition by the oral drug imatinib is highly effective for the treatment of most GISTs. By histologic examination, responsive GISTs typically show dramatically decreased cellularity and stromal changes, including marked hyalinization and even myxoid features. Similarly, by cross-sectional imaging, responsive GISTs frequently demonstrate measurable tumor shrinkage. In fact, in the landmark study of imatinib treatment in GIST by Demetri et al., significant tumor shrinkage (=clinical benefit) was noted in more than half of all patients [2]. The ability to shrink tumors with imatinib, even partially, may be highly beneficial in the subset of patients with locally advanced disease.

This chapter will discuss the available data for the use of imatinib in the preoperative or neoadjuvant setting, followed by surgical resection. This strategy is applicable to patients with locally advanced GIST arising from the stomach (most common site, 60–70 %), but may also be particularly relevant to those with GIST arising from the esophagus, duodenum, and rectum (5 % each), in which complete resection may be associated with a high morbidity. As we will highlight, there is good evidence to support the use of neoadjuvant imatinib for locally advanced disease; however, the true efficacy needs to be confirmed in larger, prospective multicenter trials. Moreover, the use of neoadjuvant imatinib raises several issues that warrant further investigation.

2 Benefits of Neoadjuvant Therapy

Neoadjuvant therapy has many advantages in the treatment of solid cancers, including GIST. As discussed, the delivery of therapy to an intact tumor prior to surgery may potentially shrink the tumor to facilitate complete resection as well as promote a decrease in vascular and friability enabling less morbid resection. Neoadjuvant therapy can also be used to theoretically eliminate, upfront, potential local and distant microscopic disease. For systemic therapies such as imatinib, neoadjuvant delivery also offers the unique opportunity to assess in situ tumor sensitivity to drug, which can help guide future treatment decision making (e.g., in the setting of recurrence).

3 Retrospective Data for Neoadjuvant Imatinib in GIST

The first reports of the use of preoperative imatinib for GIST patients were in small retrospective series that included patients with locally advanced primary disease as well as those with recurrent, multifocal, and metastatic disease. Andtbacka et al. reported on 46 patients who underwent surgery after the receipt of imatinib (400 mg daily) [3]. Among these patients, only 11 had primary disease. After receiving imatinib for a median duration of 11.9 months, eight of these patients (73 %) had at least partial tumor response, including one with complete tumor response. All patients received complete resection and were found to be free of disease at a median follow-up of 19.5 months. Raut et al. and Mearadji et al. also described their series of patients who had surgery after imatinib; however, the actual number of patients with localized, primary disease was smaller [4, 5].

Fiore et al. reported on 15 patients with GIST who received neoadjuvant imatinib [6]. After a median duration of treatment of 9 months, all patients had some degree of tumor shrinkage with 1 complete response and 11 with partial response (12/15 = 80 % objective response rate by RECIST criteria). In addition, all patients had morphologic response as assessed by the change in tumor necrosis and density by cross-sectional imaging (Choi criteria [7]). The authors reported that all patients had an improvement in their originally planned procedure, including four patients who were initially deemed high risk for tumor rupture and hemorrhage. These events did not occur, the authors imply, as a result of neoadjuvant treatment with imatinib.

The benefits of neoadjuvant imatinib in GIST continue to be supported by more recent retrospective studies. Tielen et al. reported the largest series to date, to our knowledge, which encompassed 57 patients with locally advanced, nonmetastatic GIST from four centers in the Netherlands [8]. Patients received imatinib for a median of 8 months prior to surgery. Median tumor size decreased from 12.2 to 6.2 cm after neoadjuvant treatment. Complete resection was achieved in 84 % of these patients many of whom were initially deemed unresectable. Interestingly, however, 14 patients still required multiorgan resection to achieve complete resection. In their discussion, the authors noted that "a less extensive resection rate was not clearly demonstrated" in this study.

4 Prospective Data for Neoadjuvant Imatinib in GIST

McAuliffe et al. reported data for a small, single institution (MD Anderson Cancer Center) phase 2 study of 19 patients with GIST in which the goal was to evaluate the safety as well as pathologic and radiologic response [9]. In the neoadjuvant setting, patients received only three doses of imatinib (600 mg daily) at days 7, 5, and 3 prior to surgery. The authors found that with this regimen, there was no difference in surgical morbidity compared to historical controls. Response as assessed by tumor cell apoptosis on histologic examination and tumor shrinkage/metabolic change on CT and PET scan was seen in 69 % and 71 % of patients, respectively. These responses were seen early, within the first week prior to surgery.

To date, the RTOG 0132/ACRIN 6665 is the largest reported multicenter phase 2 study of neoadjuvant imatinib in GIST. In this study, conducted from 2002 to 2006, patients received neoadjuvant imatinib (600 mg daily) for 8–12 weeks. After treatment, patients with disease progression came off protocol, whereas those with stable disease or better (e.g., partial response) went on to resection. After surgery, patients also continued to receive imatinib (400 mg daily) for 2 years. In total, 63 patients were enrolled into two groups, one of which consisted of 30 patients with locally advanced, primary GIST. Eligibility criteria for these patients with primary disease included tumor size ≥5 cm; in fact, median tumor size was 9 cm. Interestingly, in contrast to the data from the retrospective studies, only 7 % had objective response (all partial response) within 8–12 weeks by strict RECIST criteria (Figs. 1 and 2). Complete resection was achieved in 77 % of patients. In the initial report by Eisenberg et al., 2-year progression-free survival (PFS) was 83 % and 2-year overall survival (OS) was 93 % [10]. More recently, Wang et al. reported long-term outcomes of this study with a median follow-up of 5.1 years [11]. The authors found that 5-year PFS was 57 % and 5-year OS was 77 %. Interestingly, the updated data seem to suggest that a high percentage of

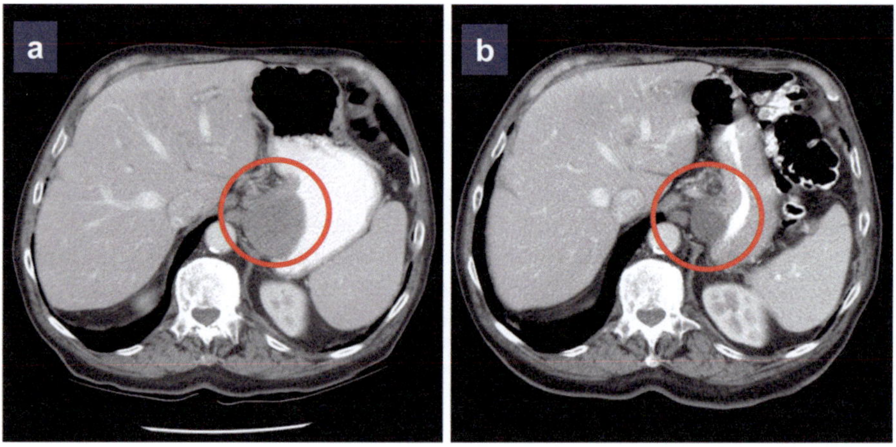

Fig. 1 CT scans in a patient with gastroesophageal junction GIST (*red circle*) before (**a**) and after (**b**) 3 months of neoadjuvant imatinib, showing partial response

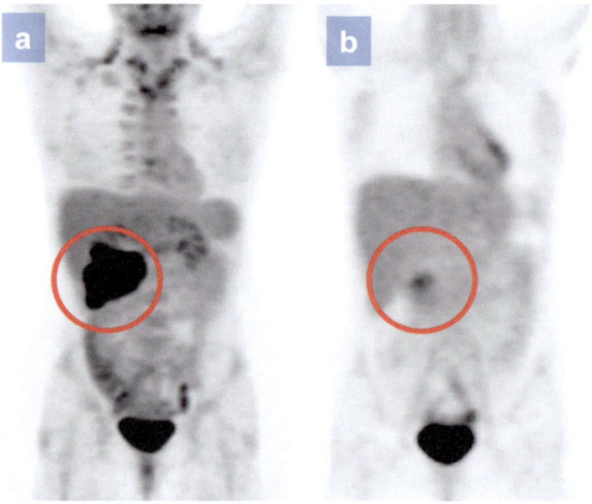

Fig. 2 PET scans in a patient with duodenal GIST (*red circle*) before (**a**) and after (**b**) 1 month of neoadjuvant imatinib, showing decrease in tumor size and metabolic response

patients experience disease progression only after the 2-year discontinuation of imatinib in the postoperative or adjuvant setting.

Currently, there is one ongoing prospective multicenter phase 2 study, the CST1571-BDE43 or APOLLON study. In this trial, patients receive imatinib (400 mg daily) for 6 months, and, similar to the RTOG study, those with either stable disease or better undergo surgical resection. In contrast to the RTOG study, however, adjuvant imatinib is not part of the study protocol. The final results of the APOLLON study have not yet been formally reported.

To date, there are no active or planned phase 3 studies of neoadjuvant imatinib for GIST, to our knowledge. Of note, however, Blesius et al. performed a retrospective subgroup analysis of patients with only localized, nonrecurrent, nonmetastatic disease who received imatinib as part of the larger, prospective phase 3 trial, BFR14 (interruption versus continuation of imatinib after 1 year of treatment) [12]. In this subgroup of 25 patients (434 total for the trial), 15 (60 %) had partial response to imatinib after a median 7.3 months of treatment; however, only nine of these patients (36 %) underwent surgical resection after imatinib. As expected, patients who had surgery had better PFS and OS; in fact, survival rates for patients with localized disease who did not undergo surgery were similar to those with metastatic disease.

5 Specific Anatomic Site: Esophagus, Duodenum, and Rectum

In the previously discussed studies, at least half, if not the majority, of patients had GIST of stomach origin. At the more rare sites, esophagus, duodenum, and rectum, the ability to achieve complete resection is made more challenging by anatomic constraints, resulting in potentially morbid operations. In the esophagus, esophagectomy is frequently needed, which requires entry into the abdomen, chest, and in most cases, the neck. In the duodenum, depending on the tumor location and the extent of involvement, pancreaticoduodenectomy (Whipple procedure) may be needed. In the rectum, tumors may require abdominoperineal resection, which removes the anal sphincter and involves the creation of a permanent colostomy. For GIST at these specific anatomic sites, neoadjuvant imatinib is an attractive strategy to enable complete and potentially less morbid resection (e.g., sphincter-preserving excision in the rectum).

For esophageal GIST, case reports of neoadjuvant imatinib have been published [13–15]. In the majority of these studies and depending upon the author's clinical judgment, patients still required esophagectomy. However, the benefit of neoadjuvant treatment in these studies seemed to be in converting patients from unresectable to resectable and preventing tumor rupture for large, bulky tumors.

Marano et al. recently reviewed the literature for duodenal GIST [16]. These tumors actually appear to have a better overall prognosis compared to GIST at other gastrointestinal tract sites, including the stomach. The authors point out that duodenal GIST, despite their location, typically displace rather than invade surrounding structures. Tumors tend to grow opposite the duodenal lumen and toward the abdominal cavity. In support of this concept, Colombo et al. reported data from a multi-institutional cohort of patients with duodenal GIST and found that the type of resection (conservative duodenal resection versus Whipple) does not impact the clinical outcome [17]. In this series, 11 patients actually received neoadjuvant imatinib (400 mg daily) for a median of 8 months. Similar to other retrospective data, nine of these patients (80 %) demonstrated objective response. In 6 of the 11 patients (55 %), pancreaticoduodenectomy was avoided and conservative resection was feasible.

For rectal GIST, several case reports and small case series have shown that neoadjuvant GIST can indeed downsize tumors to allow for sphincter-preserving surgery. Jakob et al. described 39 patients with rectal GIST of which 16 received neoadjuvant imatinib [18]. The authors found a higher rate of margin-negative complete resection in those who received neoadjuvant therapy compared to those who did not. Tielen et al. also had similar findings with 12 rectal GIST patients who received neoadjuvant imatinib, although five patients still required abdominoperineal resection and two patients required posterior exenteration, an even more extensive operation [8].

6 Consensus Guidelines

In part as a result of some of the data discussed, consensus guidelines do recognize the potential value of neoadjuvant imatinib in the management of locally advanced GIST. The European Society of Medical Oncology (2010) recommends preoperative imatinib as a treatment option if this results in “less mutilating surgery and lower risk of tumor bleeding/rupture” [19]. The National Comprehensive Cancer Network (NCCN, STS Guidelines 1.2015) recommends neoadjuvant imatinib in patients with resectable GIST but with the risk of significant morbidity. This includes patients who may require multivisceral resection or abdominoperineal resection due to locally advanced disease. Interestingly, these guidelines also suggest that if these patients have disease progression, surgery should be considered for salvage, if feasible.

7 Risk of Resistance and Other Histologic Changes with Imatinib

It is important to note that the tumor response to imatinib is rarely complete. By cross-sectional imaging, imatinib rarely results in complete tumor regression with no measurable disease. Similarly, under the microscope, histologic response to imatinib rarely induces complete necrosis without any viable tumor cells. In fact, tumor response by histology is frequently quite variable even at different components within the same tumor, ranging from 10 to 90 % reduction in tumor cellularity [20, 21].

The presence of any residual, viable tumor cells after prolonged imatinib treatment implies the possible risk of development of resistant clones. This was highlighted in a case report by Haller et al. [22]. This patient had initially unresectable GIST, received 10 months of imatinib (400 mg daily) with tumor response followed by surgical resection. Detailed histologic examination of the resected tumor specimen identified multiple remnant tumor microfoci, each measuring less than 0.3 cm. Surprisingly, in comparison to the KIT mutation status on the pre-imatinib biopsy, analysis of the resected tumor specimen identified the additional new point mutations.

The potential detrimental effect of prolonged neoadjuvant imatinib was shown recently in a study by Bednarski et al. [23] This retrospective review of patients included 41 patients with locally advanced, primary GIST who had undergone preoperative imatinib for a median duration of 315 days (10.5 months) prior to surgical resection. In this group of patients, neoadjuvant therapy greater than 365 days (12 months) was associated with a higher risk of recurrence.

Interestingly, GIST treated with imatinib can also exhibit a variety of other histologic changes. Although GISTs are more commonly spindle shaped, treated tumors may develop a purely epithelioid morphology and even a tubulopapillary growth pattern [24]. The expression of CD117 may also be reduced or even lost after treatment, a characteristic found to be associated with disease recurrence by Mearadji et al. These CD117-negative GISTs include high-grade, anaplastic sarcomas, which have been observed in both imatinib-treated and treatment-naïve tumors [25]. In rare cases, imatinib treatment may also result in the development of other histologic lineages within the tumor, including rhabdomyoblastic, cartilaginous, and osseous transdifferentiation [26, 27]. The clinical significance of transdifferentiation in imatinib-treated GIST is currently unknown.

8 Conclusion and Future Directions

Complete surgical resection is the goal of treatment for patients with localized primary GIST. In the subset of patients with locally advanced, borderline resectable or unresectable tumors, the ability of imatinib to induce measurable tumor shrinkage may offer the renewed opportunity to achieve complete resection. In support of this, several retrospective studies seem to suggest a high rate of objective response (70–80 %), allowing for resection in these patients and in many cases less morbid and function-sparing surgery (e.g., rectal GIST). Prospective studies such as the RTOG 0132/ACRIN 6665 also support the use of neoadjuvant imatinib, however, the data are not as robust. The results of the CST1571-BDE43 or APOLLON trial will hopefully provide more data to further assess the efficacy of neoadjuvant imatinib.

Several issues arise regarding the use of neoadjuvant imatinib in locally advanced, primary GIST. First, selection of appropriate candidates should be better defined.

An important component of this decision should be tumor genotyping, including mutation status. Tumors with a KIT exon 9 mutation will be more sensitive to a higher dose of imatinib (800 mg) [28]; tumors with a PDGFR-alpha mutation in D842V (exon 18) will likely be resistant to imatinib [29, 30]. Second, a key question is the appropriate duration of imatinib therapy to capture the window of opportunity between maximal tumor response and disease progression or development of resistance. Gold and DeMatteo proposed surgery within 6 months of therapy [31] and based on the data from Bednarski et al., this should certainly be not more than 12 months [23]. We advocate that in all cases, this decision to discontinue neoadjuvant treatment for surgery should be personalized to the individual patient and made in the setting of a multidisciplinary discussion (e.g., radiologist, medical oncologist, surgical oncologist). Third, adequate biomarkers of response are lacking. Metabolic response, as measured by decrease in FDG avidity by PET, has been explored by Goh et al. and Van den Abbeele et al. with somewhat conflicting results [32, 33]. We would favor other response biomarkers, including histologic and even molecular (e.g., GLUT4) [33]. Fourth, the efficacy of other targeted therapies (e.g., sunitinib, regorafenib) should be explored in the neoadjuvant setting, especially for patients who have tumors with evidence of imatinib resistance. We also support investigation of combination therapies and inclusion of novel therapies (e.g., immunotherapy) in the neoadjuvant setting.

In conclusion, in patients with locally, advanced primary GIST, neoadjuvant imatinib is a promising treatment option, which may allow complete resection in an otherwise unresectable or potentially morbid situation. Further investigation is needed to resolve the important issues involved with this treatment option.

References

1. Eisenberg BL, Trent JC. Adjuvant and neoadjuvant imatinib therapy: current role in the management of gastrointestinal stromal tumors. Int J Cancer. 2011;129:2533–42.
2. Demetri GD, von Mehren M, Blanke CD, et al. Efficacy and safety of imatinib mesylate in advanced gastrointestinal stromal tumors. N Engl J Med. 2002;347:472–80.
3. Andtbacka RH, Ng CS, Scaife CL, et al. Surgical resection of gastrointestinal stromal tumors after treatment with imatinib. Ann Surg Oncol. 2007;14:14–24.
4. Raut CP, Posner M, Desai J, et al. Surgical management of advanced gastrointestinal stromal tumors after treatment with targeted systemic therapy using kinase inhibitors. J Clin Oncol. 2006;24:2325–31.
5. Mearadji A, den Bakker MA, van Geel AN, et al. Decrease of CD117 expression as possible prognostic marker for recurrence in the resected specimen after imatinib treatment in patients with initially unresectable gastrointestinal stromal tumors: a clinicopathological analysis. Anticancer Drugs. 2008;19:607–12.
6. Fiore M, Palassini E, Fumagalli E, et al. Preoperative imatinib mesylate for unresectable or locally advanced primary gastrointestinal stromal tumors (GIST). Eur J Surg Oncol. 2009;35:739–45.
7. Choi H, Charnsangavej C, Faria SC, et al. Correlation of computed tomography and positron emission tomography in patients with metastatic gastrointestinal stromal tumor treated at a single institution with imatinib mesylate: proposal of new computed tomography response criteria. J Clin Oncol. 2007;25:1753–9.

8. Tielen R, Verhoef C, van Coevorden F, et al. Surgical treatment of locally advanced, non-metastatic, gastrointestinal stromal tumours after treatment with imatinib. Eur J Surg Oncol. 2013;39:150–5.
9. McAuliffe JC, Hunt KK, Lazar AJ, et al. A randomized, phase II study of preoperative plus postoperative imatinib in GIST: evidence of rapid radiographic response and temporal induction of tumor cell apoptosis. Ann Surg Oncol. 2009;16:910–9.
10. Eisenberg BL, Harris J, Blanke CD, et al. Phase II trial of neoadjuvant/adjuvant imatinib mesylate (IM) for advanced primary and metastatic/recurrent operable gastrointestinal stromal tumor (GIST): early results of RTOG 0132/ACRIN 6665. J Surg Oncol. 2009;99:42–7.
11. Wang D, Zhang Q, Blanke CD, et al. Phase II trial of neoadjuvant/adjuvant imatinib mesylate for advanced primary and metastatic/recurrent operable gastrointestinal stromal tumors: long-term follow-up results of Radiation Therapy Oncology Group 0132. Ann Surg Oncol. 2012;19:1074–80.
12. Blesius A, Cassier PA, Bertucci F, et al. Neoadjuvant imatinib in patients with locally advanced non metastatic GIST in the prospective BFR14 trial. BMC Cancer. 2011;11:72.
13. Neofytou K, Costa Neves M, Giakoustidis A, et al. Effective downsizing of a large oesophageal gastrointestinal stromal tumour with neoadjuvant imatinib enabling an uncomplicated and without tumour rupture laparoscopic-assisted Ivor-Lewis oesophagectomy. Case Rep Oncol Med. 2015;2015:165736.
14. Yanagawa S, Tanabe K, Suzuki T, et al. A large esophageal gastrointestinal stromal tumor that was successfully resected after neoadjuvant imatinib treatment: case report. World J Surg Oncol. 2014;12:47.
15. Staiger WI, Ronellenfitsch U, Kaehler G, et al. The Merendino procedure following preoperative imatinib mesylate for locally advanced gastrointestinal stromal tumor of the esophagogastric junction. World J Surg Oncol. 2008;6:37.
16. Marano L, Boccardi V, Marrelli D, Roviello F. Duodenal gastrointestinal stromal tumor: from clinicopathological features to surgical outcomes. Eur J Surg Oncol. 2015;41:814–22.
17. Colombo C, Ronellenfitsch U, Yuxin Z, et al. Clinical, pathological and surgical characteristics of duodenal gastrointestinal stromal tumor and their influence on survival: a multi-center study. Ann Surg Oncol. 2012;19:3361–7.
18. Jakob J, Mussi C, Ronellenfitsch U, et al. Gastrointestinal stromal tumor of the rectum: results of surgical and multimodality therapy in the era of imatinib. Ann Surg Oncol. 2013;20:586–92.
19. Casali PG, Blay JY. Experts ECECPo: Gastrointestinal stromal tumours: ESMO Clinical Practice Guidelines for diagnosis, treatment and follow-up. Ann Oncol. 2010;21 Suppl 5:v98–102.
20. Loughrey MB, Mitchell C, Mann GB, et al. Gastrointestinal stromal tumour treated with neoadjuvant imatinib. J Clin Pathol. 2005;58:779–81.
21. Agaram NP, Besmer P, Wong GC, et al. Pathologic and molecular heterogeneity in imatinib-stable or imatinib-responsive gastrointestinal stromal tumors. Clin Cancer Res. 2007;13:170–81.
22. Haller F, Detken S, Schulten HJ, et al. Surgical management after neoadjuvant imatinib therapy in gastrointestinal stromal tumours (GISTs) with respect to imatinib resistance caused by secondary KIT mutations. Ann Surg Oncol. 2007;14:526–32.
23. Bednarski BK, Araujo DM, Yi M, et al. Analysis of prognostic factors impacting oncologic outcomes after neoadjuvant tyrosine kinase inhibitor therapy for gastrointestinal stromal tumors. Ann Surg Oncol. 2014;21:2499–505.
24. Pauwels P, Debiec-Rychter M, Stul M, et al. Changing phenotype of gastrointestinal stromal tumours under imatinib mesylate treatment: a potential diagnostic pitfall. Histopathology. 2005;47:41–7.
25. Antonescu CR, Romeo S, Zhang L, et al. Dedifferentiation in gastrointestinal stromal tumor to an anaplastic KIT-negative phenotype: a diagnostic pitfall: morphologic and molecular characterization of 8 cases occurring either de novo or after imatinib therapy. Am J Surg Pathol. 2013;37:385–92.

26. Liegl B, Hornick JL, Antonescu CR, et al. Rhabdomyosarcomatous differentiation in gastrointestinal stromal tumors after tyrosine kinase inhibitor therapy: a novel form of tumor progression. Am J Surg Pathol. 2009;33:218–26.
27. Corless CL. Gastrointestinal stromal tumors: what do we know now? Mod Pathol. 2014;27 Suppl 1:S1–16.
28. Gastrointestinal Stromal Tumor Meta-Analysis Group (MetaGIST). (MetaGIST) GSTM-AG: Comparison of two doses of imatinib for the treatment of unresectable or metastatic gastrointestinal stromal tumors: a meta-analysis of 1,640 patients. J Clin Oncol. 2010;28:1247–53.
29. Corless CL, Schroeder A, Griffith D, et al. PDGFRA mutations in gastrointestinal stromal tumors: frequency, spectrum and in vitro sensitivity to imatinib. J Clin Oncol. 2005;23:5357–64.
30. Weisberg E, Wright RD, Jiang J, et al. Effects of PKC412, nilotinib, and imatinib against GIST-associated PDGFRA mutants with differential imatinib sensitivity. Gastroenterology. 2006;131:1734–42.
31. Gold JS, Dematteo RP. Neoadjuvant therapy for gastrointestinal stromal tumor (GIST): racing against resistance. Ann Surg Oncol. 2007;14:1247–8.
32. Goh BK, Chow PK, Chuah KL, et al. Pathologic, radiologic and PET scan response of gastrointestinal stromal tumors after neoadjuvant treatment with imatinib mesylate. Eur J Surg Oncol. 2006;32:961–3.
33. Van den Abbeele AD, Gatsonis C, de Vries DJ, et al. ACRIN 6665/RTOG 0132 phase II trial of neoadjuvant imatinib mesylate for operable malignant gastrointestinal stromal tumor: monitoring with 18F-FDG PET and correlation with genotype and GLUT4 expression. J Nucl Med. 2012;53:567–74.

Part II
Advanced Disease

Prognostic Factors for Advanced GIST

Christian F. Meyer

1 Clinicopathologic Prognostic Factors

Prior to immunohistochemical identification of gastrointestinal stromal tumors (GISTs) utilizing CD117 and CD34 [1], many surgical reviews analyzing prognostic factors of gastrointestinal sarcomas included leiomyosarcomas in retrospective series that stretched over long periods of time [9–12]. In 2000, a retrospective analysis of GIST analyzed a 200 patient cohort at a single institution [8]. This cohort mixed primary, recurrent, and metastatic patients. Forty-seven percent of the patients presented with metastatic disease. Overall survival (OS) for those with metastatic disease was 19 months. One hundred fourteen of the 200 patients had surgery including 28 patients with metastatic disease. Multivariate analysis revealed that male sex, tumor size (>5 cm), and incomplete or unresectable tumors were poor prognostic signs. Although this analysis did not differentiate prognostic factors among the cohorts, it established a baseline representation of median overall survival in metastatic disease.

This baseline analysis of prognostic factors was further refined in the subsequent publication of several clinical trials of advanced and metastatic GIST patients. The B2222 trial, a phase II trial of advanced GIST patients treated with either 400 or 600 mg of imatinib daily, produced a clinical benefit (complete and partial response plus stable disease) in 80 % of the patients at a median follow-up of 24 weeks [13]. Given the initial robust response, a 4-year extension study and analysis was performed [7]. Of the initial 147 patients on the study, 56 of them were in the extended analysis with 46 of them taking imatinib for 5 years and 41 on treatment at the time of data analysis. With this longer follow-up, the clinical

C.F. Meyer, MD, PhD
Medical Oncology, Sidney Kimmel Cancer Center Johns Hopkins,
1650 Orleans Street, CRB1 G89, Baltimore, MD, USA
e-mail: cmeyer13@jhmi.edu

© Springer International Publishing Switzerland 2017

C.R. Scoggins et al. (eds.), *Gastrointestinal Stromal Tumors*,
DOI 10.1007/978-3-319-42632-7_12

benefit rate was 83.7 %. Multivariate analysis of prognostic factors indicated worse outcomes for males, hypoalbuminemia (<3 g/dL), and patients with absolute neutrophil counts $>4.5 \times 10^9$/L.

Two large phase III clinical trials in metastatic GIST and their subsequent meta-analysis also supported and extended these results [6, 14, 15]. The S0033 trial enrolled 746 patients who received imatinib either 400 mg daily or twice daily. Statistically significant worse prognostic factors identified by multivariate analysis included older age, poorer eastern cooperative oncology group (ECOG) performance status [2, 3], male sex, high absolute neutrophil counts (ANCs), and a low albumin (<3.5 g/dL) [15].

Early clinical trials of metastatic GIST noted that a small cohort of patients exhibited initial resistance to imatinib as defined as occurring in the first 3 months [13, 16]. The phase III trial run by the European Organization for Research and Treatment of Cancer, Italian Sarcoma Group and Australian Gastrointestinal Trials Group (EORTC-ISG-AGITG) 62005 identified prognostic factors in these initial and late resistance groups. Multivariate analysis revealed that lung but not liver metastases, a low hemoglobin level (<7 mmol/L), and a high granulocyte count characterized worse prognosis in the 116 patients with initial resistance to imatinib, while the 818 late resistance patients had a high baseline granulocyte count ($>5.1 \times 10^9$/L), a larger tumor size (>12 cm), a 400-mg imatinib dose, and nongastric primary GIST [17]. The meta-GIST analysis combined both of these phase III trials identifying seven adverse prognostic factors for OS: hypoalbuminemia, male sex, larger tumor size, high ANC, older age, prior chemotherapy, and poor ECOG performance status [14]. A recent analysis of the EORTC-ISG-AGITG 62005 developed a nomogram for OS at 3 years on those patients who had KIT and platelet-derived growth factor receptor A (PDGFRA) genotyping available [18]. Five predictors for OS in this subset were identified: mitotic count per 50 high-powered fields (HPF) of the primary tumor, hemoglobin concentration, and ANC at the start of imatinib treatment, diameter of the largest metastasis, and tumor genotype. The nomogram was validated in a large data set of 236 patients spread over six international GIST referral centers and helped identify high-, intermediate-, and low-risk groups.

2 Treatment Prognostic Factors

2.1 *Tyrosine Kinase Inhibitors*

2.1.1 Imatinib Dose

The use of imatinib itself, though never formally compared to traditional chemotherapy in a randomized trial, clearly improves median overall survival. Previous traditional regimens performed poorly with one multiagent regimen having a median overall survival (OS) of 16.7 months [5]. In the EORTC-ISG-ATIGT 62005 study, a comparison between the two imatinib doses and historical controls from the

EORTC database of GIST patients treated with doxorubicin revealed an approximate 10-month median OS with doxorubicin compared to a median OS that was not reached with both imatinib doses out to 30 months [6].

The dose of imatinib chosen can affect progression-free survival (PFS), but not OS in GIST patients. The initial phase I study of imatinib established a mean tolerated dose (MTD) of 400 mg twice daily (BID) with 82 % of the patients achieving a clinical benefit [16, 19]. Early phase clinical trials established a dose range of imatinib from 400 mg or 600 mg daily to 400 mg twice per day [13, 19]. The B2222 trial noted no difference in OS between the 400 and 600 mg daily dosing with a median overall survival of 57 months [7]. Further planning led to two separate phase III clinical trials testing 400 mg daily vs. 400 mg twice a day [15, 17] with a preplanned meta-analysis of these two trials, meta-GIST [14]. The S0033 trial did not find an OS difference between 400 mg daily and twice per day with a median survival of 55 or 51 months, respectively. The EORTC-ISG-ASG 62005 study tested progression-free survival (PFS) at those same doses and initially found a PFS benefit for the high-dose arm with the late resistance data favoring better outcomes with high-dose imatinib for small bowel GISTs. However, further analysis at a median follow-up of 40 months revealed no difference in PFS or OS. The meta-GIST analysis confirmed the findings showing no difference in OS between the high dose (800 mg) and standard dose (400 mg) arms.

Imatinib resistance in metastatic patients develops in approximately 20 months. Questions arose regarding an interrupted treatment strategy as a means of prolonging the duration of effectiveness and reducing resistance in advanced patients on imatinib. The French Sarcoma Group tested this hypothesis in the multicenter BRF14 trial interrupting treatment in a subset of patients after 1, 3, or 5 years of imatinib therapy. Fifty-eight patients were randomized between continuation ($n=26$) and interruption ($n=32$) groups after 1 year yielding progression in 26 of the 32 in the interruption group [20]. In the 3-year cohort, interruption led to a 2-year PFS of 16 % and in the 5-year cohort progression after 1 year of follow-up in 5 of the 11 patients [21, 22]. Analysis of the 1- and 3-year cohorts demonstrated that reintroduction of imatinib produced tumor control and similar mean times to secondary resistance without a difference in OS between continuation and interruption groups [20, 21]. Longer follow-up of the 71 patients with documented progressive disease (PD) who had interrupted and restarted therapy was carried out. Rechallenge with imatinib resulted in better PFS in those patients with longer imatinib-free intervals as well as those with a complete response (CR). However, this exploratory analysis was not powered to determine effects of OS [23]. Given the poor PFS with imatinib interruption, this is not recommended in metastatic patients stable on imatinib therapy.

2.1.2 Imatinib Trough Levels (C_{min})

Imatinib has excellent oral bioavailability and a 20-h half-life with 400 mg achieving expected pharmacodynamic effects [24, 25]. However, as indicated above in the EORTC-ISG-ASG 62005 study of metastatic GIST patients, dosing of imatinib influenced PFS though not OS. Furthermore, interpatient plasma imatinib levels fluctuate greatly [26]. Variability in plasma levels could influence response to therapy. An observational study of 38 GIST patients found that the imatinib-free drug levels (AUC_u) significantly predicted response with an odd ratio (OR) of 2.6 (±1.1) [27]. A pharmacokinetic analysis of imatinib in metastatic patients done on 73 patients from the B2222 study evaluated imatinib C_{min} levels at day 29. Those patients with concentrations below 1,100 ng/mL had reduced clinical benefit as measured by tumor response and time to progression (TTP) though it did not reach statistical significance [28]. C_{min} levels were divided into quartiles (Q) for analysis and those with the lowest C_{min} levels, Q1, had a TTP of 11.3 months compared to 30.6 months for Q2–3 and 33.1 months for Q4. Responders had C_{min} levels of 1,446 ng/mL, while nonresponders were lower at 1,155 ng/mL. To apply C_{min} levels prospectively in a clinical setting, 96 patients with advanced GIST treated were evaluated in an observational study. A C_{min} level of 760 ng/mL predicted statistically significant differences in PFS whether stomach or small bowel in location [29]. Utilization of imatinib trough levels remains an area of active research without a defined role in routine clinical practice.

2.1.3 Sunitinib

After failure of imatinib in metastatic disease, sunitinib and regorafenib are indicated therapies in the second- and third-line setting, respectively [30, 31]. In the pivotal phase III GIST clinical trial of sunitinib, patients were randomized in a 2:1 design to sunitinib or placebo with sunitinib administered in a 4 weeks on, 2 weeks off, 50-mg dose regimen. Sunitinib produced a time to tumor progression (TTP) of 27 weeks compared with 6 weeks for placebo. Final analysis of the trial with conventional statistics revealed no difference between treatment and placebo arms in OS given the crossover design of the trial. However, an exploratory statistical analysis estimated a doubling of OS for sunitinib versus placebo of 73 versus 39 weeks. Multivariate analysis identified tumor size as a prognostic factor in this group of patients [32]. This overall survival endpoint is supported by further analysis of sunitinib in an international treatment-use trial of 1,124 patients, which revealed a similar OS time [33].

2.1.4 Regorafenib, Nilotinib, and Sorafenib

A number of other oral tyrosine kinase inhibitors have been utilized in GIST patients without prognostic factors identified to date. Regorafenib was recently approved in the third-line setting providing a PFS but not OS survival benefit. Further long-term follow-up is needed to determine if an OS benefit emerges [30]. Nilotinib in the third line did not show significant survival advantages in the intention-to-treat population though post hoc subgroup analysis suggested an OS benefit in a true population of patients who had received only two prior tyrosine kinase inhibitors [34].

Given prior earlier potential benefit, nilotinib was also tested as a first-line therapy against imatinib in the ENESTg1 trial. This trial was halted early for futility as it did not match imatinib efficacy [35]. Sorafenib was tested in the second and third line in an early phase trial demonstrating a progression-free survival of 5 months with most having stable disease [36]. Effectiveness was then studied in a larger community cohort of 124 patients. Sorafenib treatment in this third- or fourth-line line setting achieved 6.4 months [37]. Interestingly, a retrospective analysis of 223 GIST patients treated in the third-line setting revealed a PFS of 3.6 months and OS of 9.2 months. Factors associated with poor OS in this analysis were performance status ≥ ECOG 2 and albumin levels <35 g/L. Despite the advanced nature of GIST in these patients, further treatment with other tyrosine kinase inhibitors improved overall survival significantly compared to best supportive care in this study [38].

2.2 *Circulating Factors*

2.2.1 KIT/VEGF

Imatinib targets the KIT and platelet-derived growth factor receptors (PDGFRs), while sunitinib targets several receptors including KIT, fms-like tyrosine kinase-3 receptor (FLT-3), RET, PDGFRs, and the three vascular endothelial growth factor receptor (VEGFR) isoforms. Both therapies have been evaluated for mechanisms of resistance as well as molecular biomarkers for response to therapy. Soluble c-KIT (sKIT) and its ligand, stem cell factor (SCF), are present in the normal serum. sKIT results from proteolytic cleavage from the extracellular membrane and can bind circulating SCF, therefore possibly modulating its signaling [39, 40]. Preclinical data supported a role for sunitinib inhibiting multiple human and xenograft tumor models [41]. Further work supported its inhibition of angiogenesis, promotion of apoptosis in lung cancer and glioblastoma multiforme murine xenograft tumor models, and reduction of metastases in lung xenograft models. Analysis of its angiogenesis effects revealed the inhibition of neovascularization rather than the direct inhibition of existing tumor vasculature [42, 43]. Because sunitinib targets angiogenesis pathways, various VEGF and VEGFR proteins have been studied in clinical trials as potential biomarkers in a number of different cancers. VEGF levels tended to increase while soluble VEGFR-2 (sVEGFR-2), soluble VEGFR-3 (sVEGFR-3), and soluble cKIT (sKIT) levels decreased in renal cell carcinoma, hepatocellular carcinoma, and breast cancer [44–46].

As c-KIT plays a critical role in much of GIST pathogenesis and GISTs characteristically have increased vascularity, GIST trials evaluated these markers in metastatic patients. The B2222 imatinib trial measured VEGF, sKIT, and SCF levels in 66 of the 147 enrolled patients. While increases in SCF, VEGF, and the ratio between SCF and sKIT levels were observed, no prognostic information emerged between responders and nonresponders to imatinib. The analysis was hampered by imatinib's success as there were only nine nonresponders in the population of sera analyzed [47].

These hypothesis-generating findings were subsequently analyzed in three sunitinib trials. In the phase I/II study of sunitinib, sKIT increases correlated with non-responders while decreased sKIT correlated with responders [48, 49]. This was also supported by an open-label continuous daily dosing (CDD) sunitinib trial with an increasing statistical correlation between decreasing sKIT levels and OS [50]. The phase III trial testing sunitinib treatment at 50 mg/day for 4- of 6-week cycles originally showed a reduction of sKIT levels in the treatment arm during the first two cycles, which were a significant predictor of time to progression [51]. However, in the final analysis of this trial, sKIT levels did not correlate with OS. That correlation was found only with sVEGFR-2 baseline values and the sVEGFR-2 cycle 1, day 14 ratio to baseline.

2.2.2 Circulating Tumor Cells

Circulating Plasma DNA

Over the past two decades, novel advances in the direct detection of solid tumors through blood and plasma analysis reached clinical trial testing notably in the monitoring of circulating tumor cells (CTCs) and circulating tumor DNA (ctDNA). Intense interest in these assays as biomarkers has been championed in multiple tumor types as possibly heralding earlier detection of residual disease after surgery, earlier identification of disease resistance, and effectiveness of neoadjuvant or adjuvant therapy long before radiographic detection [52–55]. Hematologic malignancies have shown both diagnostic and clinical values in ctDNA assays in various settings such as acute promyelocytic leukemia (APL), acute lymphoblastic leukemia (ALL), and chronic myelogenous leukemia (CML) [56–58]. Indeed, the detection of minimal residual disease (MRD) in ALL and early molecular response (EMR) in CML serve as strong prognostic markers in patients [59–61].

GISTs are ideal candidates for this analysis given the known mutations, effective targeted therapy, and onset of resistance in metastatic patients. However, the analyses are in the early stages of development. Maier et al. prospectively analyzed 291 plasma samples among 38 patients for ctDNA in a phase IIIb nonintervention trial [62]. Primary tumor samples were sequenced for the identification of candidate mutations and these were then evaluated in plasma samples by allele-specific ligation polymerase chain reaction (L-PCR). Eighteen patients had active disease and 20 had a postsurgical complete response (CR). Nine of the 18 patients with active disease and 6 of 17 postsurgical patients with an increased relapse risk had ctDNA carrying the mutation identified from the primary tumor. Furthermore, those patients with active disease had a high ratio of ctDNA to wild-type DNA. Lastly, they detected increases in ctDNA in patients whose active therapy was failing or in postsurgical CR patients prior to their relapse radiographically as well as decreases in ctDNA in some patients with responses to imatinib or sunitinib.

In the phase III GRID, ctDNA was analyzed by BEAMing technology in 163 baseline samples detecting mutations in approximately 60 % of samples [63].

Importantly, the ctDNA analysis led to detection of secondary kinase mutations in 47 % of the samples as compared to 12 % of the tumor samples. The group with secondary mutations had a shorter PFS than those in the study receiving placebo. This study demonstrated the feasibility and utility of ctDNA sample collection over repetitive tumor biopsies as a means of capturing the development of resistance in GIST.

This approach has been replicated in other studies. Two small case series evaluating three and four GIST patients, respectively, looked at ctDNA in primary and resistant settings in the context of imatinib and sunitinib treatment [64, 65]. They identified both primary and secondary mutations in the ctDNA. A serum biomarker analysis of samples collected from a phase II dovitinib study in TKI-refractory GIST, detected 5 primary and 11 secondary KIT mutations among 30 patients. The absence of secondary mutations in the serum of patients correlated significantly ($P=0.02$) with a better median OS of 9.8 months [66, 67]. A similar study evaluating ponatinib in TKI-resistant GIST found ctDNA in 15 of 23 patients analyzed with associations found between decreased ctDNA and radiographic response [68].

2.3 *Molecular Prognostic Factors*

2.3.1 Mutational Landscape

KIT and PDGFRα are transmembrane receptor tyrosine kinase signaling molecules that play a fundamental role in the pathogenesis of most GISTs. Both c-KIT and PDGFRα signal through receptor homodimerization caused by binding of their ligands, SCF and PDGF, respectively [69, 70]. Gain of function mutations primarily in c-KIT and the PDGFRα drive tumorigenesis in GISTs and are mutually exclusive [2, 3, 71, 72]. The mutations occur in discrete regions of the receptors all of which result in receptor autophosphorylation and ligand-independent signaling. KIT mutations occur most often in exon 9 in the extracellular domain and exon 11 in the juxtamembrane (JM) domain, with decreased mutational frequencies in exons 13 and 17 of the kinase domains. In contrast, PDGFRα mutations occur infrequently in the juxtamembrane domain (exon 12), rarely in the first tyrosine kinase domain (exon 14) and most often in the activation loop of the second kinase domain (exon 18) [2, 71, 73].

The various KIT and PDGFRα mutations described above also correlate with morphology and anatomical location in several studies. KIT exon 11 mutations and PDGFRα exon 18 mutants occur with greatest frequency in gastric GISTs, while KIT exon 9, exon 17, and exon 13 mutations arise more often in GISTs of the small intestine. Exon 11 GISTs tend to have a spindled morphology while those with exon 9 have an epithelioid appearance [70, 71, 74–76]. The landscape of specific GIST mutations is quite broad. Exon 11 mutations tend to cluster at the 5′ end of the juxtamembrane (JM) region and include deletions between codons 550 and 561, missense mutations, point mutations, and internal tandem duplications (ITDs)

[77–80]. Less frequently, ITDs represent three prime JM mutations [81]. Deletion mutations predicted worse survival outcomes than did missense mutations [82]. Exon 9 included ITDs and missense mutations and were associated with worse prognosis in early studies [2, 75, 83] while exons 13 and 17 exhibited substitution mutations [2, 80] that occur most frequently as resistance mechanisms to imatinib treatment [84]. PDGFRα harbors similar types of mutations. The exon 18 kinase domain and exon 12 JM domain contain missense mutations and deletions while exon 14 kinase domain has missense mutations [71–73, 85, 86]. The exon 18 mutations involve codons from 841 to 848 with a high percentage involving the D842V mutation [71, 85].

Further analysis of GIST mutational heterogeneity in the context of treatment led to correlations between specific mutations and response to therapy. In the B2222 study described above, both c-KIT and PDGFRα mutations were correlated for clinical outcome. Partial response rates to imatinib in exon 11 mutations ($n=85$) were 83.5 % versus 48 % for those with exon 9, PDGFRα, or no mutations ($n=44$). This translated into a longer OS in multivariate modeling at 29 months of follow-up. Although exon 9 was worse than exon 11 prognostically, it did show improved OS compared to GISTs with PDGFRα or no mutations. Furthermore, recapitulating in vitro modeling, patients with the PDGFRα D842V mutation were found to be unresponsive to imatinib [73]. Subsequent analysis at 63 months of follow-up maintained the association of exon 11 mutational status with overall survival [7].

These mutational data were confirmed in three phase III analyses. First, the S0033 study determined that the exon 11 genotype had improved responses to imatinib, longer TTP, and better OS when compared with exon 9 or wild-type GIST genotypes. Exon 9 genotype had improved responses to a higher imatinib dose but this did not correlate with OS [87]. Second, the EORTC-ISG-AGITG trial demonstrated that KIT exon 9 mutations were the worst prognostic factor when compared with exon 11 mutations decreasing both PFS and OS outcomes. Exon 9 mutations treated at the higher dose of imatinib had improved PFS [88]. Last, in the meta-GIST analysis of the two prior phase III studies, patients with exon 11 mutations had better OS than those with exon 9, wild-type, or other mutations. Furthermore, analysis of the patients on the high-dose imatinib arm revealed better PFS for exon 9 mutations though this did not translate to better overall survival [14]. Therefore, exon 11 mutations denote better prognostic significance in the context of imatinib treatment.

Consideration of genotype on sunitinib effects in the phase I/II study revealed improved benefit for specific mutational subsets as well. Fifty-eight percent of patients with primary exon 9 mutations had clinical benefit as opposed to 34 % with primary exon 11 mutations. This translated into PFS and OS benefit in the second-line setting. Furthermore, when analyzing sunitinib response based on secondary resistance genotype in imatinib-treated patients, secondary mutations in exon 13 or 14 of KIT, which correspond to the ATP binding pocket, correlated with a significantly longer PFS and OS than those secondary mutations in the kinase activation loop. Similar to imatinib treatment, the PDGFRα exon 18 mutation D842V was resistant to sunitinib therapy [89].

3 Conclusion

Since the use of imatinib in the first metastatic GIST patient, a number of advances have prolonged the life of patients with metastatic disease [4]. Our knowledge of the fundamental molecular underpinnings have resulted in a diverse pipeline of therapeutic choices with many others on the horizon. Our understanding of GIST tumor biology has led to the investigation of a number of biomarkers that may ultimately serve to supplant tissue biopsy as a means of predictive and prognostic evaluation. The emergence of ctDNA analysis has shown great promise as a means of tracking resistance and might ultimately contribute to therapeutic decisions. The study of GISTs has become a gateway for application of new technologies in cancer biology.

References

1. Fletcher CD, Berman JJ, Corless C, Gorstein F, Lasota J, Longley BJ, et al. Diagnosis of gastrointestinal stromal tumors: a consensus approach. Hum Pathol. 2002;33(5):459–65.
2. Rubin BP, Singer S, Tsao C, Duensing A, Lux ML, Ruiz R, et al. KIT activation is a ubiquitous feature of gastrointestinal stromal tumors. Cancer Res. 2001;61(22):8118–21.
3. Hirota S. Gain-of-function mutations of c-kit in human gastrointestinal stromal tumors. Science. 1998;279(5350):577–80.
4. Joensuu H, Roberts PJ, Sarlomo-Rikala M, Andersson LC, Tervahartiala P, Tuveson D, et al. Effect of the tyrosine kinase inhibitor STI571 in a patient with a metastatic gastrointestinal stromal tumor. N Engl J Med. 2001;344(14):1052–6.
5. Edmonson JH, Marks RS, Buckner JC, Mahoney MR. Contrast of response to dacarbazine, mitomycin, doxorubicin, and cisplatin (DMAP) plus GM-CSF between patients with advanced malignant gastrointestinal stromal tumors and patients with other advanced leiomyosarcomas. Cancer Invest. 2002;20(5–6):605–12.
6. Verweij J, Casali PG, Zalcberg J, LeCesne A, Reichardt P, Blay J-Y, et al. Progression-free survival in gastrointestinal stromal tumours with high-dose imatinib: randomised trial. The Lancet. 2004;364(9440):1127–34.
7. Blanke CD, Demetri GD, von Mehren M, Heinrich MC, Eisenberg B, Fletcher JA, et al. Long-term results from a randomized phase II trial of standard- versus higher-dose imatinib mesylate for patients with unresectable or metastatic gastrointestinal stromal tumors expressing KIT. J Clin Oncol. 2008;26(4):620–5.
8. DeMatteo RP, Lewis JJ, Leung D, Mudan SS, Woodruff JM, Brennan MF. Two hundred gastrointestinal stromal tumors: recurrence patterns and prognostic factors for survival. Ann Surg. 2000;231(1):51–8.
9. Ng EH, Pollock RE, Romsdahl MM. Prognostic implications of patterns of failure for gastrointestinal leiomyosarcomas. Cancer. 1992;69(6):1334–41.
10. McGrath PC, Neifeld JP, Lawrence Jr W, Kay S, Horsley 3rd JS, Parker GA. Gastrointestinal sarcomas. Analysis of prognostic factors. Ann Surg. 1987;206(6):706–10.
11. Conlon KC, Casper ES, Brennan MF. Primary gastrointestinal sarcomas: analysis of prognostic variables. Ann Surg Oncol. 1995;2(1):26–31.
12. Evans HL. Smooth muscle tumors of the gastrointestinal tract. A study of 56 cases followed for a minimum of 10 years. Cancer. 1985;56(9):2242–50.
13. Demetri GD, von Mehren M, Blanke CD, Van den Abbeele AD, Eisenberg B, Roberts PJ, et al. Efficacy and safety of imatinib mesylate in advanced gastrointestinal stromal tumors. N Engl J Med. 2002;347(7):472–80.

14. Gastrointestinal Stromal Tumor Meta-Analysis G. Comparison of two doses of imatinib for the treatment of unresectable or metastatic gastrointestinal stromal tumors: a meta-analysis of 1,640 patients. J Clin Oncol. 2010;28(7):1247–53.
15. Blanke CD, Rankin C, Demetri GD, Ryan CW, von Mehren M, Benjamin RS, et al. Phase III randomized, intergroup trial assessing imatinib mesylate at two dose levels in patients with unresectable or metastatic gastrointestinal stromal tumors expressing the kit receptor tyrosine kinase: S0033. J Clin Oncol. 2008;26(4):626–32.
16. van Oosterom AT, Judson IR, Verweij J, Stroobants S, Dumez H, di Donato di Paola E, et al. Update of phase I study of imatinib (STI571) in advanced soft tissue sarcomas and gastrointestinal stromal tumors: a report of the EORTC Soft Tissue and Bone Sarcoma Group. Eur J Cancer. 2002;38 Suppl 5:S83–7.
17. Van Glabbeke M, Verweij J, Casali PG, Le Cesne A, Hohenberger P, Ray-Coquard I, et al. Initial and late resistance to imatinib in advanced gastrointestinal stromal tumors are predicted by different prognostic factors: a European Organisation for Research and Treatment of Cancer-Italian Sarcoma Group-Australasian Gastrointestinal Trials Group study. J Clin Oncol. 2005;23(24):5795–804.
18. Lee CK, Goldstein D, Gibbs E, Joensuu H, Zalcberg J, Verweij J, et al. Development and validation of prognostic nomograms for metastatic gastrointestinal stromal tumour treated with imatinib. Eur J Cancer. 2015;51(7):852–60.
19. van Oosterom AT, Judson I, Verweij J, Stroobants S, di Paola ED, Dimitrijevic S, et al. Safety and efficacy of imatinib (STI571) in metastatic gastrointestinal stromal tumours: a phase I study. The Lancet. 2001;358(9291):1421–3.
20. Blay JY, Le Cesne A, Ray-Coquard I, Bui B, Duffaud F, Delbaldo C, et al. Prospective multicentric randomized phase III study of imatinib in patients with advanced gastrointestinal stromal tumors comparing interruption versus continuation of treatment beyond 1 year: the French Sarcoma Group. J Clin Oncol. 2007;25(9):1107–13.
21. Le Cesne A, Ray-Coquard I, Bui BN, Adenis A, Rios M, Bertucci F, et al. Discontinuation of imatinib in patients with advanced gastrointestinal stromal tumours after 3 years of treatment: an open-label multicentre randomised phase 3 trial. Lancet Oncol. 2010;11(10):942–9.
22. Ray-Coquard IL, Bui BN, Adenis A, et al. Risk of relapse with imatinib (IM) discontinuation at 5 years in advanced GIST patients: results of the prospective BRF14 randomised phase III study comparing interruption versus continuation of IM at 5 years of treatment: a French Sarcoma Group Study. J Clin Oncol. 2010;28(15s).
23. Patrikidou A, Chabaud S, Ray-Coquard I, Bui BN, Adenis A, Rios M, et al. Influence of imatinib interruption and rechallenge on the residual disease in patients with advanced GIST: results of the BFR14 prospective French Sarcoma Group randomised, phase III trial. Ann Oncol. 2013;24(4):1087–93.
24. Peng B, Lloyd P, Schran H. Clinical pharmacokinetics of imatinib. Clin Pharmacokinet. 2005;44(9):879–94.
25. Peng B, Hayes M, Resta D, Racine-Poon A, Druker BJ, Talpaz M, et al. Pharmacokinetics and pharmacodynamics of imatinib in a phase I trial with chronic myeloid leukemia patients. J Clin Oncol. 2004;22(5):935–42.
26. von Mehren M, Widmer N. Correlations between imatinib pharmacokinetics, pharmacodynamics, adherence, and clinical response in advanced metastatic gastrointestinal stromal tumor (GIST): an emerging role for drug blood level testing? Cancer Treat Rev. 2011;37(4):291–9.
27. Widmer N, Decosterd LA, Leyvraz S, Duchosal MA, Rosselet A, Debiec-Rychter M, et al. Relationship of imatinib-free plasma levels and target genotype with efficacy and tolerability. Br J Cancer. 2008;98(10):1633–40.
28. Demetri GD, Wang Y, Wehrle E, Racine A, Nikolova Z, Blanke CD, et al. Imatinib plasma levels are correlated with clinical benefit in patients with unresectable/metastatic gastrointestinal stromal tumors. J Clin Oncol. 2009;27(19):3141–7.
29. Bouchet S, Poulette S, Titier K, Moore N, Lassalle R, Abouelfath A, et al. Relationship between imatinib trough concentration and outcomes in the treatment of advanced gastrointestinal stromal tumours in a real-life setting. Eur J Cancer. 2016;57:31–8.

30. Demetri GD, Reichardt P, Kang YK, Blay JY, Rutkowski P, Gelderblom H, et al. Efficacy and safety of regorafenib for advanced gastrointestinal stromal tumours after failure of imatinib and sunitinib (GRID): an international, multicentre, randomised, placebo-controlled, phase 3 trial. Lancet. 2013;381(9863):295–302.
31. Demetri GD, van Oosterom AT, Garrett CR, Blackstein ME, Shah MH, Verweij J, et al. Efficacy and safety of sunitinib in patients with advanced gastrointestinal stromal tumour after failure of imatinib: a randomised controlled trial. The Lancet. 2006;368(9544):1329–38.
32. Demetri GD, Garrett CR, Schoffski P, Shah MH, Verweij J, Leyvraz S, et al. Complete longitudinal analyses of the randomized, placebo-controlled, phase III trial of sunitinib in patients with gastrointestinal stromal tumor following imatinib failure. Clin Cancer Res. 2012;18(11):3170–9.
33. Reichardt P, Kang YK, Rutkowski P, Schuette J, Rosen LS, Seddon B, et al. Clinical outcomes of patients with advanced gastrointestinal stromal tumors: safety and efficacy in a worldwide treatment-use trial of sunitinib. Cancer. 2015;121(9):1405–13.
34. Reichardt P, Blay JY, Gelderblom H, Schlemmer M, Demetri GD, Bui-Nguyen B, et al. Phase III study of nilotinib versus best supportive care with or without a TKI in patients with gastrointestinal stromal tumors resistant to or intolerant of imatinib and sunitinib. Ann Oncol. 2012;23(7):1680–7.
35. Blay JY, Shen L, Kang YK, Rutkowski P, Qin S, Nosov D, et al. Nilotinib versus imatinib as first-line therapy for patients with unresectable or metastatic gastrointestinal stromal tumours (ENESTg1): a randomised phase 3 trial. Lancet Oncol. 2015;16(5):550–60.
36. Wiebe L, Kasza KE, Maki RG, et al. Activity of sorafenib (SOR) in patients (pts) with imatinib (IM) and sunitinib (SU)-resistant (RES) gastrointestinal stromal tumors (GIST): a phase II trial of the University of Chicago Phase II Consortium. JCO (meeting abstract). 2008;26(10502).
37. Montemurro M, Gelderblom H, Bitz U, Schutte J, Blay JY, Joensuu H, et al. Sorafenib as third- or fourth-line treatment of advanced gastrointestinal stromal tumour and pretreatment including both imatinib and sunitinib, and nilotinib: a retrospective analysis. Eur J Cancer. 2013;49(5):1027–31.
38. Italiano A, Cioffi A, Coco P, Maki RG, Schoffski P, Rutkowski P, et al. Patterns of care, prognosis, and survival in patients with metastatic gastrointestinal stromal tumors (GIST) refractory to first-line imatinib and second-line sunitinib. Ann Surg Oncol. 2012;19(5):1551–9.
39. Broudy VC. Stem cell factor and hematopoiesis. Blood. 1997;90(4):1345–64.
40. Dahlen DD, Lin NL, Liu YC, Broudy VC. Soluble Kit receptor blocks stem cell factor bioactivity in vitro. Leuk Res. 2001;25(5):413–21.
41. Mendel DB, Laird AD, Xin X, Louie SG, Christensen JG, Li G, et al. In vivo antitumor activity of SU11248, a novel tyrosine kinase inhibitor targeting vascular endothelial growth factor and platelet-derived growth factor receptors: determination of a pharmacokinetic/pharmacodynamic relationship. Clin Cancer Res. 2003;9(1):327–37.
42. Osusky KL, Hallahan DE, Fu A, Ye F, Shyr Y, Geng L. The receptor tyrosine kinase inhibitor SU11248 impedes endothelial cell migration, tubule formation, and blood vessel formation in vivo, but has little effect on existing tumor vessels. Angiogenesis. 2004;7(3):225–33.
43. Schueneman AJ, Himmelfarb E, Geng L, Tan J, Donnelly E, Mendel D, et al. SU11248 maintenance therapy prevents tumor regrowth after fractionated irradiation of murine tumor models. Cancer Res. 2003;63(14):4009–16.
44. Deprimo SE, Bello CL, Smeraglia J, Baum CM, Spinella D, Rini BI, et al. Circulating protein biomarkers of pharmacodynamic activity of sunitinib in patients with metastatic renal cell carcinoma: modulation of VEGF and VEGF-related proteins. J Transl Med. 2007;5:32.
45. Burstein HJ, Elias AD, Rugo HS, Cobleigh MA, Wolff AC, Eisenberg PD, et al. Phase II study of sunitinib malate, an oral multitargeted tyrosine kinase inhibitor, in patients with metastatic breast cancer previously treated with an anthracycline and a taxane. J Clin Oncol. 2008;26(11):1810–6.
46. Harmon CS, DePrimo SE, Raymond E, Cheng AL, Boucher E, Douillard JY, et al. Mechanism-related circulating proteins as biomarkers for clinical outcome in patients with unresectable hepatocellular carcinoma receiving sunitinib. J Transl Med. 2011;9:120.

47. Bono P, Krause A, von Mehren M, Heinrich MC, Blanke CD, Dimitrijevic S, et al. Serum KIT and KIT ligand levels in patients with gastrointestinal stromal tumors treated with imatinib. Blood. 2004;103(8):2929–35.
48. Maki RG, Fletcher JA, Heinrich MC, Morgan JA, George S, Desai J, Scheu K, Fletcher CDM, Baum C, Demetri GD. Results from a continuation trial of SU11248 in patients (pts) with imatinib (IM)-resistant gastrointestinal stromal tumor (GIST). JCO. 2005;23(16S (supplement)):9011.
49. DePrimo SE, Wong LM, Nicholas SL, et al, editor. Decreases in circulating levels of soluble KIT in patients with imatinib-resistant gastrointestinal stromal tumor (GIST) receiving the novel kinase inhibitor SU11248: correlative analysis of blood and plasma biomarkers. Proc Am Assoc Cancer. 2003;2003.
50. George S, Blay JY, Casali PG, Le Cesne A, Stephenson P, Deprimo SE, et al. Clinical evaluation of continuous daily dosing of sunitinib malate in patients with advanced gastrointestinal stromal tumour after imatinib failure. Eur J Cancer. 2009;45(11):1959–68.
51. Deprimo SE, Huang X, Blackstein ME, Garrett CR, Harmon CS, Schoffski P, et al. Circulating levels of soluble KIT serve as a biomarker for clinical outcome in gastrointestinal stromal tumor patients receiving sunitinib following imatinib failure. Clin Cancer Res. 2009;15(18):5869–77.
52. Diehl F, Schmidt K, Choti MA, Romans K, Goodman S, Li M, et al. Circulating mutant DNA to assess tumor dynamics. Nat Med. 2008;14(9):985–90.
53. Leary RJ, Kinde I, Diehl F, Schmidt K, Clouser C, Duncan C, et al. Development of personalized tumor biomarkers using massively parallel sequencing. Sci Transl Med. 2010;2(20):20ra14.
54. Goebel G, Zitt M, Zitt M, Muller HM. Circulating nucleic acids in plasma or serum (CNAPS) as prognostic and predictive markers in patients with solid neoplasias. Dis Markers. 2005;21(3):105–20.
55. Diaz Jr LA, Bardelli A. Liquid biopsies: genotyping circulating tumor DNA. J Clin Oncol. 2014;32(6):579–86.
56. Grimwade D, Jovanovic JV, Hills RK, Nugent EA, Patel Y, Flora R, et al. Prospective minimal residual disease monitoring to predict relapse of acute promyelocytic leukemia and to direct pre-emptive arsenic trioxide therapy. J Clin Oncol. 2009;27(22):3650–8.
57. Cazzaniga G, Biondi A. Molecular monitoring of childhood acute lymphoblastic leukemia using antigen receptor gene rearrangements and quantitative polymerase chain reaction technology. Haematologica. 2005;90(3):382–90.
58. Akard LP, Cortes JE, Albitar M, Goldberg SL, Warsi G, Wetzler M, et al. Correlations between cytogenetic and molecular monitoring among patients with newly diagnosed chronic myeloid leukemia in chronic phase: post hoc analyses of the Rationale and Insight for Gleevec High-Dose Therapy study. Arch Pathol Lab Med. 2014;138(9):1186–92.
59. Cave H, van der Werff ten Bosch J, Suciu S, Guidal C, Waterkeyn C, Otten J, et al. Clinical significance of minimal residual disease in childhood acute lymphoblastic leukemia. European Organization for Research and Treatment of Cancer--Childhood Leukemia Cooperative Group. N Engl J Med. 1998;339(9):591–8.
60. van Dongen JJ, Seriu T, Panzer-Grumayer ER, Biondi A, Pongers-Willemse MJ, Corral L, et al. Prognostic value of minimal residual disease in acute lymphoblastic leukaemia in childhood. Lancet. 1998;352(9142):1731–8.
61. Hughes TP, Saglio G, Kantarjian HM, Guilhot F, Niederwieser D, Rosti G, et al. Early molecular response predicts outcomes in patients with chronic myeloid leukemia in chronic phase treated with frontline nilotinib or imatinib. Blood. 2014;123(9):1353–60.
62. Maier J, Lange T, Kerle I, Specht K, Bruegel M, Wickenhauser C, et al. Detection of mutant free circulating tumor DNA in the plasma of patients with gastrointestinal stromal tumor harboring activating mutations of CKIT or PDGFRA. Clin Cancer Res. 2013;19(17):4854–67.
63. George D. Demetri MJ, Peter Reichardt, Yoon-Koo Kang, Jean-Yves Blay, Piotr Rutkowski, Hans Gelderblom, Peter Hohenberger, Michael Gordon Leahy, Margaret von Mehren, Heikki Joensuu, Giuseppe Badalamenti, Martin E. Blackstein, Axel Le Cesne, Patrick Schoffski, Robert G. Maki, Jian-Ming Xu, Toshirou Nishida, Iris Kuss, Paolo Giovanni Casali. Mutational analysis of plasma DNA from patients (pts) in the phase III GRID study of regorafenib (REG)

versus placebo (PL) in tyrosine kinase inhibitor (TKI)-refractory GIST: correlating genotype with clinical outcomes. J Clin Oncol. 2013;31:Abstract 10503.
64. Kang G, Bae BN, Sohn BS, Pyo JS, Kang GH, Kim KM. Detection of KIT and PDGFRA mutations in the plasma of patients with gastrointestinal stromal tumor. Target Oncol. 2015;10(4):597–601.
65. Wada N, Kurokawa Y, Takahashi T, Hamakawa T, Hirota S, Naka T, et al. Detecting secondary C-KIT mutations in the peripheral blood of patients with imatinib-resistant gastrointestinal stromal tumor. Oncology. 2016;90(2):112–7.
66. Changhoon Yoo M-HR, Baek-Yeol Ryoo, Sook Ryun Park, Shinkyo Yoon, Young-Soon Na, Yoon-Koo Kang. Analysis of serum protein biomarkers and circulating tumor (ct) DNA for activity of dovitinib in patients (pts) with tyrosine kinase inhibitor (TKI)-refractory gastrointestinal stromal tumors (GIST). J Clin Oncol. 2014;32(5s):Abstract 10550.
67. Yoo C, Ryu MH, Na YS, Ryoo BY, Park SR, Kang YK. Analysis of serum protein biomarkers, circulating tumor DNA, and dovitinib activity in patients with tyrosine kinase inhibitor-refractory gastrointestinal stromal tumors. Ann Oncol. 2014;25(11):2272–7.
68. Michael C. Heinrich, Graeme Hodgson J, Margaret von Mehren, George D. Demetri, Jonathan A. Fletcher, Jichao G Sun, Justin R Pritchard, Sen Zhang, Victor M. Rivera, Suzanne George. Detection of KIT mutants in circulating tumor DNA (ctDNA) and their association with ponatinib anti-tumor activity in patients (pts) with advanced gastrointestinal stromal tumors (GIST). J Clin Oncol. 2015;33:abstract 10517.
69. Heinrich MC, Rubin BP, Longley BJ, Fletcher JA. Biology and genetic aspects of gastrointestinal stromal tumors: KIT activation and cytogenetic alterations. Hum Pathol. 2002;33(5):484–95.
70. Corless CL, Fletcher JA, Heinrich MC. Biology of gastrointestinal stromal tumors. J Clin Oncol. 2004;22(18):3813–25.
71. Corless CL, Schroeder A, Griffith D, Town A, McGreevey L, Harrell P, et al. PDGFRA mutations in gastrointestinal stromal tumors: frequency, spectrum and in vitro sensitivity to imatinib. J Clin Oncol. 2005;23(23):5357–64.
72. Heinrich MC, Corless CL, Duensing A, McGreevey L, Chen CJ, Joseph N, et al. PDGFRA activating mutations in gastrointestinal stromal tumors. Science. 2003;299(5607):708–10.
73. Heinrich MC, Corless CL, Demetri GD, Blanke CD, von Mehren M, Joensuu H, et al. Kinase mutations and imatinib response in patients with metastatic gastrointestinal stromal tumor. J Clin Oncol. 2003;21(23):4342–9.
74. Lasota J, Corless CL, Heinrich MC, Debiec-Rychter M, Sciot R, Wardelmann E, et al. Clinicopathologic profile of gastrointestinal stromal tumors (GISTs) with primary KIT exon 13 or exon 17 mutations: a multicenter study on 54 cases. Mod Pathol. 2008; 21(4):476–84.
75. Lasota J, Wozniak A, Sarlomo-Rikala M, Rys J, Kordek R, Nassar A, et al. Mutations in exons 9 and 13 of KIT gene are rare events in gastrointestinal stromal tumors. A study of 200 cases. Am J Pathol. 2000;157(4):1091–5.
76. Antonescu CR, Sommer G, Sarran L, Tschernyavsky SJ, Riedel E, Woodruff JM, et al. Association of KIT exon 9 mutations with nongastric primary site and aggressive behavior: KIT mutation analysis and clinical correlates of 120 gastrointestinal stromal tumors. Clin Cancer Res. 2003;9(9):3329–37.
77. Miettinen M, Majidi M, Lasota J. Pathology and diagnostic criteria of gastrointestinal stromal tumors (GISTs): a review. Eur J Cancer. 2002;38 Suppl 5:S39–51.
78. Miettinen M, Furlong M, Sarlomo-Rikala M, Burke A, Sobin LH, Lasota J. Gastrointestinal stromal tumors, intramural leiomyomas, and leiomyosarcomas in the rectum and anus: a clinicopathologic, immunohistochemical, and molecular genetic study of 144 cases. Am J Surg Pathol. 2001;25(9):1121–33.
79. Taniguchi M, Nishida T, Hirota S, Isozaki K, Ito T, Nomura T, et al. Effect of c-kit mutation on prognosis of gastrointestinal stromal tumors. Cancer Res. 1999;59(17):4297–300.
80. Wardelmann E, Neidt I, Bierhoff E, Speidel N, Manegold C, Fischer HP, et al. c-kit mutations in gastrointestinal stromal tumors occur preferentially in the spindle rather than in the epithelioid cell variant. Mod Pathol. 2002;15(2):125–36.

81. Lasota J, Dansonka-Mieszkowska A, Stachura T, Schneider-Stock R, Kallajoki M, Steigen SE, et al. Gastrointestinal stromal tumors with internal tandem duplications in 3′ end of KIT juxtamembrane domain occur predominantly in stomach and generally seem to have a favorable course. Mod Pathol. 2003;16(12):1257–64.
82. Singer S, Rubin BP, Lux ML, Chen CJ, Demetri GD, Fletcher CD, et al. Prognostic value of KIT mutation type, mitotic activity, and histologic subtype in gastrointestinal stromal tumors. J Clin Oncol. 2002;20(18):3898–905.
83. Sakurai S, Oguni S, Hironaka M, Fukayama M, Morinaga S, Saito K. Mutations in c-kit gene exons 9 and 13 in gastrointestinal stromal tumors among Japanese. Jpn J Cancer Res. 2001;92(5):494–8.
84. Heinrich MC, Corless CL, Blanke CD, Demetri GD, Joensuu H, Roberts PJ, et al. Molecular correlates of imatinib resistance in gastrointestinal stromal tumors. J Clin Oncol. 2006;24(29):4764–74.
85. Lasota J, Dansonka-Mieszkowska A, Sobin LH, Miettinen M. A great majority of GISTs with PDGFRA mutations represent gastric tumors of low or no malignant potential. Lab Invest. 2004;84(7):874–83.
86. Medeiros F, Corless CL, Duensing A, Hornick JL, Oliveira AM, Heinrich MC, et al. KIT-negative gastrointestinal stromal tumors: proof of concept and therapeutic implications. Am J Surg Pathol. 2004;28(7):889–94.
87. Heinrich MC, Owzar K, Corless CL, Hollis D, Borden EC, Fletcher CD, et al. Correlation of kinase genotype and clinical outcome in the North American Intergroup Phase III Trial of imatinib mesylate for treatment of advanced gastrointestinal stromal tumor: CALGB 150105 Study by Cancer and Leukemia Group B and Southwest Oncology Group. J Clin Oncol. 2008;26(33):5360–7.
88. Debiec-Rychter M, Sciot R, Le Cesne A, Schlemmer M, Hohenberger P, van Oosterom AT, et al. KIT mutations and dose selection for imatinib in patients with advanced gastrointestinal stromal tumours. Eur J Cancer. 2006;42(8):1093–103.
89. Heinrich MC, Maki RG, Corless CL, Antonescu CR, Harlow A, Griffith D, et al. Primary and secondary kinase genotypes correlate with the biological and clinical activity of sunitinib in imatinib-resistant gastrointestinal stromal tumor. J Clin Oncol. 2008;26(33):5352–9.

Advances on Molecular Characterization and Targeted Therapies on GIST

Gabriel Tinoco, Guozhi Hu, Ana Paz-Mejía, and Jonathan Trent

1 Introduction

Gastrointestinal stromal tumors (GIST) are the most common mesenchymal gastrointestinal (GI) neoplasms, yet accounting for less than 1 % of all GI malignancies [1]. They are considered to originate from the interstitial cells of Cajal (ICC) or its progenitor cell [2]. These tumors are characterized by the presence of the CD117 (KIT) [3] and/or DOG-1 [4]. Around 3300–6000 new cases of GIST are diagnosed every year in the United States. The reported annual incidence varies by country, ranging from 6.8 per million in the United States to 19.6 in Hong Kong [5]. However, the real incidence is not known, in part due to lack of standardization for KIT and PDGFRA mutation analysis in some institutions and the fact that small GIST are often not included in cancer registries [6–8].

The highest incidence of GIST occurs between the fifth and sixth decades of life, and rarely occurs before the age of 20. A slight male predominance (53.5 % men and 46.5 % women) has been reported [9]. Around 60 % of GIST occur in the stomach, 25 % in the small intestine, and 10 % in the large bowel, rectum, appendix, and esophagus, and rarely in the extra-intestinal sites such as the gallbladder, omentum, and mesentery [10]. Some of these mesenchymal neoplasms do not cause symptoms and are discovered incidentally. More commonly, they are linked to nonspecific symptoms, except if they ulcerate, bleed, or grow large enough to produce pain or obstruction [11].

Tumors are staged based on the tumor size, number of mitoses, and presence of metastasis (to lymph nodes or other sites). Tumors smaller than 5 cm with fewer than five mitoses per 50 high-power microscopic fields (HPF) have lower risk of recurrence. Tumors larger than 10 cm with more than five mitoses per 50 HPF or ruptured GIST

G. Tinoco, MD • G. Hu, MD • A. Paz-Mejía • J. Trent, MD, PhD (✉)
Department of Medicine, Division of Hematology Oncology, University of Miami, Sylvester Cancer Center, 1475 NW 12th Ave., Miami, FL 33136, USA
e-mail: Jtrent@med.miami.edu

© Springer International Publishing Switzerland 2017

C.R. Scoggins et al. (eds.), *Gastrointestinal Stromal Tumors*,
DOI 10.1007/978-3-319-42632-7_13

have a high risk of recurrence after complete resection [10]. Gastric GIST have a better prognosis than extragastric GIST [12]. The common metastatic sites for GIST include the liver and omentum, less frequently lung, regional lymph nodes, and bone [13].

There are several entities with increased incidence of GIST: The Carney–Stratakis syndrome (familial paraganglioma and GIST) and the Carney's triad (pulmonary chondroma, GIST, and paraganglioma) are affected with nonsporadic GIST. The patients are typically younger than their sporadic GIST counterparts [14]. Patients with neurofibromatosis type 1 (NF1) have an increased risk of developing GIST [15]. NF-associated GIST commonly arise on the small intestine, frequently presenting with a low mitotic activity and lacking *KIT* and *PDGFRA* mutations [16, 17].

Surgery remains the mainstay of therapy for patients with primary GIST with no evidence of metastasis, and this should be initial therapy if the tumor is technically resectable and associated with acceptable risk for morbidity [18]. Currently, the NCCN guidelines [18] recommend that risk stratification after surgical resection should be based on tumor mitotic rate, size, and location. The nomogram developed by Gold and colleagues accurately predicts RFS after surgery and might be useful for patient care, interpretation of trial results, and selection of patients for adjuvant therapy [19].

Imatinib mesylate (Gleevec, Novartis, Basel, Switzerland) revolutionized the treatment of patients with GIST. Imatinib has been proven to have substantial effect in patients with GIST in the adjuvant, neoadjuvant, and palliative setting. It constitutes the primary medical therapy for GIST [18]. More recently, newer generations of tyrosine kinase molecules are being used in specific settings on patients with advanced GIST [18].

2 Histopathology

Sarlomo-Rikali and associates discovered that GIST stained positive for CD117 almost universally [3]. Nearly 95 % of GIST stain for CD117. Other significant immunohistochemical markers include CD34 (70 %), smooth muscle actin (35 %), S-100 (10 %), and rarely desmin (5 %) [20]. DOG-1 (Discovered on GIST-1) has been shown to be highly expressed in GIST [21] and has a very high sensitivity and specificity [4]. A recent study showed that DOG-1 immunostaining was positive in 96.3 % of GIST. From all the cases stained with CD117 and DOG-1, 98.4 % were positive for at least one of these antibodies, suggesting a combination of CD117 and DOG1 immunostaining is sufficient to confirm the histological diagnosis [22]. Moreover, DOG-1 is expressed in 36 % of cases of KIT-negative GIST tumors, making it useful in correctly identifying the rare GIST subgroups that lack KIT mutations [4].

3 Pathophysiology and Molecular Markers

The KIT tyrosine kinase receptor, when activated by its native ligand, the stem cell factor (SCF), triggers multiple signal transduction molecules involved in cellular proliferation, differentiation, maturation, survival, chemotaxis, and adhesion. The transmission of these various processes is mediated through the dimerization of KIT tyrosine kinase. Dimerization of the KIT receptor leads to phosphorylation and activation of several transduction pathways, including the phosphoinositide 3′ kinase (PI3K), JAK–STAT, Ras-ERK, and phospholipase C pathways [23].

Genetic mutations affecting *c-KIT* have been detected in 95 % of GIST [24]. Mutations in specific exons of the *KIT* genome lead to a gain of function of this tyrosine kinase receptor in GIST. KIT is constitutively active in the absence of stimulation by SCF or via homodimerization. This process ultimately induces oncogenesis [23]. Most mutations occur in the juxtamembrane region encoded by exon 11 (71 %) or extracellular region encoded by exon 9 (14 %) and less frequently in exon 13 (4 %) or exon 17 (4 %) that encode the tyrosine kinase domain [25].

Other mutations mainly affect platelet-derived growth factor receptor alpha (PDGFRα), present in around 5–8 % of GIST. A minority of GIST are c-KIT negative and PDGFRα-negative [24]. These so-called "wild-type" GIST are seen most commonly in children (around 90 % of the pediatric GIST cases) [26]. The BRAFV600E substitution is seen in about 13 % of wild-type GIST [27, 28]. This has led to a phase II clinical trial using dabrafenib (a newer generation BRAF inhibitor) [29]. It has been also reported that in naive GIST cell lines carrying activating mutations in KIT or PDGFRα, a concomitant activating mutation is present in KRAS (5 %) or BRAF (about 2 %) genes [30].

4 Tyrosine Kinase Inhibitor Therapy

Tyrosine kinase inhibitors (TKI) constitute the main medical treatment of patients with GIST. Before the year 2000 (pre-TKI era), the only available therapeutic option for patients with localized GIST was surgical resection. Unfortunately, even when excised in negative surgical margins, the recurrence rate for lesions larger than 3 cm was high [31]. The overall response rates for conventional systemic chemotherapy were very low (0–5 %), and the median survival was less than 2 years [32–34]. Furthermore, GIST are largely radioresistant, making radiation therapy ineffective [35]. It was this lack of effective treatment options that led investigators to seek alternative treatment strategies. Discovery of c-KIT overexpression sparked interest in TKI therapy for advanced GIST.

Imatinib (Gleevec) is an orally bioavailable 2-phenylpyrimidine derivative developed in the 1990s as therapy for chronic myelogenous leukemia (CML). Imatinib occupies the ATP-binding pocket of the ABL kinase domain inhibiting the oncogenic signaling. ABL shares considerable homology with the type III receptor tyrosine kinase family, which includes c-KIT [5]. Imatinib was first used as compassionate therapy in March 2000 in a patient with advanced GIST, and the patient reached partial response within few weeks [36]. These dramatic results led to a series of trials investigating the role of imatinib for patients with advanced disease.

4.1 Neoadjuvant TKI Therapy

There are situations where resection of a primary GIST might be aided with the downsizing of the tumor. For example, large GIST arising low in the rectum might require sphincter-sacrificing surgical procedures (i.e., abdominoperitoneal resection); however, if the tumor shrank and pulled away from the sphincter, local resection with sphincter preservation might be possible. In this way, neoadjuvant imatinib may provide several advantages: it will provide valuable in vivo evidence of the tumor's sensitivity to imatinib, potentially downsize the tumor, and "reduce" the surgical procedure necessary (or facilitate complete tumor extirpation). It may also work as conversion therapy for initially unresectable GIST. On the other hand, a potential downfall of the use of neoadjuvant imatinib may be that it precludes the accurate assessment of risk recurrence using any of the risk-classification models, as none of the current prognostic systems account for neoadjuvant therapy.

The largest retrospective study (to date) of neoadjuvant imatinib therapy published evaluated 126 patients who all received neoadjuvant imatinib for initially unresectable GIST; 17 patients subsequently had surgical resection. These patients received imatinib for a median of 10 months. The radiographic overall response rate was 76 % (1 CR, 12 PR). Two patients were found to have no viable tumor at the time of surgical resection [37]. In a different study, neoadjuvant imatinib improved resectability and reduced surgical morbidity in patients with locally advanced or unresectable primary GIST. The median tumor size reduction was 34 %, and the estimated PFS at 3 years was 77 % [38]. Currently, the NCCN guidelines recommend considering preoperative imatinib on an individual basis for patients in whom surgical morbidity may be improved by reducing the size of the tumor [18].

4.2 Adjuvant TKI Therapy

Despite successful primary tumor resection, GIST have a high risk for recurrence. Stemming from the initial success of imatinib therapy for metastatic disease, several trials were designed to determine the efficacy of adjuvant imatinib in patients with primary GIST after complete surgical resection.

The ACOSOG Z-9001, an intergroup randomized, double-blind, placebo-controlled trial compared imatinib (at a dose of 400 mg daily for 1 year) versus placebo in 713 patients. The study reported a recurrence-free survival (RFS) of 98 % (95 % CI 96–100) in the imatinib group versus 83 % (CI 78–88) in the placebo group (hazard ratio [HR] 0.35 [0.22–0.53], $p<0.0001$), but did not reveal an overall survival (OS) benefit [39]. Interestingly, the slopes of the disease-free survival curves become parallel after cessation of imatinib therapy. This suggests that imatinib might provide "growth suppression" of radiographically occult, micrometastatic disease. The similar OS between the study groups was likely an effect of the crossover design of the study that permitted patients assigned to the placebo group to get imatinib on tumor recurrence. This trial clearly showed, however, that the risk of recurrent disease is directly linked to TKI therapy, and suggested that the duration of therapy might play an important role.

Accordingly, the SSG XVIII/AIO study, a randomized, open-label Phase III trial, compared the administration of imatinib (400 mg daily) for 1 year versus 3 years as adjuvant therapy. Four hundred KIT-positive, high-risk patients were recruited. The results clearly demonstrated that adjuvant imatinib given for 3 years improved RFS compared to that for 1 year only (hazard ratio [HR], 0.46; 95 % CI, 0.32–0.65; $p = 0.001$; 5-year RFS, 65.6 % vs. 47.9 %, respectively) [40]. Moreover, the 3 years of imatinib arm had a better overall survival (HR, 0.45; 95 % CI, 0.22–0.89; $p = 0.02$; 5-year survival, 92.0 % vs. 81.7 %) [40]. Based on these findings, 3 years of adjuvant therapy is currently the recommended duration of therapy for patients deemed at high risk for recurrence in the United States [18].

Currently, there are several ongoing trials that aim to clarify the role and duration of imatinib as an adjuvant treatment for GIST. The EORTC 62024 is a Phase III, randomized, open-label study, which aims to compare the effect of adjuvant imatinib mesylate (400 mg daily) for 2 years versus observation on the prognosis of patients with completely resected localized GIST at intermediate/high risk of relapse and to compare overall survival among patients in both arms [41]. Preliminary results of the first interim analysis were reported at the 2013 ASCO Annual Meeting. Five-year imatinib failure-free survival (IFS) was 87 % in the imatinib arm compared to 84 % in the control arm (HR 0.80, 95 % CI 0.51–1.26); 3-year RFS was 84 % versus 66 %; and 5-year overall survival was 100 % versus 99 % [42]. Finally, the PERSIST 5 trial is a Phase II, nonrandomized, open-label multicenter study of 5-year adjuvant imatinib in patients at significant risk for recurrence following complete resection of primary GIST. This study is ongoing but not recruiting patients at this time [43].

4.3 Adjuvant/Neoadjuvant Combined TKI Therapy

The RTOG S0132/ACRIN (American College of Radiology Imaging Network) 6665 trial enrolled patients with primary GIST (≥5 cm, group A) or resectable metastatic/recurrent GIST (≥2 cm, group B) who received neoadjuvant imatinib (600 mg/day) for approximately 2 months and maintenance postoperative imatinib for 2 years [44]. Thirty patients had locally advanced primaries and 22 had locally recurrent or metastatic disease. In the localized primary disease group, 7 % (2 patients) had an objective response to preoperative imatinib, but stable disease was achieved in 83 % (25 patients). In patients with recurrent or metastatic GIST, partial response and stable disease were observed in 4.5 % and 91 % of patients, respectively [44]. The most recent update at a median follow-up of 5.1 years demonstrated that the estimated 5-year progression-free survival was 57 % in group A versus 30 % in group B, and overall survival was 77 % in group A versus 68 % in group B. Median time to progression has not been reached for group A, and was 4.4 years for group B [45]. Long-term analysis suggested that a high percentage of patients experienced disease progression after discontinuation of 2-year maintenance imatinib therapy after surgery. For that reason, they concluded that longer treatment duration should be studied in intermediate- to high-risk GIST patients [45]. These results added further evidence in support of longer treatment times. Similarly, the phase III BFR14 trial conducted by the French Sarcoma Group explored the effect of interrupting therapy after 1, 3, and 5 years of treatment with 400 mg/daily of imatinib in patients with advanced GIST. A subgroup analysis of patients with locally advanced primary GIST was associated with a 60 % partial response rate, and 36 % of patients underwent surgical resection after a median of 7.3 months of therapy. With a median follow-up of 53.5 months, there was a significant improvement in progression-free survival and overall survival for patients who underwent surgical resection versus those who did not (median not reached vs. 23.6 months, $p = 0.0318$ for PFS and median not reached vs. 42.2 months, $p = 0.0217$ for OS). In the group of patients who underwent resection followed by imatinib, the 3-year PFS and OS rates were 67 % and 89 %, respectively [46]. These data clearly demonstrate that adjuvant therapy with imatinib provides both disease-free and overall survival benefit to patients who have high-risk GIST.

4.4 *TKI for Advanced/Metastatic Disease*

Imatinib is the primary systemic therapy for patients with advanced/metastatic GIST [18]. The standard dose of imatinib was established in an EORTC phase I trial led by Van Oosterom and associates [47]. Utilizing a dose escalation schema, they concluded that a dose of 400 mg/day had the most favorable clinical benefit–side effect profile, including edema, nausea, diarrhea, malaise, and fatigue. Other rare side effects included myelosuppression, hemorrhage, and elevated transaminases, which required interruption or discontinuation in treatment [47]. Several phase II and III clinical trials were designed to assess the efficacy of imatinib in the metastatic setting. These studies reported an imatinib response ranging from 48 to 71 % and disease stabilization in 70–85 % of patients. The median progression-free survival ranges from 20 to 24 months [13, 48–50]. The B2222 trial reported an overall survival of 35 % at 9 years, and 38 % for those with complete response or partial response [51]. These data demonstrated the possibility of durable survival benefit for those patients who responded to imatinib.

Two large international studies randomized patients with metastatic GIST to standard dose or high-dose imatinib (400 versus 800 mg/daily, respectively) [13, 48]. The EORTC 62005 reported that after 760 days of follow-up, 56 % of the patients in the 400 mg daily dose had progression compared to 50 % in the 800 mg daily dose [13]. As one might expect, the lower dose cohort had fewer side effects. The North American Sarcoma Intergroup study, S0033, was an open-label phase III trial on patients with unresectable or metastatic GIST. Patients were randomized to receive the 400 mg daily dose (standard dose) versus 400 mg twice daily (high dose). At a median follow-up of 4.5 years, the median progression-free survival was nearly identical between the two dosing regimens. Similarly, the median overall survival was essentially identical. Interestingly, after progression on standard dose imatinib, 33 % of patients who crossed over to the high-dose imatinib regimen achieved either an objective response or stable disease [48]. These data were hypothesis-generating, including raising the possibility that some GIST require higher dosing to achieve therapeutic benefit.

One important concept regarding imatinib dosing is that different mutations in the *KIT* gene require different doses. The EORTC designed a phase III trial in which patients with GIST were randomized to receive imatinib at a dose of either 400 mg daily or 800 mg daily. The presence of KIT exon 9 mutations increased the relative risk of progression by 171 % and the relative risk of death by 190 % when compared with KIT exon 11 mutants [52]. Interestingly, patients whose tumors expressed an exon 9 KIT mutation did better with the higher dosing scheme [52]. It was concluded that tumor genotype is of major prognostic significance for patients treated with imatinib for advanced GIST. Interestingly, the relative risk of progression was also increased by 108 % and the relative risk of death by 76 % in patients without detectable KIT or PDGFRA mutations [52]. Typically, patients are started on 400 mg/day of imatinib, and after a short period, the dose is gradually escalated up to 800 mg/day. This seems to minimize some of the side effects when compared to starting out de novo with the 800 mg/day dosing.

A correlation study of the kinase genotype and clinical outcomes done along with the CALGB 150105 trial reported that patients with KIT exon 9 mutations treated with 800 mg daily dose of imatinib had better response rates compared to that with 400 mg daily dose (67 % vs. 17 %) [53]. Nevertheless, the survival outcomes for patients with exon 9-mutant, exon 11-mutant, or wild-type GIST were not affected by the imatinib dose. Furthermore, CD117-negative GIST patients had a similar time to tumor progression but inferior overall survival compared to CD117-positive patients. Those outcomes suggest that CD 117-negative GIST patients may also benefit from imatinib therapy [53]. The Gastrointestinal Stromal Tumor Meta-Analysis Group (MetaGIST) reviewed the data of two doses of imatinib (400 mg daily versus twice daily) in 1640 patients with advanced GIST. Patients with wild-type, KIT exon 9 mutations, and patients with other mutations had worse progression-free survival and overall survival than patients with KIT exon 11 mutations [54]. In addition to proper dosing, interruption of therapy seems to impact outcome. Patients who continuously take their imatinib seem to have a more durable response, while patients whose therapy is interrupted develop progression sooner [55]. Reinstitution of therapy for patients who experience progression can result in control of the tumor in most patients. In one study, nearly one-half of patients who had achieved an initial response and subsequently progressed following discontinuation of imatinib were able to respond to restarting therapy [56]. Thus, interruption of imatinib causes rapid progression in most patients with advanced GIST and cannot be recommended unless there is significant toxicity.

4.5 Imatinib-Resistant GIST

For some patients, resistance to imatinib develops during therapy. Several mechanisms of resistance had been proposed, including inadequate imatinib plasma levels, specific types of mutations (BRAF mutation, PDGFRA D842V mutation, NF-1, SDH complex loss), accumulation of secondary mutations, KIT gene amplification, or loss of the wild-type allele. Some patients will develop clones that become resistant, while other tumor nodules remain sensitive. In practice, imatinib resistance is divided into primary and secondary.

Primary resistance (PR) PR is defined as development of progression within the first 6 months of imatinib therapy. Approximately 10–14 % of patients with GIST have primary resistance [24, 57]. Now, it is well known that primary resistance is driven by tumor biology and genotype [25, 52, 53]. It is particularly remarkable that strong imatinib resistance is seen in the presence of the PDGRFA D842V mutation [25, 58, 59]. NF-1, SDH, RAS, and BRAF mutations also predict primary resistance to imatinib [24]. For patients with these mutations, a different therapeutic strategy would be indicated, and the use of BRAF, MEK, and VEGFR inhibitors would be logical options.

Secondary resistance (SR) SR is defined as the development of resistance to imatinib while on therapy (more than 6 months). This resistance develops as a result of acquired mutations which tend to evolve within the first 2 years of treatment [13, 60]. Most mutations that lead to SR affect KIT and PDGFRA [61–64]. In patients with imatinib-naïve GIST, most mutations occur in the juxtamembrane (exon 11) or extracellular domain (exon 9). In patients with acquired resistance, the mutations are predominantly located in two regions of the intracellular kinase domain; one in the ATP-binding pocket (exons 13 and 14), which directly interferes with the drug binding, and the second one in the activation loop (exons 17 and 18), where mutations can stabilize KIT in the active conformation and hinder drug interaction [24].

Multiple authors have reported the presence of heterogeneity of resistance within the different lesions but also within the same tumor [63–66]. Liegl et al. studied KIT and PDGFRA mutations in 53 GIST metastases obtained from 14 patients who underwent surgical debulking after progression on imatinib or sunitinib. Primary KIT oncogenic mutations were found in 11/14 patients (79 %). Of these, 9/11 (83 %) had secondary drug-resistant KIT mutations, including six (67 %) with two to five different secondary mutations in separate metastases, and three (34 %) with two secondary KIT mutations in the same metastasis. FISH analyses revealed KIT amplicons in 2/10 metastases lacking secondary KIT mutations. This study demonstrates extensive intralesional and interlesional heterogeneity of resistance mutations and gene amplification in patients with clinically progressing GIST [65]. Other mechanisms of survival of imatinib-resistant GIST cells like PI3k/AKT pathway activation and AXL or IGF1R overexpression are being studied at this time. The mechanisms of development of additional genetic mutations is poorly understood.

4.6 TKI Therapy for Imatinib-Resistant Metastatic GIST

Once there is progression of disease on standard dosage imatinib, the initial approach is typically to maximize the dose of imatinib to 800 mg daily [18]. Dose escalation does provide some patients with meaningful response, with up to one-third experiencing disease stability with this approach. In addition, the median survival for patients who require dose escalation due to progression on the standard dosing regimen is approximately 19 months [67]. After progression on the maximum tolerated dose of imatinib, patients should be switched to another therapy, including sunitinib [18]. Sunitinib is a tyrosine kinase inhibitor that has both anti-angiogenic and antioncogenic properties, since it inhibits the vascular endothelial growth factor receptor and the KIT receptor, respectively. Sunitinib has been shown to provide clinical benefit in over one-half of patients with imatinib-resistant/intolerant GIST patients [68]. In a phase III randomized trial investigating, sunitinib at a 50 mg daily dose (4 weeks on and 2 weeks off per cycle) versus placebo in metastatic, imatinib-resistant GIST, patients receiving placebo had a much worse time to progression compared to those who received sunitinib (6.4 weeks vs. 27.3 weeks; $p<0.0001$). There was a greater estimated overall survival, and the therapy was reasonably well tolerated [69]. Because of results like these, the FDA approved sunitinib for the treatment of GIST after disease progression on or intolerance to imatinib [18].

4.7 GIST Resistant to Imatinib and Sunitinib (GRIS)

Patients with GRIS may have a poor prognosis, and their treatment is challenging. Following established mechanisms of action, various TKIs have been studied in patients with GRIS, including sorafenib, nilotinib, dasatinib, and most recently regorafenib. Regorafenib is a multikinase inhibitor, with activity against KIT, PDGFR, and VEGFR, that was recently approved by the FDA for the treatment of patients with locally advanced, unresectable, or metastatic GIST previously treated with imatinib and sunitinib [18].

A multicenter phase II study in GRIS patients reported a clinical benefit rate of 79 % and a median progression-free survival of 10 months [70]. Most recently, a double-blind, phase III trial (GRID trial) randomized patients to regorafenib versus placebo (PL). The median progression-free survival was 4.8 months for REG versus 0.9 months for PL ($p<0.0001$). In addition, disease control was achieved in half of the patients in the regorafenib arm [71]. These data established regorafenib as a viable option for patients with GRIS.

Sorafenib is a multityrosine and serine/threonine kinase inhibitor, with activity against RAF, PDGFR, VEGFR, and KIT. Several studies have established the potential benefit of sorafenib for patients with GRIS. The University of Chicago phase II consortium trial examined the use of sorafenib 400 mg twice daily in

GRIS patients. The study showed an overall disease control rate of 68 %. The median progression-free survival and overall survival were 5.2 months and 11.6 months, respectively. Interestingly, one-third of patients with primary sunitinib resistance had either a partial response or stable disease for greater than 6 months on sorafenib [72]. Others have shown that sorafenib is not only effective in patients with GRIS, but has a reasonable toxicity profile [73]. Toxicity has been reported in 56 % of the patients, and many will require a dose reduction [74, 75].

Nilotinib is a multikinase inhibitor with activity against KIT, BCR/ABL, PDGFRB, and DDR1/2. The clinical activity of nilotinib, given either as a single agent or in combination with imatinib in patients with refractory GIST, was established in a phase I clinical trial [76]. This led the way for a phase II study of nilotinib as third-line therapy for patients with GRIS, which reported disease control rate of 29 % at week 24 and a median progression-free survival of 3.5 months. The median overall survival was 310 days [77]. These data demonstrated that nilotinib has efficacy in patients with resistant GIST. A subsequent phase III trial provided further evidence on the efficacy of nilotinib in patients with advanced GIST following prior imatinib and sunitinib failure [78].

Dasatinib is a multikinase inhibitor that has activity against KIT, PDGFR, BCR/ABL, and SRC. It has demonstrated activity against the PDGFRA D842V mutation which confers the maximum resistance to imatinib, and it may be an effective treatment alternative for this group of patients [79]. A phase II study of dasatinib at a dose of 70 mg twice daily in patients with GRIS showed that 32 % of patients had a partial response, and 21 % patients were progression-free for over 6 months [80]. Therefore, dasatinib represents a viable treatment option for patients with this challenging mutation.

Several other tyrosine inhibitors are currently being evaluated. Pazopanib is a multityrosine kinase inhibitor of VEGFR, PDGFR, cytokine receptor, and interleukin-2. In a multicenter phase II study of patients with advanced GIST following failure of at least imatinib and sunitinib, pazopanib showed promising results with a 24-week nonprogression rate of 17 % and an overall survival of 10.7 months [81]. Masitinib mesylate is a highly selective TKI with comparable activity to imatinib against wild-type and mutant KIT (exons 9 and 11) [82, 83]. Initial phase I data [84] led to the design of a prospective, multicenter, randomized, open-label, phase II study, evaluating the safety and efficacy of masitinib versus sunitinib for the treatment of advanced imatinib-resistant GIST [85]. Interestingly, mastitinib seems to be better tolerated than sunitinib with fewer side effects. Results of this trial demonstrate a median overall survival that was significantly longer for patients receiving masitinib followed by postprogression addition of sunitinib when compared against patients treated directly with sunitinib as second-line therapy following progression on imatinib [85]. A phase III trial designed to determine the clinical use of masitinib in patients with imatinib-resistant GIST is currently ongoing [86]. These preliminary data are encouraging and suggest that mastitinib might play a role following progression on first-line imatinib.

5 Conclusions

Treatment of gastrointestinal stromal tumors represents one of the paradigms of modern oncology. The development of selective inhibitors based on specific mutational status provides many patients with promising treatment options. Multiple tyrosine kinase inhibitors exist and show various activities against GIST. Further research and drug development will no doubt result in more options for patients afflicted with GIST.

References

1. Judson I, Demetri G. Advances in the treatment of gastrointestinal stromal tumours. Ann Oncol. 2007;18 Suppl 10:x20–4.
2. Kindblom LG, Remotti HE, Aldenborg F, Meis-Kindblom JM. Gastrointestinal pacemaker cell tumor (GIPACT): gastrointestinal stromal tumors show phenotypic characteristics of the interstitial cells of Cajal. Am J Pathol. 1998;152(5):1259–69.
3. Sarlomo-Rikala M, et al. CD117: a sensitive marker for gastrointestinal stromal tumors that is more specific than CD34. Mod Pathol. 1998;11(8):728–34.
4. Liegl B, et al. Monoclonal antibody DOG1.1 shows higher sensitivity than KIT in the diagnosis of gastrointestinal stromal tumors, including unusual subtypes. Am J Surg Pathol. 2009;33(3):437–46.
5. Corless CL, Heinrich MC. Molecular pathobiology of gastrointestinal stromal sarcomas. Annu Rev Pathol. 2008;3:557–86.
6. Kawanowa K, et al. High incidence of microscopic gastrointestinal stromal tumors in the stomach. Hum Pathol. 2006;37(12):1527–35.
7. Agaimy A, et al. Minute gastric sclerosing stromal tumors (GIST tumorlets) are common in adults and frequently show c-KIT mutations. Am J Surg Pathol. 2007;31(1):113–20.
8. Goettsch WG, et al. Incidence of gastrointestinal stromal tumours is underestimated: results of a nation-wide study. Eur J Cancer. 2005;41(18):2868–72.
9. Kukar M, et al. Gastrointestinal stromal tumors (GISTs) at uncommon locations: a large population based analysis. J Surg Oncol. 2015;111(6):696–701.
10. Fletcher CD, et al. Diagnosis of gastrointestinal stromal tumors: a consensus approach. Int J Surg Pathol. 2002;10(2):81–9.
11. DeMatteo RP, et al. Two hundred gastrointestinal stromal tumors: recurrence patterns and prognostic factors for survival. Ann Surg. 2000;231(1):51–8.
12. Miettinen M, Sobin LH, Lasota J. Gastrointestinal stromal tumors of the stomach: a clinicopathologic, immunohistochemical, and molecular genetic study of 1765 cases with long-term follow-up. Am J Surg Pathol. 2005;29(1):52–68.
13. Verweij J, et al. Progression-free survival in gastrointestinal stromal tumours with high-dose imatinib: randomised trial. Lancet. 2004;364(9440):1127–34.
14. Foo WC, Liegl-Atzwanger B, Lazar AJ. Pathology of gastrointestinal stromal tumors. Clin Med Insights Pathol. 2012;5:23–33.
15. Andersson J, et al. NF1-associated gastrointestinal stromal tumors have unique clinical, phenotypic, and genotypic characteristics. Am J Surg Pathol. 2005;29(9):1170–6.
16. Miettinen M, et al. Gastrointestinal stromal tumors in patients with neurofibromatosis 1: a clinicopathologic and molecular genetic study of 45 cases. Am J Surg Pathol. 2006;30(1):90–6.
17. Kinoshita K, et al. Absence of c-kit gene mutations in gastrointestinal stromal tumours from neurofibromatosis type 1 patients. J Pathol. 2004;202(1):80–5.

18. 1.2015, N.C.C.N.S.T.S.G.V. http://www.nccn.org/professionals/physician_gls/pdf/sarcoma.pdf. Accessed 24 Mar 2015.
19. 3.2012, N.C.C.N.S.T.S.G.V. http://www.nccn.org/professionals/physician_gls/pdf/sarcoma.pdf. Accessed 24 Dec 2012.
20. Corless CL, Fletcher JA, Heinrich MC. Biology of gastrointestinal stromal tumors. J Clin Oncol. 2004;22(18):3813–25.
21. West RB, et al. The novel marker, DOG1, is expressed ubiquitously in gastrointestinal stromal tumors irrespective of KIT or PDGFRA mutation status. Am J Pathol. 2004;165(1):107–13.
22. Novelli M, et al. DOG1 and CD117 are the antibodies of choice in the diagnosis of gastrointestinal stromal tumours. Histopathology. 2010;57(2):259–70.
23. Lennartsson J, et al. Normal and oncogenic forms of the receptor tyrosine kinase kit. Stem Cells. 2005;23(1):16–43.
24. Corless CL, Barnett CM, Heinrich MC. Gastrointestinal stromal tumours: origin and molecular oncology. Nat Rev Cancer. 2011;11(12):865–78.
25. Heinrich MC, et al. Kinase mutations and imatinib response in patients with metastatic gastrointestinal stromal tumor. J Clin Oncol. 2003;21(23):4342–9.
26. Janeway KA, et al. Pediatric KIT wild-type and platelet-derived growth factor receptor alpha-wild-type gastrointestinal stromal tumors share KIT activation but not mechanisms of genetic progression with adult gastrointestinal stromal tumors. Cancer Res. 2007;67(19):9084–8.
27. Hostein I, et al. BRAF mutation status in gastrointestinal stromal tumors. Am J Clin Pathol. 2010;133(1):141–8.
28. Agaram NP, et al. Novel V600E BRAF mutations in imatinib-naive and imatinib-resistant gastrointestinal stromal tumors. Genes Chromosomes Cancer. 2008;47(10):853–9.
29. NCT02034110. U.S.N.I.o.H.E.a.S.o.t.C.T.o.D.a.T.i.S.W.B.V.E.-M.R.C.C.g.i.
30. Miranda C, et al. KRAS and BRAF mutations predict primary resistance to imatinib in gastrointestinal stromal tumors. Clin Cancer Res. 2012;18(6):1769–76.
31. Eisenberg BL, Judson I. Surgery and imatinib in the management of GIST: emerging approaches to adjuvant and neoadjuvant therapy. Ann Surg Oncol. 2004;11(5):465–75.
32. Ryan DP, et al. A phase II and pharmacokinetic study of ecteinascidin 743 in patients with gastrointestinal stromal tumors. Oncologist. 2002;7(6):531–8.
33. Edmonson JH, et al. Contrast of response to dacarbazine, mitomycin, doxorubicin, and cisplatin (DMAP) plus GM-CSF between patients with advanced malignant gastrointestinal stromal tumors and patients with other advanced leiomyosarcomas. Cancer Invest. 2002;20(5–6):605–12.
34. Trent JC, et al. A two-arm phase II study of temozolomide in patients with advanced gastrointestinal stromal tumors and other soft tissue sarcomas. Cancer. 2003;98(12):2693–9.
35. Siehl J, Thiel E. C-kit, GIST, and imatinib. Recent Results Cancer Res. 2007;176:145–51.
36. Joensuu H, et al. Effect of the tyrosine kinase inhibitor STI571 in a patient with a metastatic gastrointestinal stromal tumor. N Engl J Med. 2001;344(14):1052–6.
37. Scaife CL, et al. Is there a role for surgery in patients with "unresectable" cKIT+ gastrointestinal stromal tumors treated with imatinib mesylate? Am J Surg. 2003;186(6):665–9.
38. Fiore M, et al. Preoperative imatinib mesylate for unresectable or locally advanced primary gastrointestinal stromal tumors (GIST). Eur J Surg Oncol. 2009;35(7):739–45.
39. Dematteo RP, et al. Adjuvant imatinib mesylate after resection of localised, primary gastrointestinal stromal tumour: a randomised, double-blind, placebo-controlled trial. Lancet. 2009;373(9669):1097–104.
40. Joensuu H, et al. One vs three years of adjuvant imatinib for operable gastrointestinal stromal tumor: a randomized trial. JAMA. 2012;307(12):1265–72.
41. NCT00103168. U.S.N.I.o.H.I.m.o.o.o.i.t.p.w.h.u.s.f.l.g.s.t.E.C.g.I. http://clinicaltrials.gov/ct2/show/NCT00103168?term=EORTC+62024&rank=1. Accessed 24 Mar 2015.
42. Casali PG, Le Cesne A, Velasco AP, Kotasek D, Rutkowski P, Hohenberger P, Fumagalli E, Judson IR. Imatinib failure-free survival (IFS) in patients with localized gastrointestinal stromal tumors (GIST) treated with adjuvant imatinib (IM): the EORTC/AGITG/FSG/GEIS/ISG randomized controlled phase III trial. J Clin Oncol. 2013;31(15 Suppl):Abstract 10500.

43. http://clinicaltrials.gov/ct2/show/record/NCT00867113. Accessed 24 Mar 2015. U.S.N.I.o.H. F.y.a.i.m.G.i.G.s.t.P.C.g.i.N.
44. Eisenberg BL, et al. Phase II trial of neoadjuvant/adjuvant imatinib mesylate (IM) for advanced primary and metastatic/recurrent operable gastrointestinal stromal tumor (GIST): early results of RTOG 0132/ACRIN 6665. J Surg Oncol. 2009;99(1):42–7.
45. Wang D, et al. Phase II trial of neoadjuvant/adjuvant imatinib mesylate for advanced primary and metastatic/recurrent operable gastrointestinal stromal tumors: long-term follow-up results of Radiation Therapy Oncology Group 0132. Ann Surg Oncol. 2012;19(4):1074–80.
46. Blesius A, et al. Neoadjuvant imatinib in patients with locally advanced non metastatic GIST in the prospective BFR14 trial. BMC Cancer. 2011;11:72.
47. van Oosterom AT, et al. Safety and efficacy of imatinib (STI571) in metastatic gastrointestinal stromal tumours: a phase I study. Lancet. 2001;358(9291):1421–3.
48. Blanke CD, et al. Phase III randomized, intergroup trial assessing imatinib mesylate at two dose levels in patients with unresectable or metastatic gastrointestinal stromal tumors expressing the kit receptor tyrosine kinase: S0033. J Clin Oncol. 2008;26(4):626–32.
49. von Mehren M, Blanke C, Joensuu H, Heinrich M, Roberts P, Eisenberg B, et al. High Incidence of durable responses induced by imatinib mesylate (Gleevec) in patients with unresectable and metastatic gastrointestinal stromal tumors (GISTs) (abstract # 1608). Proceedings of the American Society of Clinical Oncology. 2002.
50. Demetri GD, et al. Efficacy and safety of imatinib mesylate in advanced gastrointestinal stromal tumors. N Engl J Med. 2002;347(7):472–80.
51. von Mehren M, Heinrich M, Joensuu H, et al. Follow up results after 9 years (yrs) of the ongoing, phase II B2222 trial of imatinib mesylate (IM) in patients (pts) with metastatic or unresectable kit+gastrointestinal stromal tumors (GIST). [Abstract] J Clin Oncol. 2011;29(15_Suppl): Abstract 10016.
52. Debiec-Rychter M, et al. KIT mutations and dose selection for imatinib in patients with advanced gastrointestinal stromal tumours. Eur J Cancer. 2006;42(8):1093–103.
53. Heinrich MC, et al. Correlation of kinase genotype and clinical outcome in the North American Intergroup Phase III Trial of imatinib mesylate for treatment of advanced gastrointestinal stromal tumor: CALGB 150105 Study by Cancer and Leukemia Group B and Southwest Oncology Group. J Clin Oncol. 2008;26(33):5360–7.
54. Gastrointestinal Stromal Tumor Meta-Analysis Group (MetaGIST). Comparison of two doses of imatinib for the treatment of unresectable or metastatic gastrointestinal stromal tumors: a meta-analysis of 1,640 patients. J Clin Oncol. 2010;28(7):1247–53.
55. Blay JY, et al. Prospective multicentric randomized phase III study of imatinib in patients with advanced gastrointestinal stromal tumors comparing interruption versus continuation of treatment beyond 1 year: the French Sarcoma Group. J Clin Oncol. 2007;25(9):1107–13.
56. Patrikidou A, et al. Influence of imatinib interruption and rechallenge on the residual disease in patients with advanced GIST: results of the BFR14 prospective French Sarcoma Group randomised, phase III trial. Ann Oncol. 2013;24(4):1087–93.
57. Benjamin RS, et al. Gastrointestinal stromal tumors II: medical oncology and tumor response assessment. Semin Oncol. 2009;36(4):302–11.
58. Corless CL, et al. PDGFRA mutations in gastrointestinal stromal tumors: frequency, spectrum and in vitro sensitivity to imatinib. J Clin Oncol. 2005;23(23):5357–64.
59. Biron P, e.a.O.o.p.p.w.P.D.V.m.g.s.t.G.t.w.i.I.f.a.d.J.C.O.
60. Blanke CD, et al. Long-term results from a randomized phase II trial of standard- versus higher-dose imatinib mesylate for patients with unresectable or metastatic gastrointestinal stromal tumors expressing KIT. J Clin Oncol. 2008;26(4):620–5.
61. Chen LL, et al. A missense mutation in KIT kinase domain 1 correlates with imatinib resistance in gastrointestinal stromal tumors. Cancer Res. 2004;64(17):5913–9.
62. Antonescu CR, et al. Acquired resistance to imatinib in gastrointestinal stromal tumor occurs through secondary gene mutation. Clin Cancer Res. 2005;11(11):4182–90.
63. Heinrich MC, et al. Molecular correlates of imatinib resistance in gastrointestinal stromal tumors. J Clin Oncol. 2006;24(29):4764–74.

64. Wakai T, et al. Late resistance to imatinib therapy in a metastatic gastrointestinal stromal tumour is associated with a second KIT mutation. Br J Cancer. 2004;90(11):2059–61.
65. Liegl B, et al. Heterogeneity of kinase inhibitor resistance mechanisms in GIST. J Pathol. 2008;216(1):64–74.
66. Loughrey MB, et al. Polyclonal resistance in gastrointestinal stromal tumor treated with sequential kinase inhibitors. Clin Cancer Res. 2006;12(20 Pt 1):6205–6; author reply 6206–7.
67. Rankin C, von Mehren M, Blanke CD, Benjamin R, Fletcher CD, Bramwell VH, et al. Dose effect of imatinib (IM) in patients (pts) with metastatic GIST – Phase III Sarcoma Group Study S0033. J Clin Oncol. 2004 ASCO Annual meeting proceedings (post-meeting edition). 2004;22(14S (July 15 Suppl)):9005.
68. George S, et al. Clinical evaluation of continuous daily dosing of sunitinib malate in patients with advanced gastrointestinal stromal tumour after imatinib failure. Eur J Cancer. 2009;45(11):1959–68.
69. Demetri GD, et al. Efficacy and safety of sunitinib in patients with advanced gastrointestinal stromal tumour after failure of imatinib: a randomised controlled trial. Lancet. 2006;368(9544):1329–38.
70. George S, et al. Efficacy and safety of regorafenib in patients with metastatic and/or unresectable GI stromal tumor after failure of imatinib and sunitinib: a multicenter phase II trial. J Clin Oncol. 2012;30(19):2401–7.
71. Demetri GD, et al. Efficacy and safety of regorafenib for advanced gastrointestinal stromal tumours after failure of imatinib and sunitinib (GRID): an international, multicentre, randomised, placebo-controlled, phase 3 trial. Lancet. 2013;381(9863):295–302.
72. Kindler HL, Campbell NP, Wroblewski K, et al. Sorafenib (SOR) in patients (pts) with imatinib (IM) and sunitinib (SU)-resistant (RES) gastrointestinal stromal tumor (GIST): final results of a University of Chicago Phase II consortium trial. J Clin Oncol. 2011;29(15_Suppl):Abstract 10009.
73. Park SH, et al. Sorafenib in patients with metastatic gastrointestinal stromal tumors who failed two or more prior tyrosine kinase inhibitors: a phase II study of Korean gastrointestinal stromal tumors study group. Invest New Drugs. 2012;30(6):2377–83.
74. Montemurro M, et al. Sorafenib as third- or fourth-line treatment of advanced gastrointestinal stromal tumour and pretreatment including both imatinib and sunitinib, and nilotinib: a retrospective analysis. Eur J Cancer. 2012;49(5):1027–31.
75. Kefeli U, et al. Efficacy of sorafenib in patients with gastrointestinal stromal tumors in the third- or fourth-line treatment: a retrospective multicenter experience. Oncol Lett. 2013;6(2):605–11.
76. Demetri GD, et al. A phase I study of single-agent nilotinib or in combination with imatinib in patients with imatinib-resistant gastrointestinal stromal tumors. Clin Cancer Res. 2009;15(18):5910–6.
77. Sawaki A, et al. Phase 2 study of nilotinib as third-line therapy for patients with gastrointestinal stromal tumor. Cancer. 2011;117(20):4633–41.
78. Reichardt P, et al. Phase III study of nilotinib versus best supportive care with or without a TKI in patients with gastrointestinal stromal tumors resistant to or intolerant of imatinib and sunitinib. Ann Oncol. 2012;23(7):1680–7.
79. Dewaele B, et al. Activity of dasatinib, a dual SRC/ABL kinase inhibitor, and IPI-504, a heat shock protein 90 inhibitor, against gastrointestinal stromal tumor-associated PDGFRAD842V mutation. Clin Cancer Res. 2008;14(18):5749–58.
80. Trent JC, Wathen K, von Mehren M, et al. A phase II study of dasatinib for patients with imatinib-resistant gastrointestinal stromal tumor (GIST). J Clin Oncol. 2011 ASCO Annual meeting proceedings (post-meeting edition). 2011;29(15_Suppl (May 20 Supplement)):10006.
81. Ganjoo KN, et al. A multicenter phase II study of pazopanib in patients with advanced gastrointestinal stromal tumors (GIST) following failure of at least imatinib and sunitinib. Ann Oncol. 2014;25(1):236–40.

82. Dubreuil P, et al. Masitinib (AB1010), a potent and selective tyrosine kinase inhibitor targeting KIT. PLoS One. 2009;4(9):e7258.
83. Davis MI, et al. Comprehensive analysis of kinase inhibitor selectivity. Nat Biotechnol. 2011;29(11):1046–51.
84. Soria JC, et al. Phase 1 dose-escalation study of oral tyrosine kinase inhibitor masitinib in advanced and/or metastatic solid cancers. Eur J Cancer. 2009;45(13):2333–41.
85. Adenis A, et al. Masitinib in advanced gastrointestinal stromal tumor (GIST) after failure of imatinib: a randomized controlled open-label trial. Ann Oncol. 2014;25(9):1762–9.
86. Health U.S.N.I.o. A phase 3 study to evaluate efficacy and safety of masitinib in comparison to sunitinib in patients with gastrointestinal stromal tumour after progression with imatinib. ClinicalTrials.gov identifier NCT01694277.

Multimodality Therapy for Metastatic Gastrointestinal Stromal Tumor

David A. Mahvi, Emily Z. Keung, and Chandrajit P. Raut

1 Introduction

Gastrointestinal stromal tumors (GISTs) represent approximately 80 % of sarcomas that arise from the gastrointestinal tract. The primary tumor most commonly arises from the stomach (40–60 %), with small intestine and colon being the next two most common sites of primary disease. GISTs primarily metastasize to the liver and peritoneum. Rarer sites of metastasis include lymph nodes (usually in pediatric-type GIST), lung, and bone.

As in other cancer types, prognosis and 5-year overall survival (OS) are significantly impacted by tumor extent at the time of GIST diagnosis. In the contemporary era since widespread use of targeted tyrosine kinase inhibitor (TKI) therapies, individuals with localized GIST have a 5-year OS of 91 %. In comparison, those with locally advanced disease and metastatic disease at the time of diagnosis have 5-year OS rates of 74 % and 48 %, respectively [1]. Median OS of advanced or metastatic GIST is approximately 51–57 months [2].

This chapter will begin with an overview of the role of TKIs in the treatment of metastatic GIST. Next, the roles of systemic chemotherapy, radiation therapy, and hyperthermic intraperitoneal chemotherapy (HIPEC) will be addressed. Finally, the role of surgical management in the treatment of metastatic GIST will be explored.

D.A. Mahvi, MD • E.Z. Keung, MD • C.P. Raut, MD, MSc (✉)
Department of Surgery, Brigham and Women's Hospital, Center for Sarcoma and Bone Oncology, Dana-Farber Cancer Institute, Harvard Medical School, Boston, MA, USA
e-mail: craut@partners.org

© Springer International Publishing Switzerland 2017

C.R. Scoggins et al. (eds.), *Gastrointestinal Stromal Tumors*,
DOI 10.1007/978-3-319-42632-7_14

2 Tyrosine Kinase Inhibitors

2.1 Imatinib

The treatment and outcomes of metastatic GIST changed dramatically with the introduction of imatinib (Gleevec). In 1998, Hirota and colleagues [3] reported that GISTs frequently are characterized by gain-of-function mutations in the gene encoding the c-KIT receptor tyrosine kinase (RTK). Others furthered the understanding of the disease by identifying CD117 as a sensitive marker for the disease [4] and demonstrating that the interstitial cells of Cajal were likely the cells of origin [5]. This work paved way for future therapeutic options.

Imatinib is a tyrosine kinase inhibitor (TKI) that was initially developed in the 1990s for the treatment of chronic myelogenous leukemia (CML) to target the fusion protein *BCL–ABL*. This constitutively active RTK arises as a result of a reciprocal translocation of chromosome 9 and 22 that occurs in the majority of patients with CML. Approximately 95 % of GISTs exhibit pathological overexpression of KIT (CD117) [6]. Imatinib has been found to be specific for the tyrosine kinase domain abl, c-kit, and platelet-derived growth factor receptor (PDGFR) [7]. Imatinib was first shown to have activity in vitro against a GIST cell line by Tuveson et al. [8]. These findings prompted Joensuu et al. [9] to treat a Finnish patient with the drug. This patient, who had disease progression despite repeated surgical resections and multiple lines of chemotherapy, experienced tumor regression on MRI and PET scans.

This served as the catalyst for subsequent trials to investigate the use of imatinib in advanced GIST, including two randomized controlled trials. The S0033 phase III trial [10] compared standard dose (400 mg daily) with high-dose (800 mg daily) imatinib in 746 patients with advanced GIST to assess if there was a dose–effect on progression-free survival (PFS) or OS. There was no significant difference between the two dosing regimens in terms of PFS (18 vs 20 months) or OS (55 vs 51 months). However, patients in this trial who progressed on the standard dose were allowed to crossover to the 800 mg imatinib dose. Of these patients, 3 % achieved a partial response (PR) and 28 % stable disease (SD), with a median PFS of 5 months and median OS of 19 months from the date of crossover. The 2-year OS was 70 % compared to 25 % for those historically treated with traditional systemic chemotherapy. The authors concluded it was reasonable to treat using standard dose imatinib as first-line therapy for metastatic GIST and to increase the dose at the time of disease progression.

The European Organisation of Research and Treatment of Cancer (EORTC) conducted a similar study in Europe and Australia (EORTC 62005) [11] in 946 patients. Rates of complete response (CR) (5 %), PR (47 %), and SD (32 %) were similar between the two groups; however, there was a significant increase in PFS in the higher imatinib dose group (50 % vs 44 %, $p=0.026$). This difference in PFS was not sustained at 40-month median follow-up, and no difference in OS was noted [12].

In both trials, the higher dose of imatinib was associated with higher rates of adverse events. The most common toxicities were anemia, neutropenia, cardiac, nausea/diarrhea, and hemorrhage. In S0033, there were 219 grade 3 or higher adverse events in the group receiving the higher imatinib dose compared to 149 events in the group receiving the lower dose; this included two deaths [10].

The question of whether to discontinue treatment with imatinib in patients with durable response was addressed in a French Sarcoma Group phase III trial [13] that included 50 patients with nonprogressive disease after 1, 3, and 5 years on imatinib. The 2-year PFS was 80 % in the group that continued to take imatinib daily versus only 16 % in patients that had discontinued imatinib. There was no difference in grade 3 or higher adverse events. Therefore, imatinib should be continued in patients responding to treatment, unless limited by significant side effects.

Approximately 14 % of GISTs are primarily resistant to imatinib, progressing within 6 months of starting therapy [14]. Tumors that have primary resistance (and thus are unlikely to respond to imatinib) often either have mutations in *PDGFRA* (specifically *PDGFRA* exon 18 D842V) or lack mutations in *KIT* or *PDGFRA* (so-called "wild-type") [15]. Secondary resistance is defined as the disease progression after 6 months of therapy and is usually due to clonal evolution, with the gain of a secondary mutation in the same gene. The most common secondary mutations occur in exons 13, 14, and 17 of *KIT* [16, 17]. Objective clinical responses to imatinib are associated with the genotype of the tumor. Patients with the *KIT* exon 11 mutant isoform have longer median time to treatment failure and longer median OS. Heinrich et al. [16] showed that there is a higher CR/PR rate to imatinib in patients with *KIT* exon 11 mutations (71.7 %) versus *KIT* exon 9 mutations (44.7 %, $p = .007$) and wild-type (44.6 %, $p = 0.002$). Data from a planned post hoc analysis of the S0033 and EORTC 62005 trials suggested that the 800 mg dose is more effective and thus is recommended for patients with *KIT* exon 9 mutations [18]. Genetic subgroups that may benefit more from imatinib and other TKIs will likely continue to be identified as pharmacogenomics becomes more established in clinical oncological care.

The NCCN [19] endorses continuing TKI therapy even in the face of documented disease progression. Progression may occur in only a portion of the tumor or limited foci of multifocal tumor; so, discontinuation of TKI therapy would lead to more rapid, diffuse tumor progression and shortened survival. Furthermore, imatinib should be administered up to the date of surgery and restarted when the patient can tolerate oral intake.

2.2 *Sunitinib*

The second-line treatment for metastatic GIST is sunitinib (Sutent). A phase III double-blind placebo-controlled trial [20] of sunitinib was published in 2006 of 312 patients with advanced GIST who had either progressed on or were intolerant of imatinib. They were randomized in a 2:1 ratio to receive either sunitinib or placebo.

Median time to tumor progression (primary end point) was 27.3 weeks among patients who received sunitinib versus 6.4 weeks in the placebo group. Primary adverse reactions included fatigue, nausea, and diarrhea. The study was unblinded at the first interim analysis to allow patient crossover, given the significant PFS benefit seen among the sunitinib group. Of the original 118 patients initially randomized to placebo, 103 crossed over to receive sunitinib. Median OS among patients treated with sunitinib was 72.7 weeks on long-term follow-up. Median OS in the placebo arm was 64.9 weeks with a rank-preserving structural failure time analysis estimating a corrected OS of 39.0 weeks in the placebo group when accounting for crossover [21].

The above trial used a dose of 50 mg sunitinib for 4 weeks with a subsequent 2-week drug holiday. Given the potential challenges of this intermittent dosing schedule, 60 patients with imatinib-resistant GIST or imatinib intolerance in a phase II study [22] were given continuous sunitinib 37.5 mg daily. They reported a partial response rate of 13 % with SD achieved for greater than 24 weeks in another 40 % of patients. Overall, median PFS was 34 weeks and OS was 107 weeks. There was no increase in adverse events compared to intermittent dosing. The authors concluded that continuous daily dosage was an acceptable alternative.

Responsiveness to sunitinib treatment correlates with specific pathological mutations. Acquisition of secondary *KIT* mutations is the primary mechanism of imatinib resistance in GIST [16, 17]. In a phase II trial [23–25], 97 patients who were either intolerant to or progressed on imatinib were treated with sunitinib and stratified into those with *KIT* exon 9 mutations, exon 11 mutations, and *KIT-PDGFRA* wild-type mutations. PR or SD for more than 6 months was achieved in 58 % of patients with *KIT* exon 9 mutations, 34 % with *KIT* exon 11 mutations, and 56 % with *KIT-PDGFRA* wild-type mutations. Rates of PR were 37 % versus 5 % for those with exon 9 and exon 11, respectively. PFS was 19.4 months (exon 9), 19 months (wild-type), and 5.1 months (exon 11). OS was 26.9 months (exon 9), 30.5 months (wild-type), and 12.3 months (exon 11). Among patients with exon 11 secondary mutations, those with secondary *KIT* mutations in exons 13 or 14 had median PFS of 7.8 months and OS of 13 months, whereas those with secondary mutations in exons 17 or 18 had median PFS of 2.3 months and OS of 4 months. These studies highlight the importance of GIST genotype to sunitinib responsiveness.

Sunitinib is considered standard of care for patients with GIST who have failed imatinib. NCCN guidelines recommend stopping sunitinib 5–7 days before surgery and restarting about 2 weeks after surgery [19]. However, in our experience, we find it is safe to stop sunitinib as late as 72 h prior to surgery and resume when the patient is tolerating a regular diet at home.

A Korean phase III trial [26] evaluated the resumption of imatinib versus placebo in patients with metastatic or unresectable disease after failure on imatinib and sunitinb. All 81 patients included had experienced PR or SD on first-line imatinib for at least 6 months but then progressed on imatinib and sunitinib. Median PFS was 1.8 months compared to 0.9 months for placebo for a hazard ratio (HR) of 0.46. Thus, resuming imatinib is superior to placebo, but only slows progression by approximately 1 month.

2.3 Regorafenib

The most recent TKI approved by the FDA for treatment of GIST is regorafenib (Stivarga). Regorafenib inhibits multiple targets, including KIT, RET, VEGFR 1–3, PDGFRB, and BRAF [27]. A phase III randomized double-blind, placebo-controlled trial [28] was done on 199 patients with GIST resistant to imatinib and sunitinib. Patients were randomized in a 2:1 ratio to regorafenib or placebo with crossover permitted upon disease progression on placebo. A dose of 160 mg was administered daily for 3 weeks followed by a 1-week treatment break. Median PFS was 4.8 months on regorafenib versus 0.9 months on placebo (HR 0.27). Further, PR or SD was seen in 75.9 % of patients on regorafenib versus 34.8 % on placebo. The most common grade 3 or higher adverse events were hypertension, hand–foot skin reaction, and diarrhea. Since regorafenib can result in significant liver toxicity, liver function tests are recommended prior to initiating therapy and biweekly for 2 months upon starting the drug [29]. Regorafenib is now FDA-approved and recommended as the third-line TKI for patients with metastatic and/or unresectable GIST who either have progressed on or are intolerant of imatinib and sunitinib. Hypothetically, it may also be considered second-line therapy for certain tumor genotypes. Whereas sunitinib is more effective in suppressing tumors with *KIT* exon 13 and 14 mutations, regorafenib shows a higher efficacy against tumors with *KIT* exon 17 mutations [30]. However, since genotyping of tumor recurrences is not routinely performed, sequencing of drug therapy can be imatinib, sunitinib, and then regorafenib.

2.4 Nilotinib

A phase III trial [31] of nilotinib versus imatinib as first-line therapy for unresectable or metastatic GIST was terminated early for futility when a significantly higher 2-year PFS was noted in imatinib group (59.2 % versus 51.6 % in nilotinib). Nilotinib may be of potential utility in patients with tumors containing *KIT* exon 11 mutations who cannot take imatinib, though generally it is appropriate to proceed with FDA-approved agents first before trying drugs such as nilotinib [15].

2.5 Other Tyrosine Kinase Inhibitors

There are multiple other TKIs in various stages of investigation as potential alternative targeted therapies for metastatic GIST [15, 30]. Sorafenib, vatalanib, dovitinib, pazopanib, masitinib, cedirinib, and crenolanib have all completed phase II trials. Further studies, including phase III trials for the more promising agents, are ongoing.

2.6 *Other Molecular Target Inhibitors*

While receptor tyrosine kinase inhibitors remain the primary drug class target for research in advanced GIST, other molecular targets are also being studied [30]. Heat-shock protein 90 (HSP90) is believed to help stabilize proteins required for tumor growth. BIIB021, AT13387, and AUY922 are all inhibitors of HSP90 in phase II trials presently. Ganetespib and retaspimycin were shown to have limited clinical activity and higher mortality, respectively, in trials and are no longer being actively investigated for GIST treatment. PI3K-AKT-mTOR inhibitors (perifosine, everolimus, sirolimus, temsirolimus), monoclonal antibodies (olaratumab), and insulin-like growth factor 1 receptor inhibitors (linsitinib) are additional drug classes being investigated for advanced GIST.

3 Chemotherapy

3.1 *Systemic Chemotherapy*

Numerous studies have been performed to evaluate various chemotherapeutic agents for the treatment of metastatic GIST. These trials predated the imatinib era and occurred at a time when consistently accurate diagnosis of GIST was suspected. GISTs are generally unresponsive to conventional cytotoxic chemotherapy. Combinations of doxorubicin [32–38], dacarbazine [32–34, 38], ifosfamide [33, 34, 39–42], etoposide [39], cisplatin [38], paclitaxel [43], gemcitabine [37, 40], and docetaxel [36] have all been studied in metastatic GIST. Partial response rates were less than 15 % in all but one study (3/11 patients responded to the combination of doxorubicin, dacarbazine, and ifosfamide). Additionally, many of these studies did not differentiate between GIST and leiomyosarcoma, and subgroup analysis demonstrated worse results in GIST patients treated with conventional chemotherapy. With the advent of TKI therapy, traditional systemic chemotherapy is no longer considered a standard treatment for metastatic GIST.

3.2 *Hyperthermic Intraperitoneal Chemotherapy*

Hyperthermic intraperitoneal chemotherapy (HIPEC) is the delivery of heated chemotherapy directly to the abdominal cavity as a peritoneal bath rather than an intravenous infusion. Given the potential benefit of HIPEC for peritoneal carcinomatosis seen in other cancers such as *Pseudomyxoma peritonei*, colorectal cancer, and appendiceal carcinoma, there was some interest in its potential efficacy in metastatic GIST. HIPEC is generally applied in combination with cytoreductive surgery (CRS) with a goal of complete gross (R0/R1) resection.

In the era before TKI, there were a few studies examining patients with peritoneal sarcomatosis that included GIST as a subgroup. Baratti et al. [44] included eight GIST patients who underwent CRS and HIPEC with cisplatin and doxorubicin or mitomycin-C. Seven patients achieved macroscopically complete cytoreduction. However, OS was only 18.2 months, the shortest of any sarcoma subgroup in their cohort. Rossi et al. [45] published on a series of 60 patients with peritoneal sarcomatosis who underwent cytoreductive surgery and cisplatin/doxorubicin HIPEC, 14 of whom had GIST. Median OS was 34 months, and on multivariate analysis, tumor histology was not significantly predictive of OS; however, GIST-specific OS was not reported in this series.

Bryan et al. [46] performed a retrospective analysis of a prospectively maintained database and looked at 16 patients who underwent CRS followed by HIPEC with or without mitomycin-C for peritoneal dissemination of GIST at Wake Forest between 1992 and 2012, thus spanning the introduction of TKI therapy. Two patients had an additional HIPEC procedure for recurrent disease. Thirteen of the eighteen procedures achieved an R0/R1 cytoreduction, and the median OS was 3.33 years in that subgroup. Six patients never received TKI therapy. Patients that received TKIs at any point had a median OS of 7.89 versus 1.04 years. Interestingly, even the patients that had an R0/1 resection with HIPEC but without any TKI therapy had a median OS of only 1.09 years. Of the 12 procedures where TKI therapy was given, 11 had preoperative TKI therapy and 1 did not. Five patients progressed on preoperative TKI therapy; the R0/1 resection rate was 40 % and the median OS was 1.35 years. Comparatively, the six patients that did not progress on preoperative TKI therapy had a R0/1 resection rate of 83.3 % ($p=0.24$), and the median OS was not reached ($p=0.007$). They concluded that CRS/HIPEC was neither associated with improved survival in patients treated before TKIs became standard of care nor in patients whose disease progressed despite TKIs.

A randomized trial performed by Bonvalot et al. [47] in 2005 compared cytoreduction with HIPEC versus cytoreduction alone in patients with peritoneal sarcomatosis. Ten of the thirty-eight patients had GIST. Median OS was 29 months in both groups.

The current consensus is that there is no routine role for HIPEC in the treatment of peritoneal disseminated GIST.

4 Radiation

A few studies have evaluated the potential role of radiation therapy in the treatment of GIST. In a study from Toronto [48], radiation therapy (RT) was given to two patients preoperatively for a fixed mass and to eight patients postoperatively for residual tumor. The median dose was 45 Gy in 1.8 fractions, and six of nine patients that were evaluated achieved long-term local control in the radiated field. There are a number of case reports [49–51] that suggest that RT may be a potentially useful adjunct in achieving local control for residual or recurrent GIST using between 36 and 54 Gy. For metastatic lesions, a Japanese case report [52] described a patient with an isolated 11 cm retroperitoneal metastasis who received carboplatin, epirubicin, picibanil, and 51 Gy of radiation therapy. At follow-up 6 years later, the tumor was 2 cm. It is difficult to determine how much of the potential benefit was from radiation versus other treatment modalities.

Imatinib increases radiosensitivity in vitro [53]. Two case studies have shown that it is both safe and effective to deliver RT concomitantly with imatinib. In one patient, incomplete resection of a primary pelvic GIST with concurrent metastatic liver lesions was followed by 54 Gy of pelvic irradiation and imatinib [54]. The patient's liver lesions ultimately progressed despite high-dose imatinib, but the residual pelvic tumor demonstrated radiographic complete response. The second patient had a rectal GIST that was treated with neoadjuvant imatinib and RT [55]. Radiation was terminated early due to hematological toxicity and proctitis, but a good response was achieved and the patient was able to undergo a low anterior resection. It has also been shown that radiation can be safely delivered concurrently with sunitinib, a second-line treatment for GIST. However, these studies did not specifically evaluate patients with GIST [56, 57]. A study in patients that received both sorafenib and radiation therapy for hepatocellular carcinoma showed significant hepatotoxicity which led to death in 7.5 % of the 40 patients, suggesting that this combination should likely be avoided [58].

Hurwitz et al. [59] reported a series of 12 patients with locally progressive and/or symptomatic metastatic GIST and the use of RT for palliation. Eleven of twelve patients had symptomatic improvement with reasonably low toxicity using 30 Gy in 10 fractions. Cuaron et al. [60] reported a series of 15 patients treated with palliative intent and reported a 6-month PFS of 57 %. For symptomatic tumors, they achieved partial palliation in 94.4 % and complete palliation in 44.4 %.

A recent phase II prospective trial [61] was performed in Finland in which 25 patients with progressive disease at intra-abdominal sites or the liver were treated with approximately 40 Gy of external beam RT. All patients had previously received or were unable to tolerate TKI treatment prior to study entry. Two patients achieved partial remission, twenty had stable target lesion size for >3 months (median stabilization time was 16 months), and three progressed. One grade 4 event was seen (biliary tract necrosis), but the therapy was otherwise well-tolerated. The study did not collect quality-of-life data.

Radiation therapy for GIST does show potential efficacy in select scenarios, namely recurrent disease, oligometastases, TKI-resistant disease, neoadjuvant treatment in cases with high risk of R1 or R2 resection, and palliation for symptomatic disease. As most sites of metastases are intra-abdominal, historically, there had not been much interest in RT given potential toxicity to small bowel and visceral structures. The development of intensity-modulated RT [62] and simultaneous integrated boost techniques [63] allow for higher doses of radiation to be delivered with more limited toxicity to abdominal structures and low potential for delayed complications [64].

Overall, RT does seem to have potential, albeit limited, utility in the treatment of symptomatic metastatic GIST refractory to TKI. However, as most of the reports to this point have been case reports or case series, more investigation is needed to delineate when RT should be used in metastatic GIST.

5 Surgical Management of Metastatic Disease

Surgical resection has taken on a new role in the treatment of metastatic GIST in the era of TKI therapy. The exact role of surgical management in the setting of metastatic GIST has been defined by retrospective analyses from high-volume centers. To date, there have been no randomized trials to evaluate the efficacy of metastasectomy with concurrent TKI treatment. While patients can be maintained on imatinib for a prolonged duration due to its low side effect profile and over 80 % of patients initially respond to treatment, less than 6 % of patients will experience pathological complete response [65, 66], and, overall, there is roughly a 24-month median time to progression with imatinib [67]. Hypothetically, by reducing the tumor burden and removing potentially resistant clones, surgery could delay disease progression and prolong survival.

5.1 Cytoreductive Surgery

Single-institution and multi-institutional retrospective studies document long-term disease control and longer OS for selected patients with limited metastatic disease who undergo metastasectomy (Table 1).

Raut et al. [68] published the first large study reporting survival rates of patients with metastatic or locally advanced GIST who had surgery after TKI therapy. They divided patients into three groups based on response to TKI. Twenty-three patients had PR or SD that was deemed completely resectable. Thirty-two patients had localized progression but, importantly, the tumors that did progress were resectable. Fourteen patients had metastatic disease with generalized or multifocal progression. After surgery, there was no evidence of disease in 78 %, 25 %, and 7 % of patients, respectively. The 12-month PFS was 80 %, 33 %, and 0 %, respectively. The 12-month OS was 95 %, 86 %, and 0 %, respectively. Outcomes of surgery and survival rates correlated with responsiveness to TKI therapy. Furthermore, the investigators concluded that patients with advanced GIST that exhibited SD or limited progression with resectable disease benefited from surgical resection.

Gronchi et al. [71] similarly showed in 38 patients with advanced GIST the importance of preoperative response to TKI therapy. In their cohort, 27 patients underwent metastasectomy while responding to imatinib. PFS was 96 % at 12 months and 69 % at 24 months among responders after surgery. The disease-specific survival (DSS) was 100 % at 12 months for responders. In comparison, the nonresponders all progressed by 12 months with DSS of 60 %.

Table 1 Summary of retrospective series reporting surgical management of metastatic GIST

Author, Year	Patients	TKI	R0/R1 rate	Recurrence/PFS	Survival	Predictors
Raut (2006) [68]	23 SD/PR 32 localized progression 14 generalized progression	All	SD/PR: 78 % LP: 25 % GP: 7 %	SD/PR: 80 % LP: 33 % GP: 0 %	12-month OS: SD/PR: 95 % LP: 86 % GP: 0 %	Responsiveness to TKI
Rutkowski (2006) [69]	24 SD/PR 8 progressive disease	All	SD/PR: 24/24 PD: 5/8	Median time to recurrence: 17 month (SD/PR) vs 12 month (PD)	N/A	In first 5 responders, imatinib was not continued postoperative and 4 recurred. In next 19, only 1 recurrence in median follow-up of 12 months
Bonvalot (2006) [70]	12 planned metastasectomy 5 local advanced 5 emergencies	12/12	10/12	Median: 23.4 month (included 5 locally advanced)	2-year OS: 62 % (all patients)	
Gronchi (2007) [71]	35 total 27 responding to TKI, 8 not	All	Responding: 24/27 Not responding: 4/8	12-month PFS: 96 % vs 0 % 24-month PFS: 69 %	12-month DSS: 100 % vs 60 %	TKI responsiveness
DeMatteo (2007) [72]	20 SD/PR 13 focal progression 7 multifocal progression	All	SD/PR: 17/20 FP: 6/13 MFP: 2/7	2-year PFS for SD/PR: 61 % Median TTP: 12 months for FP, 3 months for MFP	2-year OS: SD/PR: 100 % FR: 36 % 1-year OS for MFR: 36 %	TKI responsiveness
Andtbacka (2007) [73]	35 recurrent/met 11 locally advanced	All	Recurrent: 11/35 Locally advanced: 11/11	Median time to recurrence: 15.1 month	All R0 alive at 30.7 months. Median OS for incomplete: 12.0 months	Initial responsiveness to imatinib predicted complete resection (91 % vs 4 %)
Al-Batran (2007) [74]	9 FP 16 GP	All	FP: 9/9; GP got dose escalation	11.3 month (FP) vs 2.5 month (GP)	Median OS: not attained (FP) vs 22.8 month (GP)	

Author, Year	Patients	TKI	R0/R1 rate	Recurrence/PFS	Survival	Predictors
Yeh (2010) [75]	14 PR/SD 21 LP 3 GP	All	PR/SD: 42.9 % LP: 4.8 % GP: 0 %	2-year PFS PR/SD: 59.4 % LP: 35.9 % GP: 0 %	2-year OS PR/SD: 69.6 % LP: 48.4 % GP: 0 %	Trend toward more secondary mutations in *KIT* exon 17 in pts with LP vs SD
Mussi (2010) [76]	49 PR/SD 31 FP	All	PR/SD: 88 % FP: 45 %	2-year PFS: PR/SD: 64.4 % FP: 9.7 %	5-year DSS: 82.9 % vs 67.6 %	
Zaydfudim (2012) [77]	54 surgery 33 no surgery	32/54 preop	35/54	1-year PFS: 91 % PR 58 % SD 11 % DP	1-year OS: 98 % surgery vs 80 %	OS and PFS in surgical group associated with TKI response and R0 resection. Metastasectomy better than medical therapy alone (5-year OS: 65 % vs 11 %)
Bauer (2014) [78]	239	All	177 R0/R1 62 R2	Median PFS: 6.3 years vs 3.4 years	Median OS: 8.7 years vs 5.3 years	Female gender, short interval of imatinib prior to surgery, R0/R1 resection, nonprogressive disease preop, and liver mets
Park (2014) [79]	42 surgery 92 only TKI	All	Surgery: 62 %	Median PFS: 87.7 month vs 42.8 month	Median OS: not reached vs 88.8 month	Surgery group were younger, fewer peritoneal mets
Rubio-Casadevall (2015) [80]	27 surgery while PR/SD 20 surgery for PD 124 no surgery	All	PR/SD: 20/27 PD: 9/20	Median PFS: 73.4 month group 1 vs 44.6 month groups 2/3	Med OS: 87.6 months vs 59.9 month	Improved OS associated with: ECOG performance status, disease limited to one metastatic organ, metastasectomy

Abbreviations: *TKI* tyrosine kinase inhibitor, *PFS* progression-free survival, *OS* overall survival, *PR* partial response, *SD* stable disease, *LP* limited progression, *GP* generalized progression, *PD* progressive disease, *DSS* disease-specific survival, *FP* focal progression, *MFP* multifocal progression, *R0* macroscopically complete resection with negative microscopic margins, *R1* macroscopically complete with positive microscopic margins, *R2* macroscopically incomplete, *ECOG* Eastern Cooperative Oncology Group

DeMatteo et al. [72] analyzed 40 patients with metastatic GIST who underwent surgery at their center following preoperative imatinib. Patients were categorized as having responsive disease, focal resistance (one tumor growing), or multifocal resistance (multiple tumors growing). The 20 patients with responsive disease had 2-year PFS of 61 % and OS of 100 %. The 13 patients with focal resistance had a median time to progression of 12 months and 2-year OS of 36 %. The seven patients with multifocal resistance had a median time to progression of 3 months and a 1-year OS of 36 %.

Rutkowski et al. [69] reported the results of cytoreductive surgery performed on 32 patients with advanced GIST. Of these patients, 24 had complete or partial response on imatinib while 8 patients had progression, and surgery was performed as salvage therapy. All responders had R0/R1 resections. The first five patients in their series did not resume postoperative imatinib, and four recurred. The subsequent 19 patients received adjuvant imatinib, and only 1 patient recurred. Of the eight patients who did not respond to neoadjuvant TKI therapy, only two patients had R0/R1 resections and five progressed at a median of 12 months; one patient died perioperatively. When initial responders were separated by postoperative imatinib therapy, significant improvement was seen in PFS compared to initial nonresponders.

Bauer et al. [78] published the largest series to date, reporting multi-institutional EORTC-STBSG data. They examined 239 patients who underwent metastasectomy while on TKI therapy; 177 achieved R0/R1 resections, while 62 had R2 resections. The median OS was 8.7 years versus 5.3 years, respectively. The median PFS following R0/R1 resection was 6.3 years compared to 3.4 years for patients undergoing R2 resection. On multivariate analysis of OS, female gender, short interval of imatinib prior to surgery (25 months vs 8 months), R0/R1 resection, nonprogressive disease preoperatively, and liver metastases were positive prognostic factors. Incomplete resection and tumor debulking did not yield survival benefits.

Indications for resection per NCCN guidelines are as follows [19]:

1. Disease that is stable on or responding to TKI therapy when complete gross resection is possible (stable/responsive disease)
2. Isolated clones progressing on TKI therapy after initial response (indicative of secondary drug resistance), while other sites of disease remain stable (limited disease progression)
3. Emergencies including hemorrhage, perforation, obstruction, or abscess

The timing of metastasectomy is not standardized, although most experts agree with initiating TKI therapy and considering surgery depending on disease response around 6 months after TKI initiation. An et al. retrospectively reviewed primary cytoreduction versus imatinib therapy [81]. They compared 35 patients who underwent surgical cytoreduction of >75 % of tumor bulk prior to starting imatinib to 214 patients who started imatinib without surgery and showed no improvement in prognosis with cytoreduction first. Verweij et al. showed in their randomized trial comparing 400 mg of imatinib to 800 mg that the median time to best response is 3.5 months and that there is minimal incremental tumor shrinkage after 9 months

[11]. Fairweather et al. recommend operating between 6 and 12 months or at a point when there is no significant change between staging CTs [67]. NCCN guidelines recommend discussing surgery after 6–12 months of disease stability on TKI therapy [19]. Despite data from the multiple retrospective studies above, cytoreductive surgery following TKI therapy has not been shown to be superior to TKI therapy alone. This can only be answered by a randomized clinical trial; attempts at such a trial have failed due to poor accrual. Therefore, at this point, metastasectomy may be beneficial in selected individuals, but patients should be counseled that there are no data to prove it will improve survival over staying on TKI therapy alone.

One retrospective study by Raut et al. [82] reviewed 50 patients with metastatic GIST who underwent surgery following sunitinib treatment to determine if the responsiveness to sunitinib was associated with patient outcomes. Complete gross resection (R0/R1) was achieved in half of patients. The completeness of resection, PFS, and OS were not significantly correlated with response to sunitinib, likely reflecting selection biases in identifying appropriate patients for surgery on sunitinib.

In general, resection appears to benefit patients who have a PR or SD, and possibly those with isolated sites of progression. If there is isolated progression of a few individual lesions on surveillance, resection is reasonable, although there have been no studies to evaluate this versus changing TKI therapy. Surgery was generally not helpful in patients who had generalized progression on TKI therapy. When all metastatic sites can be resected, TKI therapy may prolong disease-free intervals. Incomplete resection may still potentially prolong progression-free intervals by removing drug-resistant clones; disease-free interval may still be prolonged by TKI therapy as long as the remaining disease remains drug responsive.

Importantly, surgery is not an alternative to TKI therapy. TKI therapy is generally continued until surgery (stopping imatinib 24 h, sunitinib 72 h, or regorafenib 1 week prior to surgery), and all patients undergoing surgery should resume drug therapy postoperatively indefinitely as soon as able to tolerate an oral diet.

5.2 Liver Resection

The liver is the site of metastasis in approximately 65 % of patients with relapsed GIST [83]. A few studies have examined outcomes following resection of liver metastases prior to the imatinib era. DeMatteo et al. [84] looked at 34 patients with either GIST or gastrointestinal leiomyosarcoma who underwent complete resection of hepatic metastases and found a median survival of 38 months, with 30 % of patients alive at 5 years. Nunobe et al. [85] found similar results in their series of 18 patients who underwent hepatectomy for metastatic GIST with a median survival of 36 months and 5-year survival of 34 %. Finally, Shima et al. [86] showed in a series of ten patients a median survival of 39 months following hepatectomy. Of note, de la Fuente et al. [87] compared 43 patients with isolated liver metastases (34 underwent surgery) to 16 patients with liver and peritoneal disease (13 underwent surgery). Patients with isolated liver metastases undergoing surgery trended toward longer OS (40.5 months vs 28.7, $p=0.620$) and trended toward having a lower recurrence rate after surgery (16/34 vs 8/13 $p=.08$), suggesting having liver-only disease may be a predictor of slightly better prognosis. This was further confirmed in long-term follow-up of EORTC 62005 study [72]. In patients with only liver metastases, median OS was not reached compared to 7 years in patients with only peritoneal metastases and 3.7 in patients with both. Interestingly, in the group of patients who were operated on while in remission and achieved a complete macroscopic resection, median OS was not reached again in liver-only group, 8.7 years in peritoneal-only group, and increased to 8.1 years in patients with both.

After the advent of imatinib, it has been shown that the combination of imatinib and hepatic resection can offer long-term disease control in patients with isolated hepatic metastases in multiple studies (Table 2).

Turley et al. [90] studied 39 patients that underwent hepatic resection for metastatic GIST between 1995 and 2010. Thirty-one patients received TKI therapy. Three-year OS in patients receiving TKI was 71.9 % and 0 % in the seven patients who did not receive TKI therapy. They also noted that patients who were exposed to TKI therapy for prolonged periods (median 18 months) preoperatively trended toward worsened OS, suggesting against delaying surgery indefinitely. Their median OS exceeded previous reports for treatment of metastatic GIST with hepatic resection alone of 36–47 months [84–86, 88].

Xia et al. [89]reported 39 patients with metastatic GIST to the liver treated with either 6 months of neoadjuvant imatinib followed by surgery and 2–4 weeks of adjuvant therapy or imatinib alone. The 3-year OS was 89.5 % in the surgery group and 60 % in the imatinib-alone group, which was significant. Also significant was that among patients who responded poorly to 6 months of preoperative imatinib, surgery significantly improved OS compared to those that did not undergo surgery ($p=0.04$)

Zhu et al. [93] studied 42 patients with recurrent GIST to either the liver or abdomen treated with long-term imatinib alone without surgery. They found a combined median OS of 48 months. Notably, the median time to progression was longer in the liver group (48 months versus 39 months in patients with only abdominal metastases and 33 months in patients with both), but this was not significant. Median OS was not reached in the liver-alone group with three of the ten patients dying during over 3 years of follow-up. This showed that imatinib alone is a reasonable option in patients with hepatic metastases as well as other metastatic disease.

The NCCN [19] and ESMO [94] both recommend indefinite adjuvant imatinib for patients with resected liver metastases, even if resection was complete.

6 Surveillance

There presently is no standardized follow-up regimen for patients with GIST. The NCCN guidelines [19] recommend an abdominal/pelvic CT be obtained every 3–6 months after surgical resection of GIST and within 3 months after initiating TKI

Table 2 Selected series reporting outcomes after multimodality therapy for GIST liver metastases

Author	Patients	Preop TKI	Postop TKI	R0 rate	DFS	OS	Factors
Pawlik (2006) [88]	36	15	11	N/A	1 year: 52 % 3 year 21 % 5 year 16 %	1 year 91 % 3 year 65 % 5 year 27 %	Adjuvant TKI led to longest median OS
Xia (2010) [89]	19	19	19	N/A	N/A	3-year OS: 89.5 % in surgical vs 60 % in nonsurgery groups	Significant OS benefit from surgery. Surgery also improved OS in patients who responded poorly to preoperative TKI
Turley (2012) [90]	39	19	27	92 %	1 year 63 % 3 year 34 % 5 year 26 %	1 year 97 % 3 year 67 %	Surgery and postoperative TKI improve survival
Cananzi (2014) [91]	11	11	9	64 %	1 year 87 % 2 year 62 %	1 year 81 % 2 year 71 %	R0 resection and clinical TKI response correlated with OS
Brudvik (2015) [92]	49	39 perioperative	39 perioperative	47/49	5 year 35.7 % 47.1 % with TKI vs 9.5 % without	5 year 55.3 % 10 year 52.5 %	Imatinib improved survival

Abbreviations: *TKI* tyrosine kinase inhibitor, *DFS* disease-free survival, *OS* overall survival, *R0* macroscopically complete resection with negative microscopic margins therapy for patients with advanced GIST. ESMO guidelines [94] also recommend follow-up CT or MRI every 3–6 months in patients receiving adjuvant therapy for the first 3 years. Upon cessation of adjuvant therapy, ESMO further recommends follow-up imaging every 3 months for the first 2 years followed by less frequent imaging if stable.

CT scans are the typical initial imaging modality of choice. GISTs typically appear as a solid contoured mass that enhances brightly with IV contrast on CT scans. Larger tumors can be less homogenous due to hemorrhage and necrosis within the tumor. MRI can be useful in patients that cannot receive IV contrast for CT scans. MRIs are also better at evaluating GISTs in the liver and rectum [95], which is especially important ahead of a planned surgery.

PET scans are highly sensitive for detecting GISTs, but lack specificity. While not a stand-alone imaging modality for surveillance, PET can be used for detecting an unknown primary site or resolving ambiguities from CT [16]. Another potential scenario where PET can be considered is when response to therapy must be determined quickly. Specifically, TKI responsiveness can be seen as early as 1 day after treatment is started on PET scan compared to 1–2 months on standard CT scans [96–98].

GISTs that respond to TKI therapy become more homogenous and hypodense, and sometimes will later shrink in size as well. This is important when considering the two major criteria systems for GIST follow-up: RECIST and Choi. RECIST (Response Evaluation Criteria In Solid Tumors) was developed first. which determines treatment response based upon tumor measurements [99]. However, it was known that this was not necessarily well-suited for GIST surveillance, as early response to TKI therapy often does not correlate with decrease in tumor size, and further signs of tumor progression on TKI therapy are often seen as new areas of hyperdensity before an increase in size. This led Choi et al. [100] to develop a different response evaluation system that used both tumor density and size (Table 3).

Table 3 Choi criteria for tumor responsiveness in GIST

Response	Definition
Complete response	1. Disappearance of all lesions
	2. No new lesions
Partial response	1. A decrease in size of 10 % or more; or a decrease in tumor density (HU) of 15 % or more on CT
	2. No new lesions
	3. No obvious progression of nonmeasurable disease
Stable disease	1. Does not meet criteria for complete response, partial response, or progression
	2. No symptomatic deterioration attributed to tumor progression
Progression of disease	1. An increase in tumor size of 10 % or more and does not meet criteria of partial response by tumor density (HU) on CT scan
	2. New lesions
	3. New intramural nodules or increase in the size of existing intratumoral nodules

The Choi criteria were compared to RECIST in a trial [101] of 58 patients receiving imatinib for advanced GIST who had CT scans 8 weeks after starting therapy. They found that response group assigned by RECIST did not correlate significantly with either DSS or time to tumor progression. On the other hand, the Choi response group did correlate with both end points. They also showed that the Choi criteria for CT correlated well with PET scan [100, 102].

7 Conclusion

For patients with metastatic GIST, TKIs remain the primary therapy. Imatinib is the first-line drug, followed by sunitinib and then regorafenib. Research is ongoing to develop further therapeutic options. There is no standard role for chemotherapy, HIPEC, or radiation therapy at this time. Surgery can be recommended in selective cases based on response to therapy and feasibility of complete resection. Importantly, any patient undergoing surgery should resume TKI therapy promptly afterward.

References

1. American Cancer Society: Gastrointestinal Stromal Tumor (GIST). http://www.cancer.org/acs/groups/cid/documents/webcontent/003103-pdf.pdf.
2. Joensuu H, et al. Gastrointestinal stromal tumour. Lancet. 2013;382:973–83.
3. Hirota S, et al. Gain-of-function mutations in c-kit in human gastrointestinal stromal tumors. Science. 1998;279(5350):577–80.
4. Kindblom LG, et al. Gastrointestinal pacemaker cell tumor (GIPACT): gastrointestinal stromal tumors show characteristics of the interstitial cells of Cajal. Am J Pathol. 1998;152(5):1259–69.
5. Sarlomo-Rikala M, et al. CD117: a sensitive marker for gastrointestinal stromal tumors that is more specific than CD34. Mod Pathol. 1998;11(8):728–34.
6. Corless CL, et al. Pathologic and molecular features correlate with long-term outcome after adjuvant therapy of resected primary GI stromal tumor: the ACOSOG Z9001 trial. J Clin Oncol. 2014;32(15):1563–70.
7. Pardanani A, Tefferi A. Imatinib targets other than bcr/abl and their clinical relevance in myeloid disorders. Blood. 2004;104(7):1931–9.
8. Tuveson DA, et al. STI571 inactivation of the gastrointestinal stromal tumor c-KIT oncoprotein: biological and clinical implications. Oncogene. 2001;20(36):5054–8.
9. Joensuu H, et al. Effect of the tyrosine kinase inhibitor STI571 in a patient with a metastatic gastrointestinal stromal tumor. N Engl J Med. 2001;344:1052–6.
10. Blanke CD, et al. Phase III randomized, intergroup trial assessing imatinib mesylate at two dose levels in patients with unresectable or metastatic gastrointestinal stromal tumors expressing the kit receptor tyrosine kinase: S0033. J Clin Oncol. 2008;26(4):626–32.
11. Verweij J, et al. Progression-free survival in gastrointestinal stromal tumours with high-dose imatinib: randomised trial. Lancet. 2004;264(9440):1127–34.
12. Casali PG, et al. Imatinib mesylate in advanced Gastrointestinal Stromal Tumors (GIST): survival analysis of the EORTC ISG AGITG randomized trial in 946 patients. Eur J Cancer. 2005;(Suppl 3):abstract 711.

13. Le Cesne A, et al. Discontinuation of imatinib in patients with advanced gastrointestinal stromal tumours after 3 years of treatment: an open-label multicentre randomised phase 3 trial. Lancet Oncol. 2010;11(10):942–9.
14. Demetri GD, et al. Efficacy and safety of imatinib mesylate in advanced gastrointestinal stromal tumors. N Engl J Med. 2002;347(7):472–80.
15. Vadakara J, et al. Gastrointestinal stromal tumors management of metastatic disease and emerging therapies. Hematol Oncol Clin North Am. 2013;27(5):905–20.
16. Heinrich MC, et al. Molecular correlates of imatinib resistance in gastrointestinal stromal tumors. J Clin Oncol. 2006;24(29):4764–74.
17. Debiec-Rychter M, et al. Mechanisms of resistance to imatinib mesylate in gastrointestinal stromal tumors and activity of the PKC412 inhibitor against imatinib-resistant mutants. Gastroenterology. 2005;128(2):270–9.
18. Van Glabbeke MM, et al. Comparison of 2 doses of imatinib for the treatment of unresectable or metastatic gastrointestinal stromal tumors (GIST): a meta-analysis based on 1,640 patients. Presented at: American Society of Clinical Oncology 43rd Annual Meeting; June 1–5, 2007; Chicago, IL.
19. NCCN Task Force Report. Optimal management of patients with gastrointestinal stromal tumor (GIST)—update of the NCCN clinical practice guidelines. J Natl Compr Canc Netw. 2007;5(2):S1–29.
20. Demetri GD, et al. Efficacy and safety of sunitinib in patients with advanced gastrointestinal-stromal tumour after failure of imatinib: a randomised controlled trial. Lancet. 2006;368(9544):1329–38.
21. Demetri GD, et al. Complete longitudinal analyses of the randomized, placebo-controlled, phase III trial of sunitinib in patients with gastrointestinal stromal tumor following imatinib failure. Clin Cancer Res. 2012;18(11):3170–9.
22. George S, et al. Clinical evaluation of continuous daily dosing of sunitinib malate in patients with advanced gastrointestinal stromal tumour after imatinib failure. Eur J Cancer. 2009;45(11):1959–68.
23. Heinrich MC, et al. Primary and secondary kinase geno-types correlate with the biological and clinical activity of sunitinib in imatinib- resistant gastrointestinal stromal tumor. J Clin Oncol. 2008;26:5352–9.
24. Heinrich MC, et al. Sunitinib (SU) response in imatinib- resistant (IM-R) GIST correlates with KIT and PDGFRA mutation status. J Clin Oncol. 2006;24 Suppl 18:a9502.
25. Maki RG, et al. Results from a continuation trial of SU11248 in patients (pts) with imatinib (IM)-resistant gastrointestinal stromal tumor (GIST). Proc Am Soc Clin Oncol. 2005;9011.
26. Kang YK, et al. Resumption of imatinib to control metastatic or unresectable gastrointestinal stromal tumours after failure of imatinib and sunitinib (RIGHT): a randomised, placebo-controlled, phase 3 trial. Lancet Oncol. 2013;14(12):1175–82.
27. Wilhelm SM, et al. Regorafenib (BAY 73–4506): a new oral multilines inhibitor of angiogenic, stromal, and oncogenic receptor tyrosine kinases with potent preclinical antitumor activity. Int J Cancer. 2011;129:245–55.
28. Demetri GD, et al. Efficacy and safety of regorafenib for advanced gastrointestinal stromal tumours after failure of imatinib and sunitinib: an international, multicentre, prospective, randomised, placebo-controlled phase 3 trial (GRID). Lancet. 2013;381(9863):295–302.
29. Shah RR, et al. Hepatotoxicity of tyrosine kinase inhibitors: clinical and regulatory perspectives. Drug Saf. 2013;36(7):491–503.
30. Bauer S, Joensuu H. Emerging agents for the treatment of advanced, imatinib-resistant gastrointestinal stromal tumors: current status and future directions. Drugs. 2015;75(12):1323–34.
31. Blay JY, et al. Nilotinib versus imatinib as first-line therapy for patients with unresectable or metastatic gastrointestinal stromal tumours (ENESTg1): a randomised phase 3 trial. Lancet Oncol. 2015;16(5):550–60.
32. Zalupski M, et al. Phase III comparison of doxorubicin and dacarbazine given by bolus versus infusion in patients with soft-tissue sarcomas: a Southwest Oncology Group study. J Natl Cancer Inst. 1991;83:926–32.

33. Antman K, et al. An intergroup phase III randomized study of doxorubicin and dacarbazine with or without ifosfamide and mesna in advanced soft tissue and bone sarcomas. J Clin Oncol. 1993;11:1276–85.
34. Elias A. Response to mesna, doxorubicin, ifosfamide, and dacarbazine in 108 patients with metastatic or unresectable sarcoma and no prior chemotherapy. J Clin Oncol. 1989;7:1208–16.
35. Le Cesne A, et al. Randomized phase III study comparing conventional-dose doxorubicin plus ifosfamide versus high-dose doxorubicin plus ifosfamide plus recombinant human granulocyte-macrophage colony-stimulating factor in advanced soft tissue sarcomas. A trial of European Organization Research and Treatment of Cancer/Soft Tissue and Bone Sarcoma Group. J Clin Oncol. 2000;18:2676–84.
36. Verweij J, et al. A randomized phase II study of docetaxel versus doxorubicin in first and second line chemotherapy for locally advanced or metastatic soft tissue sarcomas in adults: a study of the European Organization for Research and Treatment of Cancer Soft Tissue and Bone Sarcoma Group. J Clin Oncol. 2000;18:2081–6.
37. Goss G. Clinical and pathological characteristics of gastrointestinal stromal tumors. Proc ASCO. 2000;19:2203.
38. Edmondson J, et al. Contrast of response to D-MAP+sargramostim between patients with advance malignant gastrointestinal stromal tumors and patients with other leiomyosarcomas. Proc ASCO. 1999;18:541.
39. Blair SC, et al. Ifosfamide and etoposide in the treatment of advanced soft tissue sarcomas. Am J Clin Oncol. 1994;17:480–4.
40. Patel SR, et al. Phase II clinical investigation of gemcitabine in advanced soft tissue sarcomas and window evaluation of dose rate on gemcitabine triphosphate accumulation. J Clin Oncol. 2001;19:3483–9.
41. Nielsen OS, et al. Effect of high-dose ifosfamide in advanced soft tissue sarcomas. A multicentre phase II study of the EORTC Soft Tissue and Bone Sarcoma Group. Eur J Cancer. 2000;36:61–7.
42. Frustaci S, et al. Epirubicin and ifosfamide in advanced soft tissue sarcomas. Ann Oncol. 1993;4:669–72.
43. Balcerzak SP, et al. A phase II trial of paclitaxel in patients with advanced soft tissue sarcomas. A Southwest Oncology Group study. Cancer. 1995;76:2248–52.
44. Baratti D, et al. Peritoneal sarcomatosis: is there a subset of patients who may benefit from cytoreductive surgery and hyperthermic intraperitoneal chemotherapy? Ann Surg Oncol. 2010;17(12):3220–8.
45. Rossi CR, et al. Hyperthermic intraperitoneal intraoperative chemotherapy after cytoreductive surgery for the treatment of abdominal sarcomatosis. Cancer. 2004;100(9):1943–50.
46. Bryan ML, et al. Cytoreductive surgery with hyperthermic intraperitoneal chemotherapy in sarcomatosis from gastrointestinal stromal tumor. Am Surg. 2014;80(9):890–5.
47. Bonvalot S, et al. Randomized trial of cytoreduction followed by intraperitoneal chemotherapy versus cytoreduction alone in patients with peritoneal sarcomatosis. Eur J Surg Oncol. 2005;31(8):917–23.
48. Crosby JA, et al. Malignant gastrointestinal stromal tumors of the small intestine: a review of 50 cases from a prospective database. Ann Surg Oncol. 2001;8(1):50–9.
49. Knowlton C, et al. Radiotherapy in the treatment of gastrointestinal stromal tumor. Rare Tumors. 2011;3(4):e35.
50. Pollack J, et al. Adjuvant radiotherapy for gastrointestinal stromal tumor of the rectum. Dig Dis Sci. 2001;46:268–72.
51. Ricca L, et al. Tumori stromali gastrointestinali (GIST) a localiz-zazione rettale. Un nuovo caso e revisione della letteratura. Chir Ital. 2002;54:709–16.
52. Shioyama Y, et al. Long-term control for a retroperitoneal metastasis of malignant gastrointestinal stromal tumor after chemoradiotherapy and immunotherapy. Acta Oncol. 2001;40:102–4.
53. Choudhury A, et al. Targeting homologous recombination using imatinib results in enhanced tumor cell chemosensitivity and radiosensitivity. Mol Cancer Ther. 2009;8(1):203–13.

54. Boruban C, et al. Metastatic gastrointestinal stromal tumor with long-term response after treatment with concomitant radiotherapy and imatinib mesylate. Anticancer Drugs. 2007;18:969–72.
55. Ciresa M, et al. Molecularly targeted therapy and radiotherapy in the management of localized gastrointestinal stromal tumor (GIST) of the rectum: a case report. Tumori. 2009;95:236–9.
56. Tong CC, et al. Phase II trial of concurrent sunitinib and image-guided radiotherapy for oligometastases. PLoS One. 2012;7:e36979.
57. Kao J, et al. Phase 1 study of concurrent sunitinib and image-guided radiotherapy followed by maintenance sunitinib for patients with oligometastases: acute toxicity and preliminary response. Cancer. 2009;115:3571–80.
58. Chen SW, et al. Phase 2 study of combined sorafenib and radiation therapy in patients with advanced hepatocellular carcinoma. Int J Radiat Oncol Biol Phys. 2014;88:1041–7.
59. Hurwitz J, et al. The role of radiotherapy in metastatic gastrointestinal stromal tumour (GIST). Proceedings of the Connective Tissue Oncology Society. 2008. Abstract 35023.
60. Cuaron JJ, et al. External beam radiation therapy for locally advanced and metastatic gastrointestinal stromal tumors. Radiat Oncol. 2013;8(1):274.
61. Joensuu H, et al. Radiotherapy for GIST progressing during or after tyrosine kinase inhibitor therapy: a prospective study. Radiother Oncol. 2015;116(2):233–8.
62. Taremi M, et al. Upper abdominal malignancies: intensity-modulated radiation therapy. Front Radiat Ther Oncol. 2007;40:272–88.
63. Corbin KS, et al. Considering the role of radiation therapy for gastrointestinal stromal tumor. Onco Targets Ther. 2014;7:713–8.
64. Nour AA, et al. Intensity modulated radiotherapy of upper abdominal malignancies: dosimetric comparison with 3D conformal radiotherapy and acute toxicity. Radiat Oncol. 2013;8(1):207.
65. Scaife CL, et al. Is there a role for surgery in patients with "unresectable" cKIT+ gastrointestinal stromal tumors treated with imatinib mesylate? Am J Surg. 2003;186:665–9.
66. Bauer S, et al. Resection of residual disease in patients with metastatic gastrointestinal stromal tumors responding to treatment with imatinib. Int J Cancer Journal international du cancer. 2005;117:316–25.
67. Fairweather M, Raut CP. Surgical management of GIST and intra-abdominal visceral leiomyosarcomas. J Surg Oncol. 2015;111:562–9.
68. Raut CP, et al. Surgical management of advanced gastrointestinal stromal tumors after treatment with targeted systemic therapy using kinase inhibitors. J Clin Oncol. 2006;24:2325.
69. Rutkowski P, et al. Surgical treatment of patients with initially inoperable and/or metastatic gastrointestinal stromal tumors (GIST) during therapy with imatinib mesylate. J Surg Oncol. 2006;93:304.
70. Bonvalot S, et al. Impact of surgery on advanced gastrointestinal stromal tumors (GIST) in the imatinib era. Ann Surg Oncol. 2006;13:1596.
71. Gronchi A, et al. Surgery of residual disease following molecular-targeted therapy with imatinib mesylate in advanced/metastatic GIST. Ann Surg. 2007;245:341.
72. DeMatteo RP, et al. Results of tyrosine kinase inhibitor therapy followed by surgical resection for metastatic gastrointestinal stromal tumor. Ann Surg. 2007;245:347.
73. Andtbacka RH, et al. Surgical resection of gastrointestinal stromal tumors after treatment with imatinib. Ann Surg Oncol. 2007;14:14.
74. Al-Batran SE, et al. Focal progression in patients with gastrointestinal stromal tumors after initial response to imatinib mesylate: a three-center-based study of 38 patients. Gastric Cancer. 2007;10:145.
75. Yeh CN, et al. Surgical management in metastatic gastrointestinal stromal tumor (GIST) patients after imatinib mesylate treatment. J Surg Oncol. 2010;102:599.
76. Mussi C, et al. Post-imatinib surgery in advanced/metastatic GIST: is it worthwhile in all patients? Ann Oncol. 2010;21:403.

77. Zaydfudim Z, et al. Role of operative therapy in treatment of metastatic gastrointestinal stromal tumors. J Surg Res. 2012;177(2):248–54.
78. Bauer S, et al. Long-term follow-up of patients with GIST undergoing metastasectomy in the era of imatinib – analysis of prognostic factors (EORTC-STBSG collaborative study). Eur J Surg Oncol. 2014;40:412.
79. Park SJ, et al. The role of surgical resection following imatinib treatment in patients with recurrent or metastatic gastrointestinal stromal tumors: results of propensity score analyses. Ann Surg Oncol. 2014;21:4211.
80. Rubió-Casadevall J, et al. Role of surgery in patients with recurrent, metastatic, or unresectable locally advanced gastrointestinal stromal tumors sensitive to imatinib: a retrospective analysis of the Spanish Group for Research on Sarcoma (GEIS). Ann Surg Oncol. 2015;22:2948.
81. An HJ, et al. The effects of surgical cytoreduction prior to imatinib therapy on the prognosis of patients with advanced GIST. Ann Surg Oncol. 2013;20:4212–8.
82. Raut CP, et al. Cytoreductive surgery in patients with metastatic gastrointestinal stromal tumor treated with sunitinib malate. Ann Surg Oncol. 2010;17(2):407–15.
83. DeMatteo RP, et al. Two hundred gastrointestinal stromal tumors: recurrence patterns and prognostic factors for survival. Ann Surg. 2000;231(1):51–8.
84. DeMatteo RP, et al. Results of hepatic resection for sarcoma metastatic to liver. Ann Surg. 2001;234(4):540–8.
85. Nunobe S, et al. Surgery including liver resection for metastatic gastrointestinal stromal tumors or gastrointestinal leiomyosarcomas. Jpn J Clin Oncol. 2005;35(6):338–41.
86. Shima Y, et al. Aggressive surgery for liver metastases from gastrointestinal stromal tumors. J Hepatobiliary Pancreat Surg. 2003;10(1):77–80.
87. de la Fuente SG, et al. A comparison between patients with gastrointestinal stromal tumours diagnosed with isolated liver metastases and liver metastases plus sarcomatosis. HPB. 2013;15(9):655–60.
88. Pawlik TM, et al. Results of a single-center experience with resection and ablation for sarcoma metastatic to the liver. Arch Surg. 2006;141(6):537–43.
89. Xia L, et al. Resection combined with imatinib therapy for liver metastases of gastrointestinal stromal tumors. Surg Today. 2010;40(10):936–42.
90. Turley RS, et al. Hepatic resection for metastatic gastrointestinal stromal tumors in the tyrosine kinase inhibitor era. Cancer. 2012;118(14):3571–8.
91. Cananzi FCM, et al. Liver surgery in the multidisciplinary management of gastrointestinal stromal tumor. ANZ J Surg. 2014;84(1):937–42.
92. Brudvik KW, et al. Survival after resection of gastrointestinal stromal tumor and sarcoma liver metastases in 146 patients. J Gastrointest Surg. 2015;19:1476–83.
93. Zhu J, et al. A long-term follow-up of the imatinib mesylate treatment for the patients with recurrent gastrointestinal stromal tumor (GIST): the liver metastasis and the outcome. BMC Cancer. 2010;10:199.
94. The ESMO/European Sarcoma Network Working Group. Gastrointestinal stromal tumors: ESMO clinical practice guidelines. Ann Oncol. 2014;25 Suppl 3:iii21–6.
95. Schima W, Kurtaran A. GIST: imaging diagnosis, staging, and response assessment. Wien Med Wochenschr. 2009;159(15–16):408–13.
96. Stroobants S, et al. 18FDG-Positron emission tomography for the early prediction of response in advanced soft tissue sarcoma treated with imatinib mesylate (Glivec). Eur J Cancer. 2003;39:2012–20.
97. Antoch G, et al. Comparison of PET, CT, and dual-modality PET/CT imaging for monitoring of imatinib (STI571) therapy in patients with gastrointestinal stromal tumors. J Nucl Med. 2004;45:357–65.
98. Shankar LK, et al. Consensus recommendations for the use of 18F-FDG PET as an indicator of therapeutic response in patients in National Cancer Institute Trials. J Nucl Med. 2006;47(6):1059–66.

99. Therasse P, et al. New guidelines to evaluate the response to treatment in solid tumors. J Natl Cancer Inst. 2000;92(3):205–16.
100. Choi H, et al. Correlation of computed tomography and positron emission tomography in patients with metastatic gastrointestinal stromal tumor treated at a single institution with imatinib mesylate: proposal of new computed tomography response criteria. J Clin Oncol. 2007;25(13):1753–9.
101. Benjamin RS, et al. We should desist using RECIST, at least in GIST. J Clin Oncol. 2007;25(13):1760–4.
102. Choi H, et al. Correlation of computerized tomography (CT) and proton emission tomography (PET) in patients with metastatic GIST treated at a single institution with imatinib mesylate. Proc Am Soc Clin Oncol. 2003;22:819. Abstract 3290.

Management of Liver Metastases of Gastrointestinal Stromal Tumors

Andrew D. Morris, Shishir K. Maithel, and David A. Kooby

Abbreviations

CT	Computerized tomography
GIST	Gastrointestinal stromal tumor
MRI	Magnetic resonance imaging
NCCN	National Comprehensive Cancer Network
PET	Positron emission tomography
PFS	Progression-free survival
RFA	Radiofrequency ablation
TKI	Tyrosine kinase inhibitors
XRT	External-beam radiation therapy

1 Epidemiology of GIST Liver Metastases

Gastrointestinal stromal tumors (GIST) are low-incident tumors with approximately 3000–5000 cases reported per year in the United States [1]. The liver is the most common site of solid organ metastases from GIST [1]. GIST metastases to the liver occur both synchronously and metachronously and are present at initial diagnosis between 15 and 20 % of the time. Approximately 50 % of patients with metastatic disease have isolated liver metastases with another 10 % of patients having combined liver metastases and extrahepatic disease [1]. Around 30 % of patients with GIST liver metastases will have potentially resectable disease [1], but for these patients, 5-year overall survival still remains poor at only 50 % [2]. Given that the liver is a common site of metastatic disease, and that there are several available treatment options, a coordinated approach to managing hepatic metastases from GIST metastases is important.

A.D. Morris, MD • S.K. Maithel, MD, FACS • D.A. Kooby, MD, FACS (✉)
Division of Surgical Oncology, Department of Surgery, Winship Cancer Institute, Emory University, 1365C Clifton Road NE, 2nd Floor, Atlanta, GA 30322, USA
e-mail: dkooby@emory.edu

© Springer International Publishing Switzerland 2017

C.R. Scoggins et al. (eds.), *Gastrointestinal Stromal Tumors*,
DOI 10.1007/978-3-319-42632-7_15

2 Diagnosis/Imaging

Primary GIST tumors are usually found by endoscopic methods or incidentally with abdominal imaging. Metastatic hepatic GIST lesions are often asymptomatic and are typically discovered during diagnostic, staging, or follow-up imaging. Their appearance on CT and MRI is characterized by homogenous-appearing hypervascular lesions when small, and heterogeneous lesions with peripheral enhancement and central necrosis when larger (>3 cm) [3] (Fig. 1). Heterogeneous appearance of larger lesions results from hypodense characteristics of necrosis, hemorrhage, and myxoid degeneration. Calcifications may be present in a small percentage of cases. Progression or treatment response of disease is generally tracked using CT or MRI [3]. MRI has value for defining hepatic metastases lesions through identifying cystic changes and vascularity. Intratumoral cystic changes may suggest more aggressive tumor biology [4]. GIST liver metastases appear as low-intermediate intensity on T1 and high intensity on T2. MRI can clarify smaller lesions and differentiate cystic metastases from benign cysts, although treated lesions can resemble simple cysts in the liver. Thus, it is imperative to review comparison images prior to initiating treatment to help differentiate between a treated metastasis and a cystic lesion.

Positron emission tomography-CT (PET-CT) has also been used for diagnosis and staging of GIST. While expensive and not always available at all centers,

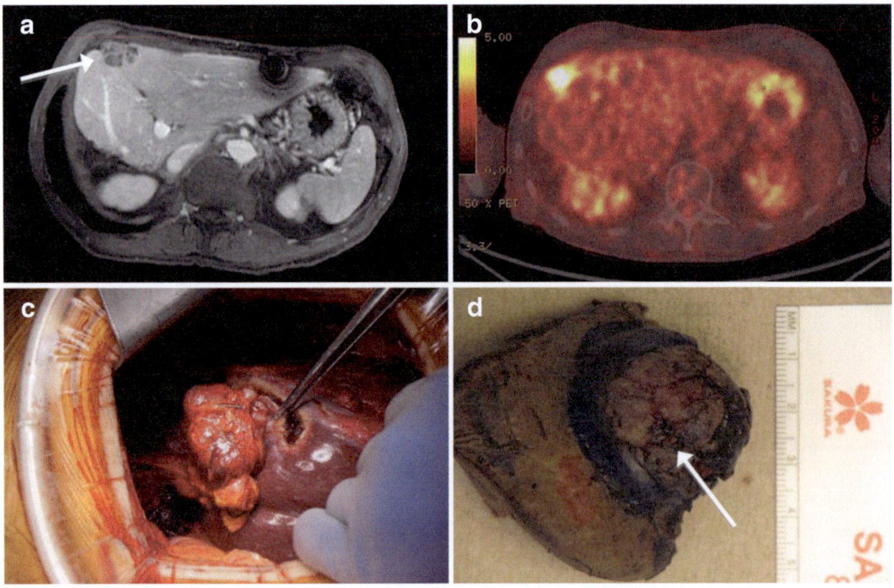

Fig. 1 Imaging, operative, gross, and histopathology of a liver GIST metastasis. (**a**) Preoperative MRI imaging of isolated peripheral liver metastasis, as noted by the *arrow*. (**b**) PET scan showing uptake and metabolic activity in liver metastasis, as noted by the *arrow*. (**c**) Intraoperative photograph of nonanatomical resection of peripheral lesion. The forceps show the planned line of transection to remove this tumor. (**d**) Gross pathology of resected GIST liver metastasis (*arrow*) with areas of necrosis and hemorrhage, with a margin of normal liver tissue

PET-CT serves a role for tracking treatment response. PET-CT is useful as it measures metabolic activity of the tumor, as opposed to only assessing size and morphology. The *Response Evaluation Criteria in Solid Tumors* (*RECIST*), which focus on tumor size changes before and after medical therapy, appear not as reliable for assessing GIST therapy response as many tumors undergo biological change (i.e., necrosis) without radiological size change (Fig. 1). PET-CT can be used to detect a subtle tumor response by noting a change in SUV activity (e.g., a drop in SUV after initiating tyrosine kinase inhibitor (TKI) therapy usually suggests response) [3].

Biopsy of GIST liver metastases carries some risk of tumor capsule rupture with subsequent peritoneal spread; however, it is common for biopsies to be performed when diagnosis is uncertain based on the clinical scenario and imaging alone [5]. Biopsy is necessary for confirming diagnosis prior to instituting targeted therapy, yet imaging confirming GIST liver metastases (in a patient with a history of primary GIST) may render this approach less imperative [6]. Percutaneous image-guided biopsy is recommended for hepatic lesions, while primary lesions are often diagnosed with an endoscopic ultrasonic biopsy. Core biopsy should be performed to aid in diagnosis and mutational analysis; biopsy of necrotic or hemorrhagic areas of the lesion should be avoided (Fig. 2). Experienced pathological assessment is necessary for these specimens owing to the complexity of categorization of GIST tumors and the relevance for therapeutic approach [6].

3 Patient Stratification for Therapy

Stratifying patients based on severity and presentation of disease facilitates identification of appropriate therapy for GIST patients with hepatic metastases. Patients can be categorized into the following groups: (1) synchronous isolated liver metastases, (2) recurrence following surgical resection, (3) disseminated

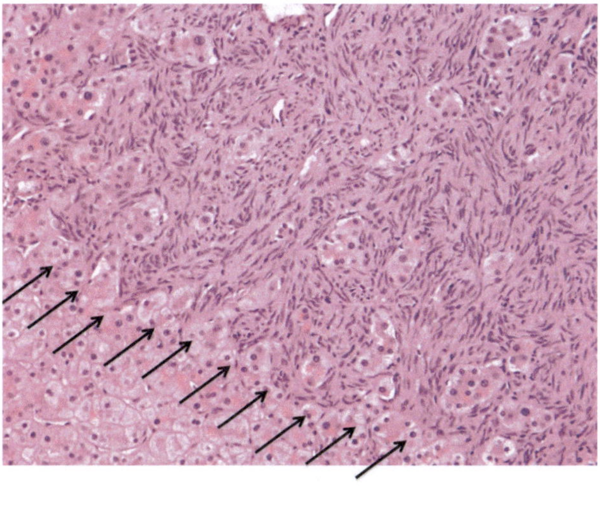

Fig. 2 Histopathology (low power) of resected GIST liver metastasis with arrows demonstrating interface of GIST tumor with normal hepatic parenchyma

disease, and (4) progression on TKI therapy. Each of these categories has varying treatment options and related survival estimates.

3.1 Synchronous Isolated Liver Metastases

Synchronous isolated liver metastases are defined as GIST tumors located in the liver that are not the primary tumor, but diagnosed at the same time, or within a year of the primary tumor [5]. These patients have not yet undergone treatment, and therefore have a wide range of medical and surgical treatment options available. This patient population also has the potential for the greatest benefit with intervention. Complete remission may be possible with surgical resection [7]. Typically, these patients undergo surgical therapy after a course of medical therapy and repeat imaging evaluation.

3.2 Recurrence Following Surgical Resection

Following operative resection of isolated primary disease, patients must be monitored for recurrence according to risk of recurrence. Identifying these patients who have subsequent metastases following R0 resection for primary GIST is typically performed by CT scanning at postoperative recommended intervals according to risk. Current National Comprehensive Cancer Network (NCCN) recommendations are repeat CT scans every 3–6 months after surgical resections or following initiation of medical treatment [8]. Various scoring systems exist to prognosticate GIST tumor recurrence. These include the National Institutes of Health (NIH), modified NIH (mNIH), and Armed Forces Institute of Pathology (AFIP) grading systems (Fig. 3) [9, 10]. Criteria demonstrated to increase risk of tumor recurrence following resection include: larger tumor size, tumor location outside the stomach, higher mitotic counts, tumor rupture, and CD117-negative immunohistochemistry. When recurrence is identified, treatment usually includes both medical and surgical components, the combined value of which is presumed to be better than each therapy alone [11, 12].

3.3 Progression on TKI Therapy

Unfortunately, there is a population of patients who have been treated with TKI without response or have progression of disease. These patients remain difficult to treat. Identifying treatment failure is crucial to successful change in management. Secondary and tertiary TKI therapies are typically initiated. Surgical intervention, however, is reserved for select cases, such as those with resectable tumors and excellent performance status (ECOG 0). Alternative nonsurgical therapies, such as ablative or transarterial therapies, should be considered in this patient population [13, 14].

	National Institutes of Health (NIH), , and NIH			modified NIH (mNIH)		
	Size/ Diameter (cm)	Mitotic Count	10-year Recurrence Free Survival	Size/ Diameter (cm)	Mitotic Count	10-year Recurrence Free Survival
Very Low Risk	<2	<5	98.3%	<2	<5	94.9%
Low Risk	2-5	<5	88.2%	2.1-5.0	<5	89.7%
Intermediate Risk	<5 5-10	6-10 <5	79.8%	<5.0 5.1-10.0	6-10 <5	86.9%
High Risk	>5 >10 Any Size	>5 Any count >10	30.4%	>10 Any size >5	Any count >5 >5	36.2%

Armed Forces Institute of Pathology (AFIP)

Group	Size	Mitotic Count	Stomach (% with progressive disease)	Duodenum(% with progressive disease)	Jejunum/Ileum(% with progressive disease)	Rectum(% with Progressive disease)
1a	<2.0	<5	0%	0%	0%	0%
2	2.1-5.0	<5	1.9%	8.3%	4.3%	8.5%
3a	5.1-10.0	<5	3.6%	-	24%	-
3b	>10	<5	10%	34%	52%	57%
4	<2.0	>5	0%	-	-	54%
5	2.1-5.0	>5	16%	50%	73%	52%
6a	5.1-10.0	>5	55%	-	85%	-
6b	>10	>5	86%	86%	90%	71%

Fig. 3 Risk stratification for primary GIST as evaluation of risk for recurrence and metastasis (Demetri et al. [8], Joensuu [9], Goh et al. [10] and Miettinen and Lasota [49])

3.4 Disseminated Disease

Widespread disease may occur either at primary diagnosis or at a later stage as disease recurrence. In this category, liver metastases are usually present, but disease in other locations (i.e., peritoneal spread) is also evident. These patients require medical treatment, most often initiated with TKI treatment [15]. The surgical options are mainly limited to debulking for palliative intent.

Each individual patient must have a well thought-out plan for treatment based on various factors. Understanding each therapeutic option and how it relates to each patient population greatly facilitates choosing the correct treatment strategy.

4 Medical Therapy

Prior to TKI therapy, surgical resection was the mainstay of treatment as cytotoxic chemotherapy has minimal effectiveness. With the advent of imatinib, medical therapy has become first-line standard of care. Initiation of TKI therapy should begin immediately following diagnosis for best response. Rates of radiological response with TKI therapy are approximately 30 % stable disease, 50 % partial response, 5 % complete response, and 15 % progressive disease [16, 17]. RECIST criteria are thought to underestimate treatment response, as there may be reductions in tumor density that are not appreciated using these criteria. Pathological analysis yields similarly poor rates of complete response, as 85–95 % of surgical specimens having residual disease after TKI therapy. Approximately 50–60 % of specimens demonstrate partial response to TKI therapy, which supports initial TKI therapy as a viable treatment strategy [18]. Progression-free survival with imatinib alone is approximately 2 years [19].

Resistance to TKI treatment can be categorized into primary resistance, which is progression of disease with initiation of imatinib therapy, and secondary resistance, a progression of disease following initial radiographic response to imatinib. Primary resistance is observed in an average of 10 % of patients, but KIT 9 and wild-type mutation can have higher rates of resistance (16 and 23 %, respectively) [20–22]. Secondary resistance is more common. Tumors often develop a secondary KIT mutation or have PDGF-R mutations that confer TKI resistance and result in imatinib failure [23]. In these circumstances, increasing the dose of imatinib is typically the first step to improve response. Second-line therapy is currently sunitinib [24], which not only is a multikinase inhibitor that preferentially targets PDGF-R and VEGF-R but also has activity against CD117. Modest response rates are attained with sunitinib salvage therapy, with an improvement in progression-free survival (PFS) with sunitinib versus placebo following imatinib failure (27.3 weeks vs. 6.4 weeks PFS, $p \leq 0.0001$). Escalation of imatinib therapy with increased dosing, as mentioned above, is also a therapeutic option as it was found to be equivalent to sunitinib. This was, however, found to be less effective in patients with exon 9 mutations (14.3 vs. 6.2 months PFS, $p = 0.037$), which emphasizes the importance of genetic mutation characterization [25]. Third-line therapy consists of regorafenib, which had a marginal increase in progression-free survival of <5 months compared to placebo [15]. Targeted medical therapy should form the backbone of treatment for patients with GIST liver metastases and surgical resection reserved for appropriately selected patients [18].

5 Patient Selection for Surgical Resection of Liver Metastases

As there are various medical and less-invasive treatments for metastatic GIST, optimization of the outcome after resection requires appropriate patient selection. The principles of selection are based on tumor biology and patient performance status. Designation of resectable, unresectable, and borderline resectable disease guides surgical approach. In the pre-imatinib era, surgical resection alone was associated with 5-year survival of 30–60 % and a median overall survival of only 16 months following complete resection. Recurrence rates upward of 60 % were noted, with the liver as the most common site [26, 27]. Discovery of imatinib and its effect on GIST affected both surgical decision-making and patient survival, especially in this patient population with advanced disease.

Additional information that is considered includes the disease-free interval, response to medical therapy, presence of extrahepatic disease, the number and size of the metastases, tumor location(s), and the patient level of fitness for surgery. Appropriate contrasted imaging (CT or MRI) of the chest, abdomen, and pelvis is necessary to adequately stage the patient. PET scanning may be useful when extra-hepatic metastases are of concern.

Assuming the patient is fit and the resection is technically sound, two factors mainly determine the success of surgical resection of GIST liver metastases: surgical margin status and TKI response. Margin-negative (R0) resection is associated with an improvement in progression-free survival as compared with margin-positive resection (29 months vs. 7 months, $p=0.002$) [28]. Overall survival at 1 year is also significantly improved for patients who undergo R0 resection (100 % vs. 37.5 %, $p=0.001$) [29]. Preoperative response to TKI therapy portends improved benefit from surgical therapy, and reduced tumor volume may improve surgical margins. NCCN guidelines recommend surgical resection to obtain microscopically negative margins, but do not specify the need for extensive margins [30]. Unlike the typical patient who undergoes hepatic resection for primary and secondary liver malignancies, GIST patients are typically noncirrhotic, cytotoxic-chemotherapy naïve, and more likely have normal background liver parenchyma. As such, they will likely tolerate more extensive hepatic resection if necessary than patients with conditions such as cirrhosis or chemotherapy-associated steatohepatitis.

Preoperative therapy for surgically resectable and borderline resectable metastatic GIST is now a standard approach. TKI therapy should be continued up until the time of surgery with resumption in the postoperative period if clinically indicated. The optimal timing of surgery continues to be an evolving target. Waiting 3–9 months after the initiation of medical therapy is recommended, since this time frame usually represents the period of greatest radiological response [31]. There are multiple studies suggesting that operating during periods of responsive disease or stable disease correlates to improved outcomes compared to progressive disease [29, 32, 33]. Additionally, delay of surgery may result in secondary mutations resulting in resistance to imatinib [16]. To successfully intervene at the time of greatest response, the surgeon must closely follow radiological response. A detailed algorithm for selecting management approach for patients with metastatic GIST is provided in Fig. 4.

6 Operative Resection

The surgical approach to GIST hepatic metastases varies based on the clinical scenario and anatomical considerations of each individual patient. As GIST liver metastases tend to be well circumscribed, there are options for both nonanatomical and anatomical resections. Additionally, when hepatic lesions are present with the primary tumor in place, a combined resection of both primary tumor and hepatic lesions may be possible in appropriately selected patients.

Either an open or minimally invasive approach can be utilized, assuming surgical skill and patient selection are appropriate. Peripheral small lesions may be more conducive to a minimally invasive resection. Nonanatomical liver resections are possible with small peripheral lesions located a distance away from major

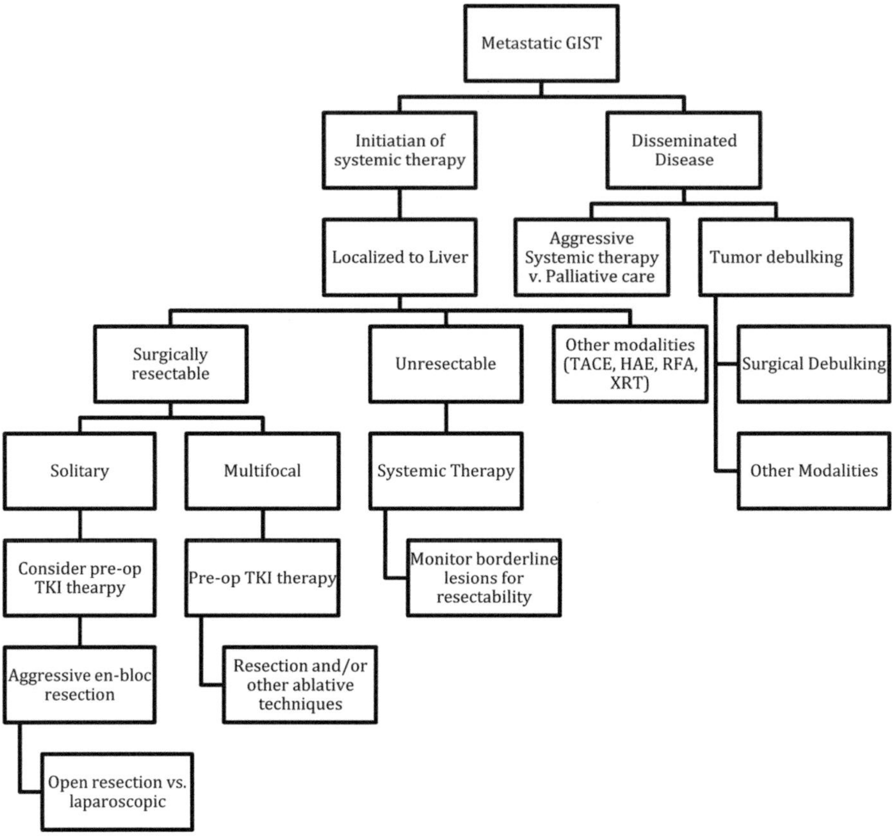

Fig. 4 Management algorithm for treatment of metastatic GIST

vascular structures (Fig. 1). Preoperative TKI therapy may reduce tumor volume making more limited resection possible, but complete radiological response does not correspond with cure, and thus liver-directed therapy should still be considered in this circumstance. The operating surgeon must review and compare the original scans to those acquired post-TKI therapy and assess for cystic change, as tumors that are initially solid may become cystic appearing after initiation of TKI therapy (Fig. 5).

For patients with extensive hepatic metastases, preoperative portal vein embolization (PVE) may allow for complete resection by preoperatively increasing the future liver remnant volume. This may apply to a select group of patients with borderline resectable disease. This approach is the accepted clinical practice for colorectal cancer metastases and other primary hepatic malignancies and can be extrapolated to the management of metastatic GIST. The decision for PVE must be made early, as timing maximal hepatic growth after PVE with the best response to TKI therapy is necessary (Fig. 6). Subsequent, repeat resections for recurrences are

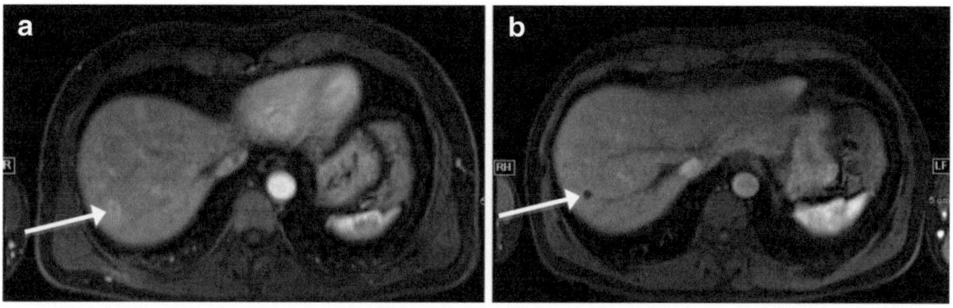

Fig. 5 (**a**). MRI imaging demonstrating small peripheral liver GIST metastasis. (**b**). Cystic changes in liver GIST metastasis seen on MRI following TKI treatment for 5 months duration as denoted by *white arrows*

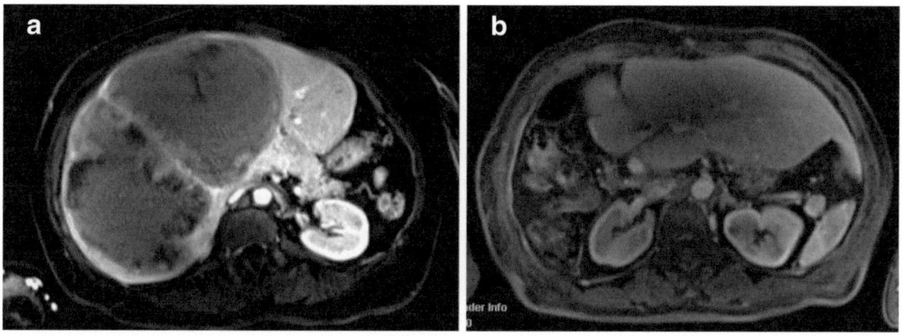

Fig. 6 (**a**). Large heterogeneous and cystic appearing GIST liver metastasis in right hepatic lobe with central necrosis. (**b**). Hepatic remnant with compensatory hypertrophy following resection of GIST liver metastasis seen in image (**a**)

possible and beneficial in appropriately selected patients with adequate liver remnant size and function [34].

Surgical debulking is also described with some success in management of GIST metastases, primarily for symptom (bleeding, pain, or obstruction) control [35, 36]. Survival estimates for selected patients undergoing hepatic resection in the presence of low-volume peritoneal disease may be similar to those for patients who undergo hepatic resection for liver-only disease (28.7 months vs. 40.5 months; $p=0.620$) [37]. Liver transplantation for metastatic GIST has been minimally employed and has limited utility [38].

Adjuvant therapy is recommended for patients with high risk of recurrence, which includes all patients who undergo resection of any kind of metastatic GIST [39]. Evidence supports the notion that suppressive therapy with TKI may be critical as there are descriptions of blossoming lesions when TKIs are stopped [40, 41]. Table 1 provides a summary of results from studies analyzing hepatic resection for GIST.

Table 1 Studies investigating effect of treatment on survival after GIST liver metastasis

Author	Date	# of pts	Investigation goal/study type	Use of TKI	Intervention	Survival
DeMatteo [46]	2007	40	Effect of progressive disease on survival, Retrospective	Pre- and post-op imatinib	Surgical resection of metastatic GIST in stable or responsive disease vs. focal progression vs. generalized progression	2-year PFS and OS of 61 % and 100 % in stable or responsive disease vs. 36 % OS in focal progression and 36 % 1-year OS with generalized progression
Gronchi [32]	2007	159	Effect of progressive disease on survival, Retrospective	Pre- and post-op imatinib	Surgical resection of metastatic GIST in patients with stable disease (SD) vs. progressive disease (PD)	PFS was 96 % at 12 months and 69 % at 24 months for responding patients, and 0 % at 12 months for progressing ones
Mussi [12]	2009	80	Effect of progressive disease on survival after resection, Retrospective cohort	Pre- and post-op imatinib	Surgical resection of metastatic GIST in patients with stable disease (SD) vs. progressive disease (PD)	Two-year PFS was 64.4 % in SD and 9.7 % in PD
Raut [11]	2010	50	Effect of progressive disease on sumatinib, Retrospective cohort	Pre- and post-op sumatinib	Surgical resection of metastatic GIST after second-line TKI therapy in responsive disease (RD) vs. limited progression (LP) vs. generalized progression (GP).	Median PFS after surgery 5.8 months, Overall survival was 16.4 months, no difference between disease responses
Turley [47]	2011	39	Effect of post-op imatinib following metastatic GIST resection, Retrospective cohort	Pre-op TKI, post-op TKI in study group	Surgical resection of metastatic GIST with post-op TKI in study group	Post-op TKI therapy improved survival (hazard ratio, 0.04, $p=0.006$)
Zaydfudim [28]	2012	87	Role of operative therapy in patients with metastatic GIST, Retrospective cohort	Pre and post-op TKI	Surgical resection of metastatic GIST	Overall survival (OS) surgery vs. systemic therapy alone (1 year OS, 98 % vs 80 % and 5-year OS, 65 % vs 11 %)

Author	Date	# of pts	Investigation goal/study type	Use of TKI	Intervention	Survival
Rubio [48]	2015	171	Effect of surgery on survival with stabilization with TKI	Pre and post-op Imatinib	Surgical resection of metastatic GIST vs. TKI treatment alone	Median survival was improved from 87.5 to 59.9 months with addition of surgery after TKI
Cao [14]	2014	45	Evaluate radioembolization vs. chemoembolization in treatment of metastatic GIST, Retrospective cohort	TKI therapy prior to procedure	Radioembolization vs. transarterial chemoembolization (TACE) in liver metastases with resistance to TKI therapy	PFS was improved with Embosphere® vs. cTACE (56.6 and 42.1 weeks, respectively; $p=0.003$)
Hakime [44]	2014	17	Evaluate responsiveness of GIST to radiofrequency ablation, Prospective study	TKI therapy based on study group	Radiofrequency ablation (RFA) of liver metastases, without adjuvant imatinib, with adjuvant imatinib, and RFA of progressive lesions	Two-year PFS after RFA was 75 % with TKI, 29 % w/o TKI, and 20 % in progressive lesion
Rathmann [13]	2015	11	Evaluate responsiveness to radioembolization, Restrospective study	TKI therapy prior to intervention	Radioembolization of liver metastases after failure of TKI therapy	Median PFI was 15.9 months (range, 4–29 months). Median survival was 29.8 months (range, 10–72 months).
Joensuu [42]	2015	25	Evaluate responsiveness of GIST to radiotherapy, Prospective trial	Continued current TKI therapy	External beam radiotherapy for progressive metastatic GIST as an adjuvant therapy after failure of other treatment	Median duration of stabilization of 16 months with XRT vs. 4 months for lesions w/o XRT

7 Other Modalities of Liver-Directed Therapy

Patients who are not surgical candidates have other options for liver-directed therapy. External beam radiation, radiofrequency or microwave ablation, transarterial chemoembolization or bland embolization, and hepatic artery radioembolization are alternatives to surgery that have been studied and supported by clinical studies.

External-beam radiation therapy (XRT) had been used for the treatment of GIST prior to TKI therapy with limited response. Small studies show that XRT can be effective in prolonging stable disease in conjunction with TKI therapy in patients with metastatic disease. Partial response with XRT is limited with ~5 % having radiological regression of disease [42]. Now that TKIs have become the mainstay of treatment, XRT has been relegated to palliative or last-line therapy.

Radiofrequency ablation (RFA) has become increasingly used in the treatment of hepatic lesions, and as such, has been adapted for treatment of GIST tumors. Small studies have shown examples of complete response following ablation of small lesions with follow-up time points out to 4 years. Progression-free survival was dependent on continued TKI treatment to slow metastatic progression [43, 44]. Microwave ablation has also been successfully combined with surgical resection for the treatment of liver metastases [34].

In patients with hepatic lesions who have failed other therapies and are not candidates for resection, radioembolization with yttrium-90 (Y-90) may be an option for treatment. Hepatic lobe radioembolization with Y-90 has been performed with good response and reasonable results. In one study, three patients showed complete response post procedure, three patients had partial response to therapy, and the last patient had stable disease. Importantly, these patients had already progressed through two lines of TKI therapy [13]. Bland embolization of GIST metastases has also been utilized with reports of a 45 % response rate by mRECIST [45]. Median overall survival was found to be almost 24 months in patients when bland embolization had been used as an adjunct third line therapy compared to 30 months with the addition of Y-90 [13]. Improved survival has also been shown with radioembolization as compared with transarterial chemoembolization (56.6 and 42.1 weeks PFS, $p=0.003$) [14].

With the application of these other modalities of therapy to metastatic GIST, there has not been adequate comparison between them to demonstrate a single superior modality. Each must be considered on an individual patient basis. Therefore, multidisciplinary discussion of these current third-line options is pivotal in providing the best treatment strategy. It is expected that these options will be increasingly utilized as we continue to push the envelop for patients with unresectable disease.

8 Conclusion

Patients with liver metastases from GIST primary tumors represent a heterogeneous population. The differential success with TKI therapy and resection indicates that the genetic composition of GIST tumors is crucial to prolonged recurrence-free and overall survival. There are still many unanswered questions regarding the optimal timing of surgery, the utility of debulking procedures, the efficacy of less-invasive therapies, and the role of novel pharmaceuticals. Currently, surgical resection in appropriately selected patients, in combination with TKI therapy, provides the best treatment strategy for potential cure and prolonged survival.

References

1. DeMatteo RP, Lewis JJ, Leung D, et al. Two hundred gastrointestinal stromal tumors: recurrence patterns and prognostic factors for survival. Ann Surg. 2000;231(1):51–8.
2. Cheung TT, Chok KS, Chan AC, et al. Analysis of long-term survival after hepatectomy for isolated liver metastasis of gastrointestinal stromal tumour. ANZ J Surg. 2014;84(11):827–31.
3. Choi H, Charnsangavej C, Faria SC, et al. Correlation of computed tomography and positron emission tomography in patients with metastatic gastrointestinal stromal tumor treated at a single institution with imatinib mesylate: proposal of new computed tomography response criteria. J Clin Oncol. 2007;25(13):1753–9.
4. Yu MH, Lee JM, Baek JH, et al. MRI features of gastrointestinal stromal tumors. AJR Am J Roentgenol. 2014;203(5):980–91.
5. Ye YJ, Gao ZD, Poston GJ, et al. Diagnosis and multi-disciplinary management of hepatic metastases from gastrointestinal stromal tumour (GIST). Eur J Surg Oncol. 2009;35(8):787–92.
6. Pisters PW, Patel SR. Gastrointestinal stromal tumors: current management. J Surg Oncol. 2010;102(5):530–8.
7. Zalinski S, Palavecino M, Abdalla EK. Hepatic resection for gastrointestinal stromal tumor liver metastases. Hematol Oncol Clin North Am. 2009;23(1):115–27, ix.
8. Demetri GD, von Mehren M, Antonescu CR, et al. NCCN Task Force report: update on the management of patients with gastrointestinal stromal tumors. J Natl Compr Canc Netw. 2010;8 Suppl 2:S1–41; quiz S42-44.
9. Joensuu H. Risk stratification of patients diagnosed with gastrointestinal stromal tumor. Hum Pathol. 2008;39(10):1411–9.
10. Goh BK, Chow PK, Yap WM, et al. Which is the optimal risk stratification system for surgically treated localized primary GIST? Comparison of three contemporary prognostic criteria in 171 tumors and a proposal for a modified Armed Forces Institute of Pathology risk criteria. Ann Surg Oncol. 2008;15(8):2153–63.
11. Raut CP, Wang Q, Manola J, et al. Cytoreductive surgery in patients with metastatic gastrointestinal stromal tumor treated with sunitinib malate. Ann Surg Oncol. 2010;17(2):407–15.
12. Mussi C, Ronellenfitsch U, Jakob J, et al. Post-imatinib surgery in advanced/metastatic GIST: is it worthwhile in all patients? Ann Oncol. 2010;21(2):403–8.

13. Rathmann N, Diehl SJ, Dinter D, et al. Radioembolization in patients with progressive gastrointestinal stromal tumor liver metastases undergoing treatment with tyrosine kinase inhibitors. J Vasc Interv Radiol. 2015;26(2):231–8.
14. Cao G, Zhu X, Li J, et al. A comparative study between Embosphere((R)) and conventional transcatheter arterial chemoembolization for treatment of unresectable liver metastasis from GIST. Chin J Cancer Res. 2014;26(1):124–31.
15. Demetri GD, Reichardt P, Kang YK, et al. Efficacy and safety of regorafenib for advanced gastrointestinal stromal tumours after failure of imatinib and sunitinib (GRID): an international, multicentre, randomised, placebo-controlled, phase 3 trial. Lancet. 2013;381(9863):295–302.
16. Sciot R, Debiec-Rychter M, Daugaard S, et al. Distribution and prognostic value of histopathologic data and immunohistochemical markers in gastrointestinal stromal tumours (GISTs): an analysis of the EORTC phase III trial of treatment of metastatic GISTs with imatinib mesylate. Eur J Cancer. 2008;44(13):1855–60.
17. Hong X, Choi H, Loyer EM, et al. Gastrointestinal stromal tumor: role of CT in diagnosis and in response evaluation and surveillance after treatment with imatinib. Radiographics. 2006;26(2):481–95.
18. Bauer S, Joensuu H. Emerging agents for the treatment of advanced, imatinib-resistant gastrointestinal stromal tumors: current status and future directions. Drugs. 2015;75(12):1323–34.
19. Demetri GD, von Mehren M, Blanke CD, et al. Efficacy and safety of imatinib mesylate in advanced gastrointestinal stromal tumors. N Engl J Med. 2002;347(7):472–80.
20. Heinrich MC, Corless CL, Demetri GD, et al. Kinase mutations and imatinib response in patients with metastatic gastrointestinal stromal tumor. J Clin Oncol. 2003;21(23):4342–9.
21. Eisenberg BL, Pipas JM. Gastrointestinal stromal tumor--background, pathology, treatment. Hematol Oncol Clin North Am. 2012;26(6):1239–59.
22. Heinrich MC, Maki RG, Corless CL, et al. Primary and secondary kinase genotypes correlate with the biological and clinical activity of sunitinib in imatinib-resistant gastrointestinal stromal tumor. J Clin Oncol. 2008;26(33):5352–9.
23. Heinrich MC, Owzar K, Corless CL, et al. Correlation of kinase genotype and clinical outcome in the North American Intergroup Phase III Trial of imatinib mesylate for treatment of advanced gastrointestinal stromal tumor: CALGB 150105 Study by Cancer and Leukemia Group B and Southwest Oncology Group. J Clin Oncol. 2008;26(33):5360–7.
24. Demetri GD, van Oosterom AT, Garrett CR, et al. Efficacy and safety of sunitinib in patients with advanced gastrointestinal stromal tumour after failure of imatinib: a randomised controlled trial. Lancet. 2006;368(9544):1329–38.
25. Hsu CC, Wu CE, Chen JS, et al. Imatinib escalation or sunitinib treatment after first-line imatinib in metastatic gastrointestinal stromal tumor patients. Anticancer Res. 2014;34(9):5029–36.
26. Nunobe S, Sano T, Shimada K, et al. Surgery including liver resection for metastatic gastrointestinal stromal tumors or gastrointestinal leiomyosarcomas. Jpn J Clin Oncol. 2005;35(6):338–41.
27. Brudvik KW, Patel SH, Roland CL, et al. Survival after resection of gastrointestinal stromal tumor and sarcoma liver metastases in 146 patients. J Gastrointest Surg. 2015;19(8):1476–83.
28. Zaydfudim V, Okuno SH, Que FG, et al. Role of operative therapy in treatment of metastatic gastrointestinal stromal tumors. J Surg Res. 2012;177(2):248–54.
29. Cananzi FC, Belgaumkar AP, Lorenzi B, et al. Liver surgery in the multidisciplinary management of gastrointestinal stromal tumour. ANZ J Surg. 2014;84(12):E1–8.
30. Demetri GD, Benjamin RS, Blanke CD, et al. NCCN Task Force report: management of patients with gastrointestinal stromal tumor (GIST)--update of the NCCN clinical practice guidelines. J Natl Compr Canc Netw. 2007;5 Suppl 2:S1–29; quiz S30.
31. Xia L, Zhang MM, Ji L, et al. Resection combined with imatinib therapy for liver metastases of gastrointestinal stromal tumors. Surg Today. 2010;40(10):936–42.

32. Gronchi A, Fiore M, Miselli F, et al. Surgery of residual disease following molecular-targeted therapy with imatinib mesylate in advanced/metastatic GIST. Ann Surg. 2007;245(3):341–6.
33. Raut CP, Posner M, Desai J, et al. Surgical management of advanced gastrointestinal stromal tumors after treatment with targeted systemic therapy using kinase inhibitors. J Clin Oncol. 2006;24(15):2325–31.
34. Maehara N, Chijiiwa K, Eto T, et al. Surgical treatment for gastric GIST with special reference to liver metastases. Hepatogastroenterology. 2008;55(82–83):512–6.
35. Pantaleo MA, Di Battista M, Catena F, et al. Surgical debulking of gastrointestinal stromal tumors: is it a reasonable option after second-line treatment with sunitinib? J Cancer Res Clin Oncol. 2008;134(5):625–30.
36. Guiteau J, Fanucchi M, Folpe A, et al. Hypoglycemia in the setting of advanced gastrointestinal stromal tumor. Am Surg. 2006;72(12):1225–30.
37. de la Fuente SG, Deneve JL, Parsons CM, et al. A comparison between patients with gastrointestinal stromal tumours diagnosed with isolated liver metastases and liver metastases plus sarcomatosis. HPB (Oxford). 2013;15(9):655–60.
38. Serralta AS, Sanjuan FR, Moya AH, et al. Combined liver transplantation plus imatinib for unresectable metastases of gastrointestinal stromal tumours. Eur J Gastroenterol Hepatol. 2004;16(11):1237–9.
39. Zhu J, Yang Y, Zhou L, et al. A long-term follow-up of the imatinib mesylate treatment for the patients with recurrent gastrointestinal stromal tumor (GIST): the liver metastasis and the outcome. BMC Cancer. 2010;10:199.
40. Zhu J, Wang Y, Hou M, et al. Imatinib mesylate treatment for advanced gastrointestinal stromal tumor: a pilot study focusing on patients experiencing sole liver metastasis after a prior radical resection. Oncology. 2007;73(5–6):324–7.
41. Joensuu H, Vehtari A, Riihimaki J, et al. Risk of recurrence of gastrointestinal stromal tumour after surgery: an analysis of pooled population-based cohorts. Lancet Oncol. 2012;13(3):265–74.
42. Joensuu H, Eriksson M, Collan J, et al. Radiotherapy for GIST progressing during or after tyrosine kinase inhibitor therapy: a prospective study. Radiother Oncol. 2015;116(2):233–8.
43. Yamanaka T, Takaki H, Nakatsuka A, et al. Radiofrequency ablation for liver metastasis from gastrointestinal stromal tumor. J Vasc Interv Radiol. 2013;24(3):341–6.
44. Hakime A, Le Cesne A, Deschamps F, et al. A role for adjuvant RFA in managing hepatic metastases from gastrointestinal stromal tumors (GIST) after treatment with targeted systemic therapy using kinase inhibitors. Cardiovasc Intervent Radiol. 2014;37(1):132–9.
45. Takaki H, Litchman T, Covey A, et al. Hepatic artery embolization for liver metastasis of gastrointestinal stromal tumor following imatinib and sunitinib therapy. J Gastrointest Cancer. 2014;45(4):494–9.
46. DeMatteo RP, Maki RG, Singer S, et al. Results of tyrosine kinase inhibitor therapy followed by surgical resection for metastatic gastrointestinal stromal tumor. Ann Surg. 2007;245(3):347–52.
47. Turley RS, Peng PD, Reddy SK, et al. Hepatic resection for metastatic gastrointestinal stromal tumors in the tyrosine kinase inhibitor era. Cancer. 2012;118(14):3571–8.
48. Rubio-Casadevall J, Martinez-Trufero J, Garcia-Albeniz X, et al. Role of surgery in patients with recurrent, metastatic, or unresectable locally advanced gastrointestinal stromal tumors sensitive to imatinib: a retrospective analysis of the Spanish Group for Research on Sarcoma (GEIS). Ann Surg Oncol. 2015;22(9):2948–57.
49. Miettinen M, Lasota J. Gastrointestinal stromal tumors: pathology and prognosis at different sites. Semin Diagn Pathol. 2006;23(2):70–83.

Surgical Palliation

Brittany A. Potz and Thomas J. Miner

1 Introduction

Common symptoms of patients with advanced GIST include pain, overt bleeding, and obstruction [1–4]. GISTs have a high incidence of (1) resistance to current treatment and (2) metastatic recurrence, making surgical resection for curative intent not possible for many patients. However, that does not mean that these patients have to live the rest of their lives with the symptoms of their disease. Palliative surgery can be offered with the intent of relieving the symptoms associated with advanced disease and improving patient's quality of life. Decisions regarding the use of surgical procedures for palliative care require the highest level of surgical judgment. Surgeons must consider the medical prognosis of the disease, the availability and success of nonsurgical treatments, and the individual patients' quality and expectancy of life [5, 6]. Optimal palliative decision making is facilitated through effective interactions among the patient, family members, and the surgeon through a dynamic relationship described by the palliative triangle [1]. While evidence suggesting successful palliative procedures for patients suffering from advanced GIST is lacking, there is evidence to suggest that palliative surgical treatment of some of the common symptoms associated with GIST can be successful in carefully selected patients. Palliation with Gleevac and radiation are potential options that require further research to explore.

B.A. Potz, MD • T.J. Miner, MD (✉)
The Department of Surgery, Alpert Medical School of Brown University, Rhode Island Hospital, Providence, Rhode Island, USA
e-mail: tminer@usasurg.org

© Springer International Publishing Switzerland 2017

C.R. Scoggins et al. (eds.), *Gastrointestinal Stromal Tumors*,
DOI 10.1007/978-3-319-42632-7_16

2 Defining the Goals and Strategies of Palliative Surgery

To truly understand the significance of palliative surgery, one must understand both the obvious and subtle distinctions between palliative and curative surgery. Surgery for curative intent generally involves complete removal of the cancer, with the primary goal of prolonging the patient's life [7–9]. These operations are sometimes complex and can involve multiple procedures to ensure removal of all diseased tissue from the patient. Although secondary gains of the procedure such as symptom improvement are welcome, the benefit of curative surgery (namely increased survival) is so high that it outweighs the risks of performing the operation. Because of this, significant risks associated with these procedures such as significant morbidity, permanent loss of function, patient discomfort, and sometimes, an increased risk of perioperative mortality might be considered acceptable (Fig. 1) [7, 9].

In contrast, surgical palliation refers to the use of a procedure with the intention of relieving symptoms, minimizing patient distress, increasing the durability of treatment, improving quality of life, decreasing pain, shortening treatment duration, minimizing treatment toxicity, and improving morbidity and mortality. During the palliative phase of care, brief gains that may be achieved in patient survival should not outweigh efforts aimed at minimizing the morbidity, the mortality, or the duration of treatment and improving patient quality of life [9–14] (Fig. 1). Standardization of palliative surgical care across the country has traditionally been difficult to achieve because of the fact that there are many variables to consider. These variables include, but are not limited to, symptom severity, the patient's preferences, the family's preferences, and the varying ability of surgeons to deal with end-of-life issues. Therefore, in 1998, the American College of Surgeons Committee on Ethics made a statement on the principles guiding care at the end of life. The following principles were included in their statement: (1) respect the dignity of both patient and caregivers; (2) be sensitive to and respectful of the patient's and family's wishes; (3) use the most appropriate measures that are consistent with their choices; (4) ensure alleviation of pain and management of other physical symptoms; (5) recognize, assess, and address psychological, social, and spiritual problems; (6) ensure

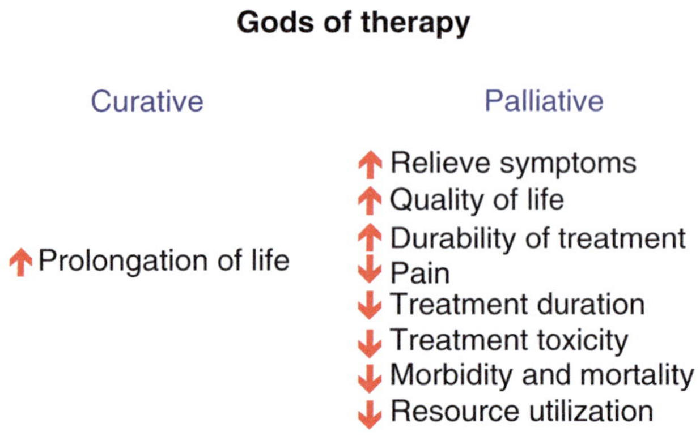

Fig. 1 Surgical palliation refers to the use of a procedure with the intention of relieving symptoms, minimizing patient distress, increasing the durability of treatment, improving quality of life, decreasing pain, shortening treatment duration, minimizing treatment toxicity, and improving morbidity and mortality

appropriate continuity of care by the patient's primary and/or specialist physician; (7) provide access to appropriate palliative care and hospice; (8) respect the patient's right to refuse treatment; and (9) recognize the physician's responsibility to forgo treatments that are futile [15].

To study this concept of performing curative versus palliative surgical procedures in end-stage cancer patients at Memorial Sloan Kettering Cancer Center, researchers looked at the outcomes of patients with advanced gastric cancer who underwent either curative or palliative surgery between 1985 and 2001. Three hundred and seven patients received noncurative gastric resection; 48 % were palliative and 53 % were nonpalliative. Palliative surgery was defined as a procedure performed to palliate symptoms or improve quality of life. The study concluded that there are important differences among patients undergoing curative versus noncurative operations for advanced cancer. Significant differences between primary tumor sites, staging, degrees of nodal and metastatic disease, and the types of procedures performed supported the differentiation between palliative and nonpalliative surgical designations. Successful symptom control preventing the need for additional palliative intervention was achieved in 76 % of the patients evaluated in the study. This study highlights the importance of making a distinction between curative and palliative intervention to improve the success of the procedure and increase patient satisfaction [14].

3 Decision Making: The Palliative Triangle

Optimal palliative decision making is facilitated through effective interactions among the patient, family members, and the surgeon via a dynamic relationship described by the palliative triangle. The three corners of the triangle are made up of the patient, the family, and the physician, and center of the triangle focuses on hope. Emphasis must be placed on those things that can realistically be delivered with the goal of providing the patient with a good quality of life, symptom resolution, technically superior palliative operations, dignity, and compassion [16] (Fig. 2).

The dynamics of the triangle allow the patients and families complaints, values, and goals to be considered against the known medical and surgical alternatives. Outcome data for palliative procedures are useful for the surgeon to be able to deliver accurate information to patients regarding chance of success, procedure-related durability, the possibility for complications, and anticipated survival. Anticipating, understanding, and addressing a patient's and/or a family's expectations about the intent of the proposed procedure are the vital aspects of the palliative triangle. The dynamics of the triangle help to moderate incongruent beliefs and guide the decision-making process toward the best possible choice for each individual patient. The palliative intent needs to be understood and explicitly agreed upon by everyone involved in the discussion. The strong relationship formed by the palliative triangle likely explains the observation of high patient satisfaction toward surgeons after palliative operations, even in patients having no demonstrable benefit from surgery and in those experiencing serious complications [5].

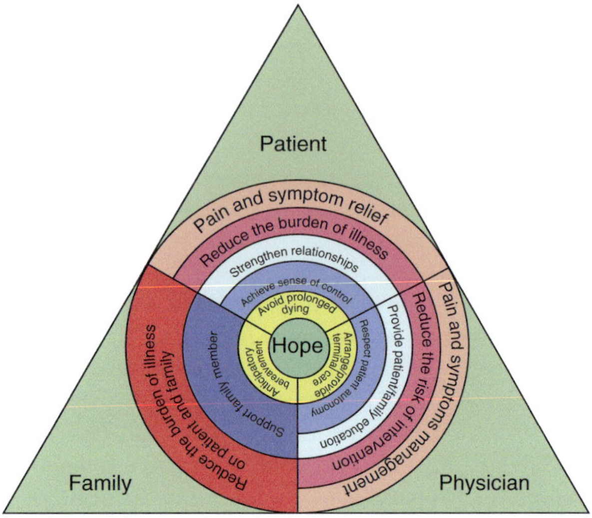

Fig. 2 The palliative triangle. Interactions between the patient, the family, and the surgeon guide decisions regarding palliative care (From Thomay et al. [10])

Patient selection is the key to performing palliative procedures on patients in order to successfully yield symptom relief at the end of life while minimizing operative morbidity and mortality [1]. A study performed at the Brown University examined the outcomes of patients managed with the palliative triangle method and evaluated the factors associated with effective patient selection. A palliative operation was performed in 106 patients or 46.0 % of patients. Complaints requiring palliative surgery included: gastrointestinal obstruction (35.8 %), local control of tumor-related symptoms (bleeding, pain, malodor) (25.5 %), jaundice (10.4 %), and other (perforation, fistula, or pulmonary/urological/neurological symptoms) (28.3 %). Of these 106 patients who underwent palliative surgery, 5 patients required procedures for recurrent symptoms and 6 for additional symptoms. One hundred and twenty-one patients (or 53.3 %) were not selected for a palliative procedure. The main reasons cited for not undergoing surgery were low symptom severity (23.9 %), decision for nonoperative palliation (19.0 %), patient preference (19.8 %), concerns about complications (15.7 %), and other (21.6 %). During the follow-up period, a palliative operation was later required in seven patients for worsening symptoms severity and in five patients for the development of significant new symptoms for a total of 129 palliative procedures performed. The results of the study revealed that patients selected for a palliative operation had better performance scores (Eastern Cooperative Oncology Group and National Cancer Institute fatigue scores) and nutritional status than those who had undergone nonoperative approach. Patient-reported symptom resolution or improvement was noted in 117 of 129 procedures (90.7 %), and this symptom relief occurred within 30 days after the operation. Palliative procedures were associated with 30-day postoperative morbidity (20.1 %) and mortality (3.9 %). Median survival was 212 days. Their research suggests that palliative operations performed on patients carefully selected by emphasizing the palliative triangle approach were associated with excellent results in terms of symptom resolution and morbidity [5]. In this study, typically either one or two meetings between the patient, family, and surgeon lasting 60–90 min took place before consensus on the appropriate palliative care intervention was achieved. This again highlights the complexity of the decision making involved in palliative procedures.

Palliative surgical treatment options are not right for every patient. Care must be individualized in a multidisciplinary manner, so that the most appropriate treatment option is chosen for each specific patient. Surgeons must be cautious never to promise an outcome that they cannot realistically expect to deliver. Recognizing those patients who are at (1) too high a risk for procedure-related complications or death or (2) those in whom a particular procedure is unlikely to provide a clear benefit is a key component to the triangle. Currently, there is no operative risk assessment tool available for patients undergoing palliative procedures. Vidri et al. looked at the data contained within the ACS-NSQIP database to evaluate its use for operative risk assessment in patients with advanced cancer. The study concluded that the data contained within ACS-NSQIP may provide results that approximate risk (morbidity and mortality outcomes at 30 days), but it lacked the critical information required to make sound decisions regarding palliative care. The authors recommend using this tool with caution, because more suitable outcome measures such as symptom relief, quality of life, pain control, cost effectiveness, and patient satisfaction, which are essential to adequately evaluate the success of a palliative operation, are not included within the data [9, 12, 17].

4 Palliative Communication

Excellent communication between providers, patients, and family is key to successful palliation, no matter whether surgery is performed or is not even offered [5]. Physicians' communication skills are associated with important patient and physician outcomes including: patient satisfaction, patient participation in care and adjustment to illness, malpractice liability, and important clinical markers of health. When doctors communicate well with their patients, clinical problems are identified more accurately, patients are more satisfied with their care, treatment plans are more likely to be followed, feelings of distress and vulnerability are lessened, and patient's well-being is improved [5]. At the end of life, patients and families seek well-developed communication and interpersonal skills from their physicians to guide them during this particularly vulnerable time [5].

While conversations regarding diagnoses, treatment options, and prognoses take place routinely between physicians and patients, effective communication between patients and physicians is often lacking. In a recent study, more than 20 % of patients felt they were told their cancer diagnosis in an impersonal manner, suggesting that many physicians are still unacquainted with or unskilled at good communication. In a significant number of patients, this communication in an impersonal manner was associated with a lack of understanding or a bad relationship with the physician and was cited as a reason for changing physicians [5, 18]. One explanation for this lack of communicative skill in physicians is that there is a shortage of training and literature on surgical palliation. Most surgical training programs have no curriculum to teach palliative care. The Brown University studied this problem by introducing a pilot curriculum in palliative surgical care to its general surgery residents. The program consisted of three 1-h sessions, which included group discussion, role-playing exercises, and instruction in advanced clinical decision making. Residents completed pretest, posttest, and 3-month follow-up surveys designed to measure the program's success. Forty-seven general surgery residents from the Brown University participated. Most residents (94 %) had "discussed palliative care with a patient or patient's family" in the past. Initially, 57 % of residents felt "comfortable speaking to patients and patients' families about end-of-life issues," whereas at posttest and at 3-month intervals, 80 % and 84 %, respectively, felt comfortable (p <0 .01). Few residents at pretest (9 %) thought that they had "received adequate training in palliation during residency," but at posttest and at 3-month follow-up, 86 % and 84 % of residents agreed with this statement (p <0.01). All residents believed that "managing end-of-life issues is a valuable skill for surgeons." Ninety-two percent of residents at 3-month follow-up "had been able to use the information learned in clinical practice." The study concluded that with a reasonable time commitment, surgical residents are capable of learning about palliative and end-of-life care [19]. This practice should be put to use by all medical residencies.

A practical and effective technique for summarizing and simplifying medical communication is the context, listening, acknowledgment, strategy, and summary (CLASS) protocol of Buchman. Another approach is the setting, patient's perception, invitation, knowledge, emotions, and strategy/summary (SPIKES) protocol, which is a variation of the CLASS protocol that focuses on communicating bad news with patients and families [5]. These techniques can be quickly and easily reviewed to help improve basic communication fundamentals. Incorporating communication skills to provide excellent perioperative palliative care into medical or surgical practice takes time, effort, experience, understanding, and compassion, but it has repeatedly proven to be essential for effective end-of-life care [5].

5 Outcomes of Palliative Surgery: Limited But Promising Data

Palliative procedures play invaluable roles in patients with disseminated malignancy. With appropriate counseling and patient selection, symptom resolution can be achieved in as many as 80 % of patients [11–13, 20] The effect on patient outcome as determined by: resolution of chief complaints, quality-of-life control, and morbidity of therapy and resource utilization should predominate decisions regarding surgical palliative care [12, 13]. Currently, there is no specific clinical data regarding the use of palliative procedures to alleviate symptoms from specific disease processes such as advanced GIST. There is a continued need for high-quality descriptive research including prospective cohort studies, as well as randomized controlled trials to define optimal management strategies.

Investigators and clinicians face numerous barriers in conducting high-quality research in the palliative patient population. These barriers include lack of funding, difficulties in identifying eligible patients, and a variety of practical and methodological challenges of designing these studies. In addition, there are a variety of ethical challenges that arise in the design and conduct of studies of palliative intent, particularly in the conduct of clinical trials. The development of palliative care research has been challenged by a persistent uncertainty about the ethics of these studies. Many providers, institutional review boards, and investigators remain uncertain about the ethical limits of research involving dying patients. However, one should consider the ethical problems inherent in decisions not to conduct research. Accepting the current standard of evidence will expose future patients to unnecessary surgery and ineffective treatments. Therefore, it is critically important to address these ethical challenges carefully and to advance the current understanding and treatment options for palliative care patients [12, 21].

A prospective analysis of over 1000 consecutive palliative procedures at the Memorial Sloan Kettering Cancer Center thoroughly evaluated the outcomes of palliative procedures for all types of cancers. Patients with advanced GIST typically present with pain, bleeding, and obstruction; therefore, we will focus on the surgical treatment of symptoms associated with the gastrointestinal tract. Four hundred and five patients (out of 1022) underwent 516 palliative procedures performed for gastrointestinal symptoms, and 82 % of these patients reported symptom resolution after the palliative procedure. One hundred and fifty-one patients underwent 206 procedures for duodenal obstruction management, and 79 % of patients experienced symptom resolution. These patients underwent endoscopic dilatation/stenting (84 % reported symptom resolution), operative or endoscopic gastrostomy (72 % reported symptom resolution), gastrojejunostomy (75 % reported symptom resolution), and gastrectomy (100 % reported symptom resolution). One hundred and fifteen patients underwent 140 procedures for small and large bowel obstruction, and 90 % of the patients reported symptom resolution. These patients underwent small bowel resection/bypass (91 % reported symptom resolution), colonic resection/bypass (24 % reported symptom resolution), colostomy (100 % reported symptom resolution), endoscopic dilatation/stenting (100 % reported symptom resolution), ileostomy (70 % reported symptom resolution), and lysis of adhesions (80 % reported symptom resolution). Sixty-four patients underwent 69 procedures for jaundice, and 92 % of patients reported symptom resolution. These patients underwent endoscopic intervention (94 % reported symptom resolution) and operative biliary bypass (90 % reported symptom resolution). Forty patients underwent 44 procedures for poor nutrition, and 77 % of patients reported symptom resolution. These patients were treated with an endoscopic feeding tube (79 % reported symptom resolution) and operative feeding tube (67 % reported symptom resolution). Forty-five patients underwent 57 procedures for "other" complaints, and 58 % patients reported symptom resolution. These patients underwent endoscopic management for bleeding/anemia (67 % reported symptom resolution), operative management for bleeding/

anemia (67 % reported symptom resolution), tumor debulking for pain (100 % reported symptom resolution), organ resection for pain (100 % reported symptom resolution), hernia repair for pain (100 % reported symptom resolution), operative management for fistula (10 % reported symptom resolution), endoscopic management for fistula (0 % reported symptom resolution), and other (33 % reported symptom resolution). All patients who experienced symptom relief did so within 30 days of the operation. There was no difference between endoscopic or operative procedures in the frequency of symptom resolution [22]. This study indicates that palliative procedures for almost all the gastrointestinal symptoms associated with advanced GIST can be successful. Interestingly, overall, it was shown that symptom resolution was achieved in 80 % of patients, although further interventions were required for new (25 %) or recurrent (25 %) symptoms. These procedures, however, were associated with significant morbidity (40 %) and mortality (10 %) and limited anticipated survival (approximately 6 months). They concluded that although predictable symptom relief following palliative procedures can be expected in carefully selected patients, recurrence or the development of additional symptoms limits the durability of the intervention [1, 22].

Temple et al. performed a study with the main purpose of characterizing outcomes following palliative intervention for patients suffering from malignant bowel obstruction in the setting of metastatic colorectal cancer. They performed a retrospective review of a prospective palliative database and identified 141 patients undergoing surgical or endoscopic procedures for symptoms of malignant bowel obstruction. Eight-four percent of patients were palliated successfully. Symptom relief of nausea, vomiting, and pain was excellent for all patients; 84 % of patients were able to eat after discharge. In patients who were treated with gastrostomy tubes, 64 % of patients were incapable of sustaining nutrition independently even though they were able to eat. Eighty-eight percent of patients who were treated operatively (those who underwent bypass and stoma creation) were able to sustain oral nutrition. Thirty percent of patients developed new symptoms requiring additional procedures or readmissions. Thirty percent of patients had complications, 10 % of which were graded as grade 3 (disability or organ resection) or grade 4 (interventional radiology, intubation, operation, therapeutic endoscopy) complications. Thirty-day postoperative mortality was 4 %; two patients died from progression of disease, and four patients had postoperative complications. Their data demonstrate that appropriate palliative intervention can be achieved for carefully selected malignant bowel obstruction patients. In their study, gastrostomy tubes were placed in 22 % of patients, stomas were created in 13 %, and 10 % of patients were relieved of their obstruction with lysis of adhesion alone [13].

Moore et al. studied surgical versus nonsurgical options for the treatment of patients with colorectal cancer who present with obstructive symptoms. Colorectal stenting has become an increasingly common alternative to surgery, secondary to the fact that it may have fewer risks. Moore et al. presented their clinical experience over an 8-year period with colorectal stenting in a tertiary Australian hospital. They looked at patients from 2000 to 2008 who underwent colorectal stenting via medical records. Clinical data collected included patient demographics, tumor type, extent of metastatic disease, stent characteristics, technical and clinical success, acute and chronic complications, and long-term follow-up status. Thirty five patients received a total of 39 stents. Technical success was achieved in 95 %, and clinical relief of obstruction was achieved in 89 % of patients. One case was complication by perforation at the time of the procedure, and three cases experienced delayed perforation. Reintervention was required in 17 % of patients, all of whom had less than 50 % hepatic volume replacement by metastatic disease. They concluded that colorectal stenting is a feasible and safe alternative for patients presenting with obstructive symptoms, but the benefit may be restricted to patients with a short expected survival [20]. Similar results were found by Chi et al. who looked at the outcomes on patients undergoing palliative operative or endoscopic procedures for malignant bowel obstruction due to recurrent ovarian cancer. These patients underwent percutaneous endoscopic gastrostomy (PEG) tube placement, colonic stent, placement intestinal bypass/resection, ileostomy procedures, and colostomy procedures. The procedures were operative in 14 (54 %) patients and endoscopic in the other 12 (46 %). Overall, symptomatic improvement or resolution within 30 days was achieved in 23 (88 %) of 26 patients, with 1 (4 %) post-procedure mortality. At 60 days, 10 (71 %) of 14 patients who underwent operative procedures and 6 (50 %) of 12 patients who had endoscopic procedures had symptom control. Median survival from the time of the palliative procedure was 191 days (range, 33–902) for those undergoing an operative procedure and 78 days (range, 18–284) for those undergoing an endoscopic procedure. The study concluded that symptoms can be successfully palliated in close to 90 % of patients [23]. These data demonstrate that both open and endoscopic procedures can provide effective palliative intervention in the carefully selected patients.

Morrough et al. evaluated the frequency and durability of palliative procedures in the setting of metastatic breast cancer. They measured symptom relief as a surrogate for improved quality of life within the context of the number of procedures performed, time spent in hospital, and perioperative morbidity/mortality risk. Among 91 patients with symptomatic metastatic breast cancer, surgical and nonsurgical means of intervention provided 30-day symptom improvement in 91 % of patients, although 25 % of patients required additional intervention for recurrent symptoms and 16 % underwent additional intervention for new symptoms, and overall 70 % of patients reported ongoing palliation for the duration of life. Their data also demonstrated a difference in outcome based on the organ system involved and the nature of the presenting complaint. They found that patients presenting with a chief complaint of pain are most likely to experience long-term benefit from palliative intervention [12].

Appropriate selection of patients with advanced cancer of any type for palliative surgery can yield several months of symptom relief at the end of life while minimizing operative morbidity and mortality. Additional benefits to palliative procedures over other treatment methods include: (1) its low cost compared to treatments that require expensive chemotherapeutic agents, multiple treatments, or need for specialized equipment; (2) immediate therapeutic results; (3) single treatment session with relatively few indications for reoperation; and (4) potential to effectively treat large tissue lesions not amenable to other treatments [11]. Despite the success of most palliative operations, approximately 25 % an average of patients will require further interventions for new or recurrent symptoms [11, 12]. Postoperative complications can present in as many as 29 % of patients and overall mortality can reach 11 %, mostly secondary to the advanced disease and associated comorbidities [11, 13, 20, 22]. Worse outcomes after palliative surgery have been associated with poor functional status, recent weight loss, and low serum albumin [1]. Given the potential risks, while medicine awaits prospective trials that focus on the quality of life using patient-reported outcome, open discussion among the physician, patients, and their families is essential for optimal palliative care.

6 Decision Making in Palliative Surgery: The Unique Case and Specific Challenges of Advanced GIST Patients

Approximately 50 % of GISTs develop recurrence even after complete resection of the primary tumor. The median time to recurrence after the initial surgery ranges from 18 to 24 months. The most common site of recurrence is within the abdomen (liver in 50 %, peritoneal surface in 50 %, and both in about 20 %) [24]. The high and diffuse incidence of recurrent and metastatic disease means that many of these patients are not candidates for curative surgical intervention. However, using the principles of the palliative triangle, many of the common symptoms reported with GIST can be relieved with surgical palliative procedures.

Resistance to imatinib therapy is common and can be of two types: (1) primary resistance (patients who do not respond to imatinib treatment) and (2) secondary resistance (patients who have disease progression after 6 months of imatinib treatment). Imatinib works best on patients with a KIT mutation in exon 11 (response rate 67–83 %) as compared to a KIT mutation in exon 9 (40 % response rate). GIST-negative for a KIT gene mutation may show a platelet derived growth factor receptor alpha (PDGFRA) mutation (3 % cases); this small subgroup of patients does show a favorable response to imatinib. Approximately 10 % of patients do not have a detectable mutation in either KIT or PDGFRA. These patients have shown a 32 % response rate to imatinib [24]. Therefore, there is a significant group of patients with primary resistance to imatinib therapy. The other group of patients resistant to Imatinib therapy is patients with secondary resistance or those patients who have disease progression of tumor after 6 months of a measurable response. These patients with secondary resistance are thought to have acquired new secondary mutations in KIT or PDGFRA that interfere with imatinib activity. Primary and secondary resistance is becoming a major clinical problem in the treatment of GIST-associated disease [1, 24]. Therefore, the high incidence of primary and secondary resistance and the high and diffuse incidence of recurrent GIST mean that many of GIST patients are not candidates for curative surgical intervention. These patients may be ideal candidates for palliative therapy.

7 Symptoms of Advanced GIST

Gastrointestinal stromal tumors are the most common mesenchymal tumors of the GI tract. They commonly arise from the stomach (50–60 %) and small bowel (30–35 %) and less frequently arise from the colon and rectum (5 %) or esophagus (<1 %) [3, 20]. Less than 5 % of GISTs are not associated with the gastrointestinal tract (omentum, mesentery, and retroperitoneum) [3]. As a result, the clinical presentation and symptoms of GIST vary widely, but the majority of patients have symptoms that involve the GI tract. Of those patients who have GIST, most patients do suffer from the symptoms of their disease. One study found that 70 % of patients with GIST are symptomatic, 20 % are asymptomatic, and 10 % are found at autopsy. GISTs tend to displace adjacent structures without invading them. Thus, GIST can grow very large before producing symptoms [24].

As discussed, the symptoms of GIST are very site-specific. The most common symptoms of gastric, small intestine, colon, and anorectal GISTs are bleeding due to mucosal ulceration. These patients present with hematemesis, melena, hematochezia, and occult bleed with signs and symptoms of anemia [24]. The next most common symptom is abdominal mass. Symptoms can sometimes be indolent, with most patients having nonspecific symptoms such as nausea, emesis, weight loss, increased abdominal girth, or abdominal discomfort. These patients can also present with intestinal obstruction. Infrequently, GIST can rupture or bleed, leading to a more emergent presentation. Retroperitoneal GIST presents as a palpable mass in the abdomen or lower extremity edema. Esophageal GIST presents with dysphagia, odynophagia, retrosternal chest pain, or hematemesis [3, 24].

Many of the symptoms associated with advanced GIST are amenable to surgical treatment in the carefully selected patient.

8 Identification of Palliative Intent and Role of Surgery for Advanced GIST: (Bleeding, Obstruction, Pain)

Evidence suggesting successful palliative procedures for patients suffering specifically from advanced GIST is essentially nonexistent. Available data described above can be extrapolated to patients with GIST, however, suggesting that that palliative treatment of common GIST symptoms can be successful in carefully selected patients. Indications for palliative procedures for patients suffering from advanced GIST generally fall into three main areas of concern: obstruction, bleeding, and perforation. However, individual patients may present with more chronic complaints which include abdominal distension, weight loss, fatigue, anorexia, back pain, hematemesis, melena, jaundice, anemia, palpable abdominal mass, and occult bleeding [2]. Palliative surgery is an appropriate option for management of some symptomatic patients, and the surgical procedure should be chosen based on the patient's symptoms and quality-of-life goals [8].

The relief of intractable pain, bleeding, and intestinal obstructions, among other debilitating symptoms, allows patients to be comfortable and retain an acceptable level of functionality. With appropriate counseling and patient selection, symptom resolution can be achieved in as many as 80 % of patients [8, 11–13, 22] Data show palliative procedures can provide effective relief of obstruction, bleeding, and pain in 89 %–100 %, 67 %, and 85 %–100 %, respectively [11–13, 20, 22]. One of the questions frequently asked by patients undergoing palliative surgery is whether or not they will end up with a "tube" (feeding tube) or a "bag" (colostomy or ileostomy). Research suggests that feeding tubes are placed in up to 33 % of patients, and stomas are required in up to 23 % of patients undergoing palliative surgery of any kind [13, 22, 23].

9 Palliation with Medication

Preliminary retrospective studies suggest that preoperative Imatinib is associated with decreased morbidity, improved surgical margins, and improved local disease-free overall survival [25]. Hunt et al. looked at the 94 patients who underwent surgical resection after neoadjuvant tyrosine kinase inhibitor (TKI) therapy. They found that neoadjuvant TKI can be effectively used for the treatment of both primary and recurrent/metastatic GIST and can help reduce tumor burden, predict disease biology, and help define a role for surgical resection in a metastatic setting [26]. Therefore, it can be extrapolated that the use of Imatinib may help with some of the symptoms caused by bulky advanced disease.

Interestingly, even though the first line of treatment of recurrent or metastatic GIST is Imatinib, there is evidence to suggest that patients with advanced (high-risk tumors according to modified NIH criteria or recurrent/metastatic disease) GIST are not getting Imatinib as often as patients with locally advanced disease. Pawlik et al. performed an international multi-institution analysis of 158 patients looking at surgical management of advanced gastrointestinal stroma tumors. Six hundred and nine patients who underwent surgery for GIST were identified from seven major cancer centers in the United States. There were 87 patients with locally advanced GIST and 71 patients with recurrent/metastatic GIST. Ninety-five percent of patients with locally advanced GIST required a multivisceral resection; most patients underwent a microscopically complete resection. Interestingly, although 82 % of patients had high-risk tumors according to modified NIH criteria or had recurrent/metastatic disease, only 56 % of patients received adjuvant TKI therapy. Among patients with locally advanced GIST, 3-year recurrence-free survival and overall survival rates were 65 % and 87 %, respectively. In contrast, 3-year recurrence-free survival and overall survival rates among patients with recurrent/metastatic GIST were 49 % and 82 %, respectively. On multivariate analysis, predictors of worse outcomes included high mitotic rate and male sex for patients with locally advanced GIST. Age and lack of adjuvant TKI therapy were associated with adverse outcomes among patients with recurrent/metastatic GIST. This suggests that among patients with advanced GIST, TKI therapy is underused [3]. Since Imatinib may help with bulky disease, it may follow that patients with advanced GIST may experience some symptoms resolution with GIST; however, further research needs to be done to confirm this theory.

10 Palliation with Radiation

Data regarding the use of radiation therapy for GIST are limited. There are case reports that indicate that radiation may reduce tumor burden and produce durable local control in locally advanced and metastatic tumors. Wu et al. investigated the role of radiation therapy in the treatment of GISTs and retrospectively analyzed their institutional experience with patients that had locally advanced or metastatic GISTs treated with radiation therapy. They found that a high rate of palliation was achieved for symptomatic tumors. Treatment was well tolerated, and concurrent use of TKI therapy was not associated with additional toxicity. Further studies need to be completed to establish the role of radiation therapy in the management of GIST [27].

11 Conclusions

Effective palliation rather than cure is often the most appropriate goal in the management of patients with advanced GIST. These patients are often not candidate for curative surgical procedures but may still require intervention for symptoms of their disease. Patients with advanced GIST often suffer from symptoms of the GI tract including obstruction, bleeding, and pain. Research suggests that both endoscopic and operative interventions can successfully palliate these symptoms and improve quality of life. However, the decision to undergo palliative surgery requires a deliberate process. Surgeons must consider the medical prognosis of the disease, the availability and success of nonsurgical treatments, and the individual patients' quality and expectancy of life [5, 28]. Optimal palliative decision making is facilitated through effective communication and dynamic interactions among the patient, family members, and the surgeon through a relationship described by the palliative triangle [1]. While evidence suggesting successful palliative procedures for patients suffering from advanced GIST is lacking, there is evidence to suggest that palliative surgical treatment of common GIST symptoms can be successful in carefully selected patients. Future work will need to be performed to identify which patients with advanced GIST benefit from which palliative procedures with the goal of increasing quality of life for each individual patient.

References

1. Miner TJ. Palliative surgery for advanced cancer: lessons learned in patient selection and outcome assessment. Am J Clin Oncol. 2005;28(4):411–4.
2. Yang F, Jin C, Du Z, Subedi S, Jiang Y, Li J, et al. Duodenal gastrointestinal stromal tumor: clinicopathological characteristics, surgical outcomes, long term survival and predictors for adverse outcomes. Am J Surg. 2013;206(3):360–7.
3. Bischof DA, Kim Y, Blazer DG, Behman R, Karanicolas PJ, Law CH, et al. Surgical management of advanced gastrointestinal stromal tumors: an international multi-institutional analysis of 158 patients. J Am Coll Surg [Internet]. Elsevier Inc.; 2014;219(3):439–49. Available from: http://dx.doi.org/10.1016/j.jamcollsurg.2014.02.037.
4. Shen C, Chen H, Yin Y, Chen J, Han L, Zhang B, et al. Duodenal gastrointestinal stromal tumors: clinicopathological characteristics, surgery, and long-term outcome. BMC Surg [Internet]. BMC Surgery. 2015;15(1):98. Available from: http://www.biomedcentral.com/1471-2482/15/98.
5. Miner TJ. Communication as a core skill of palliative surgical care. Anesthesiol Clin [Internet]. Elsevier Inc; 2012;30(1):47–58. Available from: http://dx.doi.org/10.1016/j.anclin.2011.11.004.
6. Miner TJ, Cohen J, Charpentier K, McPhillips J, Marvell L, Cioffi WG. The palliative triangle: improved patient selection and outcomes associated with palliative operations. Arch Surg. 2011;146(5):517–22.
7. Brar S, Law C, Mcleod R, Helyer L, Swallow C, Paszat L, et al. Defining surgical quality in gastric cancer : a RAND/UCLA Appropriateness Study. J Am Coll Surg [Internet]. Elsevier Inc; 2013;217(2):347–57.e1. Available from: http://dx.doi.org/10.1016/j.jamcollsurg.2013.01.067.
8. Brar SS, Mahar AL, Helyer LK, Swallow C, Law C, Paszat L, et al. Processes of care in the multidisciplinary treatment of gastric cancer: results of a RAND/UCLA Expert Panel. JAMA Surg [Internet]. 2014;149(1):18–25. Available from: http://www.ncbi.nlm.nih.gov/pubmed/24225775.
9. Miner TJ, Jaques DP, Tavaf-Motamen H, Shriver CD. Decision making on surgical palliation based on patient outcome data. Am J Surg [Internet]. 1999;177(2):150–4. Available from: http://www.ncbi.nlm.nih.gov/pubmed/10204560.
10. Thomay AA, Jaques DP, Miner TJ. Surgical palliation: getting back to our roots. Surg Clin North Am. 2009;89(1):27–41.
11. Blakely AM, Mcphillips J, Miner TJ. Surgical palliation for malignant disease requiring locoregional control. Ann Palliat Med. 2015;4(1):48–53.
12. Morrogh M, Miner TJ, Park A, Jenckes A, Seidman A, Morrow M, et al. A prospective evaluation of the durability of palliative interventions for patients with metastatic breast cancer (MBC). Cancer. 2010;116(14):3338–47.
13. Dalal KM, Gollub MJ, Miner TJ, Wong WD, Gerdes H, Schattner MA, et al. Management of patients with malignant bowel obstruction and stage IV colorectal cancer. J Palliat Med. 2011;14(7):822–8.
14. Miner TJ, Jaques DP, Karpeh MS, Brennan MF. Defining palliative surgery in patients receiving noncurative resections for gastric cancer1 1No competing interests declared. J Am Coll Surg [Internet]. 2004;198(6):1013–21. Available from: http://linkinghub.elsevier.com/retrieve/pii/S1072751504001498.
15. Listed NA. The American College of Surgeons Committee on Ethics. Statement on principles guiding care at the end of life. Bull Am Coll Surg. 1998;83(4):46.
16. Thomay AA, Jaques DP, Miner TJ. Surgical palliation: getting back to our roots. Surg Clin North Am [Internet]. 2009;89(1):27–41. Available from: http://linkinghub.elsevier.com/retrieve/pii/S0039610908001746.
17. Vidri RJ, Blakely AM, Kulkarni SS, Vaghjiani RG, Heffernan DS, Harrington DT, Cioffi WG, Miner TJ. ACS-NSQIP as a quality-measurement tool for advanced cancer patients. Ann Palliat Med. 2015;4:200–6.

18. Figg WD, Smith EK, Price DK, English BC, Thurman PW, Steinberg SM, et al. Disclosing a diagnosis of cancer: where and how does it occur? J Clin Oncol [Internet]. 2010;28(22):3630–5. Available from: http://jco.ascopubs.org/cgi/doi/10.1200/JCO.2009.24.6389.
19. Klaristenfeld DD, Harrington DT, Miner TJ. Teaching palliative care and end-of-life issues: a core curriculum for surgical residents. Ann Surg Oncol. 2007;14(6):1801–6.
20. Chouhan H, Wong CX, Maharaj P, Lawrence MJ, Hunter A, Moore JW, et al. Colorectal stenting for malignant obstruction : an 8-year clinical experience. ANZJSURG.com [Internet]. 2012;82:408–11. Available from: http://onlinelibrary.wiley.com.revproxy.brown.edu/doi/10.1111/j.1445-2197.2012.06086.x/epdf.
21. Laneader A, Angelos P, Ferrell BR, Kolker A, Miner T, Padilla G, et al. Ethical issues in research to improve the management of malignant bowel obstruction: challenges and recommendations. J Pain Symptom Manage [Internet]. 2007;34(1):S20–7. Available from: http://linkinghub.elsevier.com/retrieve/pii/S0885392407002679.
22. Miner TJ, Brennan MF, Jaques DP. A prospective, symptom related, outcomes analysis of 1022 palliative procedures for advanced cancer. Ann Surg. 2004;240(4):719–26;726–7.
23. Chi DS, Phaëton R, Miner TJ, Kardos SV, Diaz JP, Leitao MM, et al. A prospective outcomes analysis of palliative procedures performed for malignant intestinal obstruction due to recurrent ovarian cancer. Oncologist. 2009;14(8):835–9.
24. Gupta P, Tewari M, Shukla HS. Gastrointestinal stromal tumor. Surg Oncol. 2008;17(2):129–38.
25. Rutkowski P, Gronchi A, Hohenberger P, Bonvalot S, Schöffski P, Bauer S, et al. Neoadjuvant imatinib in locally advanced gastrointestinal stromal tumors (GIST): the EORTC STBSG experience. Ann Surg Oncol [Internet]. 2013;20(9):2937–43. Available from: http://link.springer.com/10.1245/s10434-013-3013-7.
26. Bednarski BK, Araujo DM, Yi M, Torres KE, Lazar A, Trent JC, et al. Analysis of prognostic factors impacting oncologic outcomes after neoadjuvant tyrosine kinase inhibitor therapy for gastrointestinal stromal tumors. Ann Surg Oncol [Internet]. 2014;21(8):2499–505. Available from: http://www.ncbi.nlm.nih.gov/pubmed/24639192.
27. Cuaron JJ, Goodman KA, Lee N, Wu AJ. External beam radiation therapy for locally advanced and metastatic gastrointestinal stromal tumors. Radiat Oncol [Internet]. 2013;8(1):274. Available from: http://www.ncbi.nlm.nih.gov/pubmed/24267287.
28. Miner TJ. Communication skills in palliative surgery: skill and effort are key. Surg Clin North Am [Internet]. Elsevier Ltd; 2011;91(2):355–66. Available from: http://dx.doi.org/10.1016/j.suc.2010.12.005.

Index

© Springer International Publishing Switzerland 2017

C.R. Scoggins et al. (eds.), *Gastrointestinal Stromal Tumors*,
DOI 10.1007/978-3-319-42632-7

MIX
Papier aus verantwortungsvollen Quellen
Paper from responsible sources
FSC® C105338

If you have any concerns about our products,
you can contact us on
ProductSafety@springernature.com

In case Publisher is established outside the EU,
the EU authorized representative is:
Springer Nature Customer Service Center GmbH
Europaplatz 3, 69115 Heidelberg, Germany

Printed by Libri Plureos GmbH
in Hamburg, Germany